DOCTORS WITH BUGGIES SNOWSHOES, AND PLANES

by
Louise Shadduck

With all good wishes,
Louise Shadduck

tamarack books inc.

1993

Dedicated to the memory of
Governor Charles Armington Robins, M.D.
Employer, Teacher, and Friend
and to his beloved
Pat, Patty, Jeannie, and Becky

COVER PHOTO:
Dr. O. A. Kellogg

Printed and bound in the United States of America

Tamarack Books, Inc.
P.O. Box 190313
Boise, ID 83719-0313
1-800-962-6657

TABLE OF CONTENTS

*These counties were served by physicians in surrounding counties.

INTRODUCTION

This book had its genesis in the minds of a group of remarkable Idaho women, all wives of doctors. Mrs. J.M. Taylor, whose husband received Medical License 237 on April 3, 1903, began to keep a journal on southern Idaho doctors, planning to eventually to put it in print. Other wives began similar files. Eventually the Idaho Medical Auxiliary was formed and members wanted to preserve its history. In 1961, the Idaho Medical Association asked the Auxiliary to compile a history for the Territorial Centennial in 1963.

Author Grace Jordan, wife of Idaho Governor and U.S. Senator Len Jordan, was asked to do the writing. At work on a book of her own, she declined, but suggested that Irene Jones, wife of Boise physician and surgeon Ralph Jones, would be equal to the task. Mrs. Jones was the first Idaho Medical Auxiliary historian. She and women throughout the state worked many years attempting to put a book together, with most of the work falling to Irene Jones.

After Mrs. Taylor's death, her notebook was given to Irene Jones by Mrs. Taylor's daughters, Alice Walters and Mary Schweibert. Questionnaires were sent to all doctors in the state. Many responded, but many did not. History committee members changed and Mrs. Jones was left an overwhelming job. Before computers, it was almost impossible.

The autumn of 1990, auxiliary friends asked if I would take on the project. I would. Ralph and Irene Jones and I loaded the back of my car with two boxes of files containing doctor biographies, numerous pages that she had typed, and clippings. Most research from the Salmon River north to Bonners Ferry fell to me and, in other areas, to implement. Here is the book. This is a fitting year, as the Idaho Medical Association was organized 100 years ago—in 1893.

No one can know the debt that I and the Idaho medical community owe to the late Irene Jones for a faith that held the material together until such time as it could be put into a book.

Although I have never stood in awe, I have admiration for most doctors I have known. Along with being the first, and still a public member on the Idaho Board of Medical Discipline, it has brought to me recognition of the responsibility each doctor holds in his or her hands with each patient treated.

As readers travel through the pages, they will recognize the part these professionals have played in the building of Idaho and its institutions. My hope is that the book is worthy of the men and women who came to the raw frontier to care for the ailing, without a hospital in sight, and stayed to build a thriving, modern state with medical care to match.

Further, I hope that blessed Irene Jones would be proud of the results after the faith she showed in handing on materials she and the IMA Auxiliary collected.

ACKNOWLEDGMENTS

Only with the help of many friends could this journal make it to publication. With a grateful heart, I mention their names. Foremost is Irene Wilson Schroeder, classmate and lifetime friend, who volunteered and input over one hundred doctor profiles to the computer. Judy Hodge appeared for the second time on a book of mine for computer input. When Judy became ill, Nancy Harmening moved into her spot and has been invaluable.

Penny Nelson Armstrong gathered together a group of nurses in Sandpoint to speed interviewing, and followed up with stories and photos. Evelyne Jensen of Boise, also a cherished and longtime friend, contributed hours to search out material and old photos. Marie Whitesell, former president of the IMA Auxiliary, made numerous calls rounding up material; and Carol Skellenger, 1993 Auxiliary president, has loaned books, videos, and helpful ideas.

Marcy Horner, director, Linda Marcy, librarian, and Joan Hust, Dr. William T. Wood Medical Library at Kootenai Medical Center; Guila Ford, finding needed information at the Idaho State Historical Library; Don Deleski, executive, Rhea Velasquez and Diane Mundlin, Idaho Board of Medicine; Arlo Grunerud, Bill Nixon, Gretchen and Don Fraser.

Elizabeth Leisk Mills, Betty Penson Ward, Linda Birdsong, Dr. Ralph Davis, Dr. Ralph Jones, Alice (Mrs. John) Walters, Velma Morrison, Edith Miller Klein, Eileen Leisk, Sally Howell, Del and Ruth Rupert, Daphne Copenhaven, Carol Horning Stacey, Sheri Pyle of the Idaho VA Hospital, Bonnie Haines of the Idaho Hospital Association; Zella Goodwin, Benewah Historical Society; Eileen (Mrs. Walter R.) Peterson, and Helen McKinney.

Others include the Honorable Robert E. Smylie, U.S. Senator Larry Craig and staff members Glady Schroeder, Sandy Patano, Steve Judy and Lisa Lallis; Patricia Robins

Yenor, Dr. Bernard Rapp, Pat Olin Elgee, Richard Ah Fong, Brenda and George Cheney, LeRoy Pope, Marcia Skinner; Steve Schenk and Mary Carr, North Idaho College; President Elisabeth Zinser, University of Idaho; Dr. Roy Schwartz of WAMI, Shirley Christensen, Bonnie Port, Pete and Rhoda Wilson, Arlene Johnson Allured, Phyllis Loehr Kline, Maxine Bradley, Les M. Shadduck Sr., Les Shadduck III, Dorothy Dahlgren and Emma Weeks of North Idaho Museum, Dora Pennington, John and Mary Shephard, Norma Sears Lee, Mary Lee Gray Shephard, Paula Ellis Stephenson, Ida Hawkins, Miriam Daugharty, Kathy Moseley, Jane Gumprecht, Eva Armitage, John and Sadie Harrison, and Barbara McKinney.

Erna Ruth Benz, Jean Vanderwell, Marsha and Mary Greenwood, Jack and Mary Fran Soltman; Dr. E.R.W. Fox, Dr. Bill and Dolores Wood, Dr. Ged and Helen Barclay; George and Norma Greene, Barbara Mossman, Jim Lyle, Jack and Elbert Stellmon, Alphons Boxleitner, Woody Bean, Marlene Johnston and administrative staff, Gritman Hospital of Moscow; and Jim Kalbus. Many thanks to Publisher Kathy Gaudry and Tamarack Books; and to Becky and Gail Ward.

There are others who gave help over the many years to the late Irene Jones and to me. Deepest apologies to those who will know they should be included, but are not. Your generous forgiveness is asked.

CHAPTER
1

THE BEGINNINGS

Other than the Indian medicine men, Meriwether Lewis of the famed Lewis and Clark Expedition, was the first doctor to practice in Idaho Territory. Lewis was secretary to President Jefferson on leave from the Infantry where he had learned to be a superior woodsman and skilled at Indian fighting. Before the trek west, the President sent Lewis to Philadelphia to buy equipment and take a special three-months course in medicine from four physicians of the College of Physicians. Among them was the famed Dr. Benjamin Rush, whose name and writings became well-known to future Idaho doctors who trained at Chicago's Rush College of Medicine.

Dr. Rush instructed Lewis in treatment of minor illnesses and hygiene. He then helped Lewis buy ninety dollars and sixty-nine cents worth of medical supplies. Lewis requested that Captain William Clark of the Infantry accompany him and to serve as supply and health officer. In 1805, they were the first white men in Idaho and before the journey was over, both young captains had doctored a number of people.

The story of the first one hundred years (and a bit beyond) of Idaho medicine is the story of adventurous and resolute men and women groping for ways and means to help the ill and ailing. It is the story of the Whitmans and the Spaldings who set out in 1836 to establish missions among the Indians. All four were missionaries for the Presbyterian Church and Dr. Marcus Whitman was, indeed, a pioneer physician. Eliza and Henry Harmon Spalding and Narcissa Whitman all had a share in tending the sick.

The first surgical operation in the Territory was performed by Dr. Whitman when he removed an arrowhead from the back of the renowned Jim Bridger at Jackson Hole, now in Wyoming. The Whitmans established their mission at Walla Walla. The Spaldings continued on to the Clearwater River to Lapwai ("The Place of the Butterflies" in Nez Perce language) to build their mission. It was considered the first permanent settlement in what is now Idaho.

Army doctors accompanied the army to Idaho posts and took care of more civilians than military personnel, with many Indians treated without charge. Dr. Clinton Wagner had entered the Union Army as an assistant surgeon after the Civil War began. He came to Boise in 1861 and liked the area so much that in 1869, he resigned from the army to establish his own practice. Dr. Junius B. Wright was Boise's first civilian doctor and while he arrived in a different wagon, he was on the scene when the first overland mail came through in 1864.

Idaho's early medicos had interesting and unusual experiences as they brought the art and science of healing to the frontier. An ever-demanding and ever-increasing field bringing longer and healthier lives to all of us, the medical care of today is due in large part to those pioneer doctors who were brave enough to keep pushing Idaho and west ahead of them as they crossed the prairies and mountains of America to tend the sick and ailing. All of that time, they kept ears and eyes alert for the possibilities of any medical improvements of their day.

With steady hands and courageous hearts in the face of hardships of sleepless nights, demanding days, and never enough help, they hammered a heritage with the covered wagon, and forged it in the fires that lighted the cabins from Thunder Mountain to Silver City, from David Thompson's Kulyspell House on the shore of Pend Oreille Lake to the Whitman Mission at Lapwai.

CHAPTER
2

THE PIONEER DOCTORS

DR. WILLIAM CARROL WHITWELL

When Nora Whitwell of Salmon, widow of the much-loved Doctor W.C. Whitwell, was ninety-two, she sat down at her desk the day after Christmas in 1961, and wrote of her memories of the faithful doctor. Dr. Whitwell had by then been dead for forty-two years, but the memories remained keen.

A genuine pioneer, William was born in Linden, Tennessee, in 1850. His early education was in Linden and medical training at Vanderbilt University in Nashville. He was graduated in the science of medicine, and received a gold medal for being the best in the study of gynecology.

The new doctor began practice in his hometown, but soon moved to Decatur, Texas, and practiced until 1887. Open to the lure of the west, Dr. Whitwell answered an appeal from the U.S. government for a doctor to fill a vacancy at the Lemhi Indian Reservation near Salmon, Idaho. He was accepted and arrived that summer.

He came to love the area and its people, so much so that he wore himself out over the period of years, traveling its rugged terrain and treating its equally rugged citizens. But when he first arrived in that long narrow strip of land along the west side of the splendor that is the Beaverhead Mountain Range, he knew he was where he wanted to be. Mountains everywhere!

He turned to the northwest and there were the Yellowjacket and Salmon River Mountains. A turn to the south, and the Lemhis. A number of creeks and small rivers all drained into the Salmon River that has its headwaters in Lemhi County. This was home.

As had former Lemhi Reservation doctors, he served the

Indians and extended his practice through the area. There was only one other doctor at the county seat of Salmon. As he traveled by horseback, he met and made friends with many. An especial one was Nora Yearian, whose parents were well-known sheep and cattle ranchers, who lived near the agency. At the end of his first two years, he and Nora were married.

Dr. Whitwell resigned as "Agency Doctor," as the physicians were called, and the young couple moved to Salmon in the fall of 1889. From Salmon the doctor answered calls from far and near. Many trips were made by horseback along the high, narrow, and circuitous trails along the ridges and down the sides of the mountains down to Salmon River canyon and over the mountain range to the gold mining town of Leesburg, and wherever a prospector needed medical help. No wonder that Dr. Whitwell was very successful in his practice. His disposition was cheery and patients and friends were met with a special southern greeting of "Howdy, howdy!" Patients often remarked, "Just to see that smile of Doc's helps."

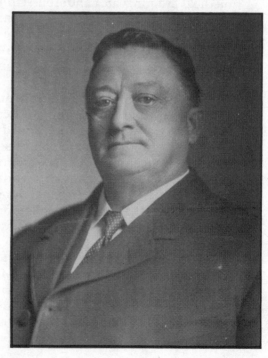

Dr. William Carroll Whitwell of Salmon first answered an appeal made by the U.S. Indian Service for a doctor to fill a vacancy at the Lemhi Reservation near Salmon. He was a true pioneer doctor, traveling by horseback, horse and buggy, and sled. He served in the Idaho Legislature, helped build a new water system and schools for Salmon.
(Courtesy Mrs. Jack McKinney)

Dr. Whitwell was dedicated to civic affairs. The water supply for Salmon was from local wells and not very good. With a few other energetic citizens, Dr. Whitwell was active in procuring a fine water system by tapping a mountain stream flowing into the Salmon River just across from town. Pure water was piped into the homes and businesses.

A new school was needed. The doctor joined others in bringing about a two-story brick building and he went on the school board, serving for nearly twenty years. He was state senator from Lemhi County for three terms. From 1901-02 he was the senator while Gilbert F. Yearian and James J. Deming served in the House. In 1903-04, he served with Chester G. Mathewson and Robert W. McBride. When he went back for the 1907-08 session, the word "city" was dropped from Salmon and only one representative, James L. Kirtley Jr., served. Prominent as a Mason and belonging to the Lemhi Lodge, Dr. Whitwell was Grand Master of the Lodge of Idaho, serving through 1908.

Because there were no facilities in Salmon for major surgeries, Dr. Whitwell sent several patients to the Mayo Clinic in Minnesota. He was a successful diagnostician. In every case that he sent them, the Mayo Brothers found his diagnosis was correct. They offered him a position as diagnostician, but he preferred to remain in Salmon, caring for his friends.

As the years sped by, other doctors arrived in Salmon and did well. But when they ran into an obscure case, they called upon Dr. Whitwell for consultation. In later years of practice, he made a specialty of chronic cases and developed a remedy for simple goiter, whereby the goiter was removed without surgery and the patient restored to health. He also had a flu remedy that was successful, and during the epidemic of 1918, he never lost a patient that he was able to treat throughout the attack.

Exhausted from overwork, he became ill with pneumonia at the end of 1918, and died. The Whitwells' four children included a son, Earl, who died at age seven; three daughters, Laura, Gladys, and Marcia, who attended grade and high school in Salmon, went on to college, and married.

DR. G. E. NOGGLE

A doctor who could remember the final resting place of three other old-timers who had been killed by Indians, was Dr. G.E. Noggle. He came to Valley County, Idaho, in 1903 and practiced until 1919, during which time he became fascinated with the history, looked up old settlers to visit and old landmarks to explore. He became a friend of John Hailey, Idaho's famous stage owner and driver, who gathered early data to write a history. Dr. Noggle helped Hailey in locating information. He pointed out the graves of Tom Hailey, George Monday and Gross Close, killed by the Indians on August 20, 1878.

Born in Bloomington, Illinois, in 1872, he was graduated from the University of Kansas with an M.D. degree in 1895. He soon started the westward trek to Valley County. He was coroner and physician of Valley and Boise counties. It is likely through his medical service that he learned of the three men who were killed by Indians.

After sixteen years in Valley and Boise counties, Dr. Noggle moved in 1919 to Caldwell to practice. He and his wife, Madien, had two sons, Warren and Francis.

DR. RAYMOND J. CLUEN

Dr. Cluen practiced in Canyon and Ada counties and took time out to serve as an X-ray specialist with the U.S. Navy during World War I. He was born February 22, 1880 in Winterset, Iowa. He was graduated from high school at sixteen as president of his class. At twenty he received his M.D. degree from Drake University. Dr. Cluen practiced in Des Moines, Chicago, and as a specialist in X-ray in Rochester, Minnesota. He came to Parma, Idaho in 1910, for seven years before entering the Navy and returned for a year.

Dr. and Mrs. Cluen, the former Neva Phillips Leib of Iowa, moved to Boise in 1920. They had one son, John Raymond. Dr. Cluen was a member of the Idaho and American Medical Associations and the American Roentgenologist Society. He was a member of the Masons, Shrine, Knights of Pythias, Elks, American Legion and active in the Methodist church.

DR. EDWIN E. WATTS

In all kinds of weather, Dr. Edwin E. Watts of Gifford, rode over the Potlatch Ridge and Gifford prairie for years, regardless of the hour called. He rode horseback, drove horse and buggy, and about fifteen years before his death in 1942, he made a few calls in his car. Feeling the car was not a safe vehicle, he gave it to his daughter. During summers in the pioneer community of Gifford, he spent most of the time on the porch, where people came for advice and treatment. Sometimes there was a lineup of people waiting for him.

He was known for unselfish devotion and many calls were made without asking for a fee. During the influenza epidemic in 1918 scores were dying and Dr. Watts worked day and night, often traveling miles in a bobsled drawn by horses.

He was born on Washington's birthday in 1854, one of twin sons of Mr. and Mrs. John Watts of Iowa. The boys were orphaned at eleven. Edwin decided early that he wanted to be a doctor and worked while in grade and high school to save money toward that day. He received his medical degree in 1875 from American University in Philadelphia and took post-graduate courses. He practiced for a few years in the midwest and came to Juliaetta, Idaho in 1888. He practiced briefly at Southwick on Potlatch Ridge before moving to Gifford, where he remained until his death in 1942. He was the oldest practicing physician in Idaho, and possibly in the United States in point of service. He had been a Mason for over sixty years. Five children survived, one of whom, Dr. Victor Watts, practiced in Smith Center, Kansas.

DR. DAILEY COOPER RAY

Traveling by horseback, horse and buggy, sleigh, and when necessary, by walking, Dr. D.C. Ray epitomized the pioneer Idaho doctor. He did surgery by kerosene lamplight on the kitchen table of a farmhouse, and on a number of calls, spent several days with critical cases or waiting out the stork. "Doc," as he was called by nearly everyone, was born February 18, 1877 on a farm in Bedford, Indiana, one of ten boys and two girls.

After grade and high schools, he had one year at

Mitchell College and three at Indiana Teachers College, taught country schools four terms to enter the hospital college of medicine, University of Kentucky, Louisville, graduating in 1902. He worked at the Indiana Reformatory Hospital in Jeffersonville his last two years.

Arriving in Malad, Idaho, November 1, 1902, he bought the equipment and good will of a doctor who "had enough of the wide, open spaces." The first year he collected $1,500 and $500 of that went to buy out his predecessor. Later he began to save money by practicing within a radius of twenty-five miles, with the nearest hospitals eighty and one hundred and twenty miles away. In 1912 he was able to buy a secondhand car which, he said, "was nothing to brag about."

Many times his car bogged down in mud or snow drifts and he waded or walked the rest of the way. The roads were unpaved and no snow plows were used. In several cases, neighboring farmers combined to keep a road open so he could reach a patient. He liked remembering that he never started on a call without completing it.

On May 20, 1920, he moved to Pocatello to practice for thirty-eight years with a brother, Dr. Fred M. Ray, who arrived in 1911, from a practice in Leadore. A third brother, Charles N., was a doctor in Salt Lake City. When "Doc" arrived in Malad he was in a rundown condition from overwork and study, and soon built himself from 145 pounds to a healthy 185. He learned to get physical exercise and his hobbies included clearing 1,000 acres of sagebrush land in Malad and Marsh Valley, where he owned two farms. He always looked for hard work to regain a good condition. Highway construction interested him and he worked on several survey crews laying out highways. He said that it rested him mentally.

He served two terms as a Democrat legislator and one as a Senator from Bannock County. He was president of the State and Southeast Idaho and a member of the American Medical Associations. After fifty years of practice, the American Academy of General Practitioners presented him with a bronze plaque honoring his devotion. He was past master of the Malad Masons, Scottish Rite, and Elks in Pocatello.

March 20, 1912, at Malad he married Martha Lewis,

whose grandfather, John Lewis, was one of the signers of the Idaho Constitution. Doctor Ray said of her, "A wonderful wife for a doctor, self-sacrificing, attractive, and preparing my meals day or night, whenever I returned from a case." They had four sons and two daughters, two of whom became doctors of medicine. Mrs. Ray served a term as president of the Idaho Medical Auxiliary.

DR. GRANT W. PENDLETON

Dr. Pendleton was born at Blackhawk, Colorado, June 3, 1864, four years after his father, James Howard Pendleton, moved his family across the plains by ox team from Iowa to Denver. Grant attended public schools in Boulder, Denver, and Idaho Springs, Colorado, and the medical college of the University of Denver, graduating with an M.D. April 3, 1888. After two months practice in Leadville, he decided to move to Idaho and arrived at the village of Eagle Rock (now Idaho Falls) while Idaho was still a territory. There were about 200 people in the village when he opened his practice on June 3, 1888.

December 18, 1896, Dr. Pendleton and Olive Eldora Johnson were married at Pocatello. They became the parents of Francis Wallene, February 23, 1898; Emerald Grantzen, March 8, 1900; Olive Howard Wallace, March 21, 1901; Harlan Douglass, June 28, 1902; Favorite, December 2, 1903; Forrest Luther, December 24, 1904; Garold Warren, May 14, 1906; and Horace Jay Wesley, February 1, 1909; and an adopted son, Alton Ross, who was born October 27, 1905.

His hours were long and arduous, traveling many miles to settlers on distant ranches during the snowstorms of winter and the heat of summer. He always answered the calls of the sick. He was a member of the Bingham County Board of Pharmacy, city physician of Eagle Rock in 1889-90; member of Woodmen of the World, Modern Woodmen, and he and his wife were members of Women of Woodcraft and Royal Neighbors. The family belonged to the Seventh Day Adventist Church.

DR. H. L. DAUSMAN

A short undated news item in the *Boise Statesman* reported that Dr. Dausman of Idaho City was called to Boise to attend Dr. Scheffert, who had suddenly become ill with diphtheria. Dr. Scheffert, himself a pioneer doctor, became ill from going without sleep or proper food, taking care of patients.

Dausman and Scheffert were close friends and when the former received the call on a Sunday evening at five o'clock, he immediately left Idaho City on horseback and rode through a blinding snowstorm to reach Boise at two the next morning. His care of Dr. Scheffert was so effective that the latter was soon up and about. Dr. Dausman remained in Boise for several days, to be sure that his friend was restored to good health.

The *Idaho Semi-Weekly World* of April 21, 1885, reported:

> Dr. H.L. Dausman of Boise City, last Wednesday received a dispatch from Kansas City, with the sad intelligence of the death of his only sister, wife of Dr. L.A. Berger. She died in Kansas City on April 15, of typhoid fever after a short illness, leaving three little children. She was thirty years. Dr. Berger and wife were residents of this place (Boise City) several years ago. Mrs. Berger's friends here will be pained to hear of her death.

DR. EDGAR LEE WHITE

Standing on the street corners, waving a newspaper with big, black headlines and shouting, "Extra, Extra, read all about it!" was only one of the ways the young Edgar L. White earned money to become a doctor. At age five, he moved to Spokane with his parents from St. Louis, Missouri, where he was born on April 21, 1883.

His father was a contractor and optimistic about the future of the Inland Northwest. His son adopted that attitude on his jobs and later as a physician and surgeon. The young "Eddie" White began selling papers when ten and continued until fifteen, adding other jobs as he went along. On Saturdays and holidays he worked with his father, learning the building business. He saved as much money as possible for medical school.

When college rolled around, he entered Washington State College at Pullman, where he shone on the football field as well as in the classroom. He was second tackle at W.S.C., and in 1905 enrolled at the University of Michigan.

He was named first captain of freshman football and track teams. Later, he was varsity fullback.

During the vacation periods, he worked as a builder in Missouri, until entering Rush Medical College in Chicago, where he received his M.D. degree in 1909. He returned to Spokane for internship in St. Luke's Hospital. In 1910, he moved to Lewiston to be assistant to Dr. Phillips and remained for more than fifty years. He died there on May 20, 1963.

Principally in the area of surgery, Dr. White built a large practice. He married Catherine Leydon Rouse, daughter of Mr. and Mrs. I.A. Rouse of Spokane on April 17, 1911. Dr. and Mrs. White shared ideals and they built a thirty two-bed hospital in Lewiston in 1916. The cost was announced as being $19,800. The hospital continued operations until 1946, when it was closed because of a shortage of nurses, due to the World War II effort. Dr. White understood the situation well, as he served in the Army Medical Corps during World War I, and remained active in the American Legion. Dr. and Mrs. White also operated a training school for nurses from 1917 to 1930.

In June of 1959, Dr. White recalled that in his fifty years of practice he had delivered 3,000 babies. Among them were three of whom he was especially proud: Dr. Joseph E. Baldeck Jr., Dr. James H. Bauman, and Dr. Oliver M. Mackey Jr.

An avid trapshooter, Dr. White served six terms as president of the Lewiston Gun Club; member of the Hi-Yu Indian and Pacific Indian Trapshooters; for many years was physician for the Lewiston Roundup, one of the great rodeo shows, and was later made an honorary member of the Roundup Board.

He was Dean of the Past Potentates of Calam Temple of the Shrine, serving as Potentate in 1919; a Masonic, Knight of Pythias, Elks; North Idaho District, Idaho State and American Medical Associations, and Idaho Academy of General Practice. Mrs. White died in 1955.

DR. FELIX FROMAN

How did they stand it? A reasonable question for Dr. and Mrs. Felix Kent Froman. It seemed that all the agonies of pioneer life fell on them.

The Fromans came from Missouri to Boise Valley in 1864.

He had exactly twenty-five cents in his pocket. They had started for California, but liked the valley and decided to stay. He was a surgeon in the Confederate Army, who returned in the summer of 1864, broken in health, to find his beautiful home burned, his stock killed or driven away, and his wife and children hiding in a Negro servant's cabin. She had suffered the fright and indignity of being forced at gunpoint to cook for the Union soldiers before they set fire to the home.

It did not take them long to decide to join a wagon train west. There were sixty wagons, and Dr. Froman was captain of the train. On the way, one child wandered away from camp and was never found. Another child, a daughter who was four when they left Missouri, lived to adulthood. Other children were buried in a family plot on Canyon Hill in Caldwell. Twenty of the couple's descendants are buried there. One daughter was the fourth person buried in the then-new cemetery.

Dr. Froman did his medical travel on horseback and his saddlebags remain in possession of the family. He was prominent in the valley and became a representative from then-Ada County to the ninth Idaho Territorial Legislature in Boise on December 4, 1876. It was a short session and he was back to his patients by January 12, 1877. He was active in the Masonic Lodge.

In failing health, Dr. Froman took up land in Oregon and lived there for sixteen years, returning to Caldwell to make his home with his son, George. He died there in January 1897.

DR. THOMAS NEWBY BRAXTAN

An amazement and a wonder was Dr. Thomas Braxtan, well known physician for forty-six of the fifty-one years he lived in Boise. He would have been the last to think he had done anything unusual in his practice, but was described as living "four lifetimes in one." He died in 1964 at age eighty-seven.

Born in Paoli, Indiana, November 2, 1876, as a boy he helped his father, a stockman, driving and selling mules in Atlanta, Georgia. He attended Paoli schools and in 1901 the University of Cincinnati granted his Doctor of Medicine degree. That same year on November 7, he married his

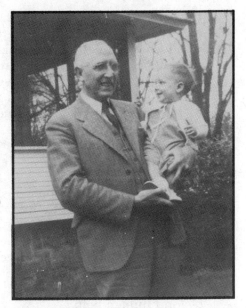

Both Grandpa-Doctor Thomas N. Braxtan and his first grandchild, Mark A. Robinson III, flash proud and happy smiles in 1942. Dr. Braxtan was a well-known Boise physician for forty-six years. He interned in Austria before he moved to Idaho in 1913. In addition to his private practice, he was Ada County Physician and Idaho Soldiers Home and Boise Children's Home doctor.
(Courtesy Mary Robinson)

hometown sweetheart, Mary Ellen Stout, a graduate of Earlham College.

An internship was not required then and from 1901 until 1909, he practiced at Loogootee, Indiana, entering post-graduate studies in New York for the 1907 summer session. Vienna University in Austria was chosen for studies in pathology and internal medicine from September 1911 to January 1912. He served an internship in the Wertheim Clinic in Vienna during 1912. In 1918, he took special work in the DeLee Clinic in Chicago and later attended special courses at Washington University in St. Louis.

Early-day physicians had unusual experiences and Dr. Braxtan had more than most. He started his practice in Loogootee, using a horse and buggy to make calls. In 1914, a year after he arrived in Boise, he bought his first car, a good used Overland, for $600.

He delivered triplets in the home of the mother. When asked about them many years later, he said, "Well, all three were still living and feeling fine when I checked on their twenty-first birthday!" The triplets, like most babies of that era, were mainly breast fed and were pacified with "sugar tits," which were made of sugar wrapped in a cloth.

He fought the big flu epidemic of 1918, and found that

the only way he could get enough rest to remain on his feet and keep doctoring was to take the telephone off the receiver. He fought other epidemics that struck the area: diphtheria, polio, smallpox, and measles.

In 1914, he drove his Overland to the high-country village of Ola, above Emmett, to deliver a baby and found a "placenta preview" case. Knowing that the mother-to-be would need hospital care, he packed her with gauze and drove over the rough mountain roads fifty miles to St. Luke's Hospital in Boise. He successfully delivered the baby.

The number of mothers losing their lives in childbirth seemed unnecessary to him, and he was determined to save mothers and babies. He delivered about four-thousand babies, many in the homes and under difficult conditions. Among them were his four children and four grandchildren. He lost only one mother, and she had not seen him until the time of delivery, and had complications beyond human help.

Accomplishments of the four children indicate up-bringing and inspiration. Ellen Braxtan (Mrs. F.F.) Carlson was graduated from the National School of Education with a Bachelor of Education degree. She took Laboratory Technician training at the University of Oregon Medical School. She lived in Spokane, and had one daughter, Judy.

John Thomas Braxtan was graduated from Harvard College and its Graduate School of Business. He became an officer of the Bemis Bag Company in St. Louis. He had two children: a son, Thomas Newby Braxtan III, and a daughter, Sharon.

Mary M.B. (Mrs. M.A.) Robinson was graduated from the University of Idaho with a Bachelor of Science degree and took Laboratory Technician training at the University of Oregon Medical School. She lives in Boise and has two sons, Mark and John, and a daughter, Carol.

Rachel S.B. (Mrs. C.L.) Barrett was graduated from the University of Idaho with a Bachelor of Science degree. She lives in Boise and is the mother of two daughters, Lynne and Marty, and one son, James L.

Dr. Braxtan was a staff member at St. Luke's and St. Alphonsus, and was staff chief at St. Lukes for two years. He was president of the Southwest Idaho Medical Society;

and was a physician in Ada County and at the Soldier's and Children's Homes in Boise for many years.

Outside of medicine and family, his interests included one or two saddle horses. For many years he was one of the few in the valley capable of training English saddle horses.

DR. WILLIAM H. JOHNSON

In the science of medicine and surgery Dr. Johnson distinguished himself as an able and energetic practitioner. During the Civil War, his father, William, enlisted with a regiment of New York volunteers serving three years in the Union Army. At war's end, he returned to New York and worked in the baggage department of the Erie Railroad Company, rising to become superintendent. He married Mary McCarrick who was born at Bally McCart, County Armagh, Ireland. William H. Johnson was born May 12, 1873, in Buffalo, New York.

William H. Johnson attended public schools of Buffalo and Baltimore Medical College getting his M.D. in 1904. He practiced in Mattoon, Wisconsin, for three years before deciding that Idaho offered more challenges and moved to Gooding. A year later he moved to Caldwell and established a practice.

Dr. Johnson remained an avid student all his life and belonged to various medical organizations. He was married to Mary Frank in 1896. They had one daughter, Viola Elizabeth.

DR. W. W. JONES

Dr. Walter William Jones, eighty-seven, known simply as "Doc Jones," died July 18, 1963 at Jordan Valley. He was well-known in southwestern Idaho and southeastern Oregon and responded to calls in the remote Owyhee Mountains for fifty-two years. Most of that time he was the only doctor in an isolated farming and ranching area. He had a heart attack and died enroute to the nearest hospital, seventy miles away in Caldwell.

Services were held in the First Methodist Church of Caldwell with the Reverend Dr. Harold N. Nye officiating. Silver City Lodge No. 13, AF&AM, of Homedale conducted services at Canyon Hill. Born in Coalfield, Iowa, February 28, 1876, he taught school for three years before graduating from the University of Iowa in 1903. He did post graduate work at Johns Hopkins University Hospital, Baltimore.

Dr. Jones was a senior medical officer in the Navy in World War I. He married Clara Mintonye in 1900 in Iowa and she died in 1929. Dr. Jones practiced in Iowa eight years before coming to Jordan Valley in 1910. He owned the Jordan Valley Pharmacy and was a member of the Idaho and Oregon Medical associations. He and Mrs. Jones had three daughters, Mrs. Eliza Azculnaga, Boise; Mrs. Pauline Evans, Portland; and Mrs. Hilda Reilly, Long Beach; three sons, Walter W. Jr., Cleveland, Ohio; Curtis C., Chico, California; and Everett E., Jordan Valley

DR. EARL D. JONES

The late Judge William Stibal Pettite of Roberts, in an article in the *Market Lake Citizen*, September 22, 1960, eulogized Dr. Earl D. Jones. The headline and parts of that article are:

No Night too Dark or Stormy,
No Road too Bad or Long.

In these words Dr. Earl D. Jones, D.O., M.D. based his life work. From 1914 to his death in 1936, Dr. Jones . . . helped thousands of patients . . . no case was too small or big, . . . too far away . . . travels—by team, horseback, even by boat . . .

From Camas Meadows to Humphrey and Monida to Birch Creek on to Menan, Roberts and Osgood . . . his paths . . . life work. Never did he complain . . . 'Doc Jones was quite a man.' . . . native of Plane, Iowa, the son of Wm. and Jennie Jones. After the death of her husband in 1917, Jennie Jones moved to Roberts to be near her son. She died . . . a few years before Dr. Jones died. Dr. Jones received his Doctor of Osteopathy degree at twenty-three at Fort Madison, Iowa, . . . further medical training at Kirksville, Missouri and Denver. After practicing in Centerville, Idaho, and Victor and Denver, Colo., he moved to Pocatello.

In 1906 he was appointed city physician, the first Osteopathic doctor in the United States so named. . . . he purchased some land in the lakebottom area of Roberts and moved there. In 1915 he received an M.D. from the Pacific Medical College in Los Angeles . . . one of the few to hold both degrees. While Dr. Jones was away, Dr. O.B. Beller had handled much of the medical work in the area.

Dr. Jones established the area's only hospital for many years at Roberts, . . . His first wife, Marie Townsend, whom he married in 1909 at Salt Lake City, died the next year in Pocatello. Ten years later, he married Bessie Bradley of Kansas. They met while she was in Roberts as business manager of the Elliston-White Chautauqua . . . They had one son, Bill, of Boise; two grandsons, Nicky and Bill, made their home in Roberts with Mrs. Jones. Granddaughter Sharon lives in Terreton.

Dr. Jones . . . was president of the Idaho Board of Osteopathic Examiners and . . . Idaho Osteopathic Association in 1910. In 1917–18 he was . . . a Democratic member of the state legislature. He was an Elk and Mason . . . He helped organize the First National Bank of Roberts . . . directors . . . chose Stibal president and Dr. Jones as vice president. Dr. Jones organized the Picture Showhouse . . . was associated with Roberts Cheese Factory . . . he delivered three babies within a short time of one another—even though one arrived near Menan, one in Osgood, and one near Roberts.

The doctor's work ended at fifty-eight, while being treated in Idaho Falls for an infected hand . . . he rests, as was his request, on his family ranch, a marker . . . states, 'No Night too Dark or Stormy, No Road too Bad or Long.'

DR. H. E. LAMB

In a fascinating letter, pioneer Doctor Harry E. Lamb of Wendell, Gooding, and Twin Falls wrote of hardships, joys, and sorrows of early day practice in southern Idaho. Parts of the letter are:

In 1909 my wife Effie, daughter, Harriett, and I boarded the train West . . . I had my degree in medicine from Creighton and practiced in Nebraska. We settled in Wendell (and) the first years were real pioneering.

My faithful horse Red, underwent hardships along with me . . . it was impossible for me to do a delivery more than two or three miles out in the country and return home before morning . . . so the farmers gave me a place to lay my weary bones for the night. Effie, earned her leather medal . . . I would not only tear my britches on barbed wire fences, but was wearing

long underwear. Always one of the officers of the
absent-minded, I often forgot to tie Red when I made
a call and much to my chagrin would find him at
home when I returned. My family increased from
three to five in Wendell . . . we moved to Gooding,
which had a larger population.

World War I was on its way, roads had not been
improved . . . an epidemic of flu broke out. The
springs of my car could not stand the rough roads . . .
one month my garage bill was $300. I called a doctor
from Boise on consultation one day and we made the
call in my Ford. Being very polished, all he said was,
'The only car I know of, that can climb telephone
poles, is a Stutz, why don't you buy one?' But I could
only afford a Ford.

During my first year at Gooding I . . . delivered a
baby by car headlights; confined another woman in a
covered wagon . . . performed a minor operation on
an extremely large woman, with nothing available but
the dining room table for operating. The wing of the
table collapsed and imagine my chagrin, for the lady
hadn't fallen asleep and was looking me straight in
the eye. Gooding did not have a hospital. When my
son had an acute attack of appendicitis I called a
surgeon from Twin Falls and again the dining room
table served the purpose.

With the flu raging . . . war progressing, a doctor's
constitution had to be made of iron. The many nights
that I sat up all night or slept in the car while my
driver drove . . . I gained about a hundred pounds,
. . . I 'pieced' between calls at night.

. . . my first car, a one-cylinder with carbide lights.
It was a honey, sounded like a threshing machine and
was as fast as an alligator. All that was necessary to
start it was to crank it for thirty or forty minutes. The
real thrill came when I approached a hill, again Effie
would come to my rescue by getting out and pushing.
As the car had no windshield, the snowy nights were
very touching when the snow dashed in and down
my shirt collar.

The war ended . . . youngest child was born,
increasing our family from five to six . . . again the
urge to migrate so . . . to Twin Falls. I pricked my
finger with a tonsil snare, developed a severe blood
poisoning . . . soon as I was out of the hospital, not
being able to work, Harriett, LeRoy, Effie and I

started for California. I was well on the road to
recovery when we reached home, but my left fore-
finger remained stiff . . . I had read Doctor Kanaval's
book on amputations, so I . . . went to Chicago and
had him amputate my finger, including the metacarpal
phalangeal joint so as to make the hand look more
normal.

From university days . . . ambitions to study in
Vienna . . . in 1929 this became possible. Previous to
this I had from four to six weeks . . . from 1914 to
1929 . . . at Mayo's, New York and Chicago.

I made farming my hobby. I started buying North
Side land . . . later most of my property was on the
South Side. Today I know every little turn and crook
in Twin Falls, but when I started practice I spent as
much time locating my patients as I did treating them.

We all know that after getting the patients, the
collections are the next hardest thing. When I first
began . . . I took livestock for pay. We started with
one lamb and ended with Effie feeding thirty by
bottle. Throughout practice I have given patients
credit and been paid with everything from jewelry to
animals. Like everything else one even gets beat on
this game occasionally. I took two bird dogs in for
twenty-five dollars apiece and the next day they both
died of distemper.

Perhaps younger doctors in Idaho will fly airplanes
on their calls, but I'll end mine by driving a twelve
cylinder Lincoln.

DR. GEORGE A. KENNEY

A life "stranger than fiction, full of dramatic incident,
climaxes, tragedy and romance," was led by Dr. George A.
Kenney, a graduate of medicine and learned at the
carpenters bench. He came to Idaho Territory and the
Lemhi Indian Agency in April 1874, and for more than
thirty years administered to the ill over a territory larger
than the state of Connecticut. It was wild and rough, and
the scattered camps of miners and cowboys were as wild
as the country. Trails led to the isolated settlements, and
the Indians were as untamed as the land over which they
roamed and claimed as their own. He always carried a six
shooter and needle gun during those early times and rode
horseback.

Dr. Kenney came to the lonely frontier in the Lemhi

Valley traveling 450 miles over Indian trails. His salary as agency doctor was fifty dollars per month, and to increase his income he started a daily selling of butter to the thinly populated section. None of the ranchmen milked cows or put up hay. Bands of cattle fed on the range the year around, and many perished during the severe winters.

It was at Dr. Kenney's ranch, which he located three miles below the Agency in 1876, now "Seventeen Mile Ranch," that Lewis and Clark camped and traded with the Indians for good horses to continue their journey. The Indian woman, Sacajawea, here met her brother in the valley where she was born.

Dr. Kenney was the only physician in that vast territory, and his practice was large. Sometimes he rode all night and day through bitter winter storms, to administer to a patient. Often he performed operations alone, with few surgical instruments, and no place for the patient to receive proper care. The doctor remembered saving the lives of many turbulent and reckless men. "Most of the trouble and the cause for many operations," said the doctor, "was liquor."

"Every one drank in those days, the cause of shootings and fights. Even at a funeral the men drank heavily, not through disrespect, but it was the way to drown troubles. Every one rode horseback, and injuries to travelers, miners on the trails, cowboys on outlaw cayuses, required many a bone to be set." Dr. Kenney had a half cup of bullets, taken from operations.

"About the worst trip I ever had," said the old doctor, "was a call by courier to Leesburg in mid-winter. Bill Luderman had been shot. I snowshoed over the mountain and learned that Luderman, who was nineteen years old and weighed 210 pounds, was building a ditch on placer ground he owned with a partner named Tim Conners. Conners would not do anything with the property, and became angry when Luderman built a ditch to convey water for mining, saying Luderman was 'trying to steal the ground.' That day the camp was having contests in ski jumping, a gala time for all. The snow was covering the cabins of the camp, and Luderman was one of the contestants, leaping the houses of the miners for the longest jump. Conners was carrying the mail between

Leesburg and Prairie Basin, thirty miles into the interior, and when he came in he was drunk, and began to quarrel with Luderman, threatening to kill him. A friend handed Luderman an old style rifle, while Conners carried a new gun. Conners got drunker and noisier, and finally shot at Luderman blowing away the thumb on his right hand, which so hindered him it seemed impossible for him to return the fire. Conners shot him again through the thigh before Luderman finally got the hammer of his gun pulled back, and shot Conners through the body. Return fire from Conners fatally wounded the young man, who was innocent of any wrong doing."

Dr. Kenney arrived and did all he could for the boy, then lashed him to a toboggan and with men to draw the sled, started for Salmon City. Conners had miraculously escaped fatal injury, the ball glancing along his breast bone and coming out the back. He was later tried by a jury and hanged.

A large part of the surgical practice of Dr. Kenney consisted in amputating legs. Lemhi Indian "Happy John" had tuberculosis of the knee and the Indians brought him to the doctor, offering a string of ponies if he would doctor him. Dr. Kenney amputated the leg out in the yard, using a razor and a very fine-tooth saw to cut the leg off near the body, as the bone was diseased. The patient got well quickly and some months later the doctor asked to see the wound, and "Happy John" charged him a dollar before he would let him make the inspection.

Dr. Kenney was coroner for years. In all the tragedies of the Salmon River Country, he had a hand in doctoring the sick, performing surgical operations, and holding inquests over the bodies of those killed. He performed surgical work that today's doctor would deem impossible, without better instruments and facilities. His services were so much in demand that he once went for thirty nights and days without having his clothes off for proper rest.

DR. CHARLES M. SHAFF

Dr. Charles M. Shaff was born at Placervillle, California, July 6, 1855. He moved to the Willamette Valley in Oregon where he lived until 1883, when he moved to the village of Lewiston. The residential area was west of what is now old

Sixth Street and extended from Main north to B. There were no hospitals and his practice took him to all of the surrounding country. Trips across the Grand Ronde River in Oregon on horseback were common. Cattle trails were followed, and it was often necessary to swim the rivers, but those conditions were willingly faced.

Dr. Shaff graduated from the University of Iowa Medical School in 1881. Although he was located in what was known as the western frontier, Dr. Shaff made frequent trips to outside hospitals and clinics. He took post-graduate work in New York in 1888; later studied in Chicago, again in New York and Harvard Medical School where he specialized in eye, ear, nose, and throat.

Dr. Shaff was president of the Idaho State Medical Society, and held a Fellowship in the American College of Surgeons. He played an important part in the early statehood of Idaho and its educational struggles. When he arrived in Lewiston, feeling was high for the annexation of Idaho to Washington. Southern Idaho offered the State University to Lewiston in the event that the fight should be dropped, but the offer was refused. A Lewiston delegation succeeded in having the Legislature pass a memorial asking Congress to approve the annexation but sentiment died before the order was acted upon.

For years Dr. Shaff was a member of the Board of Regents of the University of Idaho and the Board of Trustees at the Lewiston Normal School. He was a 33rd degree Mason. In 1888 he married Rena M. Poe, step-daughter of Judge Poe, a prominent Lewiston lawyer. They had one daughter.

DR. MOSES STEARNS

Dr. Moses Stearns, pioneer physician of Twin Falls, died at age eighty-eight. He retired from active practice in 1912.

Following graduation from Washington Medical College, St. Louis, Dr. Stearns practiced in Springdale, Arkansas, and moved to Emmett in 1906 and then to Twin Falls in 1908. He practiced in Twin Falls until 1912, associated with Dr. C. D. Weaver. Dr. Stearns rode horseback to answer his calls in the Rock Creek area.

He was born November 17, 1862, in Osceola, Missouri, and was married June 4, 1902 in Springdale. Following his retirement, he became interested in growing roses and won several prizes. He devoted much of his time to writing poetry and studying.

He was survived by his widow, Mrs. Bertha Stearns; one daughter, Mrs. Helen Coleman, Twin Falls; one son Frank Stearns, Shoshone, and one granddaughter, Marilyn Stearns, Shoshone.

DR. MAURICE H. TALLMAN

Dr. Maurice H. Tallman was born in Kalamazoo, Michigan, April 27, 1886, to James G. and Jennie B. (DeWater) Tallman, who moved to Boise in 1904. He graduated from Boise High in 1906, and entered the medical department of the University of Iowa that fall. He graduated an honor member in 1910.

Dr. Tallman opened a Boise office, specializing in diagnosis. He was in the United States Army as a heart specialist at Camp Pike, Arkansas, from February, 1918 to April, 1919. He became chief medical examiner with the rank of captain. He did post graduate work in New York City, Philadelphia, and Chicago. He had so wide a reputation in diagnosis that his patients came from all over Idaho, and northwest states. He belonged to the American and Idaho State Medical Societies, Association of Military Surgeons, Boise Commercial, Elks, and country clubs.

May 2, 1917, Dr. Tallman married Gertrude Lossi of Montana. They owned and occupied one of the attractive homes on Harrison Boulevard.

DR. HALBERT FLETCHER NEAL

Dr. Neal started medical practice in 1904 in Meridian and spent the rest of his life ministering to, and in building of, the community. Born in Peru, Nebraska, November 9, 1879, to Charles Philander and Illinois Tate Neal, he was educated in the Peru schools and Normal College. He received his M.D. from the University of Nebraska in 1903. He married Grace Louise Andrews at Indianola, Nebraska, December 28, 1904, and they moved to Meridian.

Dr. Neal specialized in obstetrics and in 1920 took a post-graduate course in New York. He assisted in organizing and became vice-president of the Meridian State Bank; was clerk and trustee of the high school from 1911 until his death. He was a Republican; member of the Idaho and American Medical associations; St. Luke's Hospital staff; Masonic, Odd Fellows, and Modern Woodmen lodges; Boise Physicians Club; and Methodist Church. Dr. and Mrs. Neal had two daughters, Carol, Louise, and one son, Charles.

DR. JOHN B. MORRIS

When the Indian war broke out in 1877, Dr. John B. Morris of Mount Idaho was in Portland, but returned at once, at considerable risk to himself in crossing hostile Indian territory. He cared for the wounded soldiers who had participated in the battle in which thirty had been killed.

Dr. Morris was born in Knoxville, Missouri, October 1, 1850, the son of Benjamin and Amanda (Hamilton) Morris. In 1872 he entered St. Louis Medical College, graduating in 1874. He earned the entire cost of his education.

Following the war's end in 1878, Dr. Morris settled in Lewiston. In 1879 he married Laura Billings, and they had two children, Cora and Benjamin. The doctor served four years as county treasurer, elected in 1894 as a Democrat. He was alderman, school director, and a 32d degree Mason.

DR. ROBERT T. WHITEMAN

Dr. Whiteman of Cambridge was the 635th doctor to be licensed to practice in Idaho, following enactment of the medical licensing act. He began practice at Council in 1911. He was the senior practicing physician in Washington County and the only physician in Cambridge at the time of his death January 22, 1964. He was born September 26, 1886 in Elkhart, Indiana, where he attended school. His M.D. was from the University Medical School at Ann Arbor in 1909.

Following internship at Kansas City, Missouri, he moved to Council. He remained there until being commissioned first lieutenant in the National Guard in 1917 and went to France. For twenty-one months he served with the Second Idaho Infantry Regiment, 41st division. On return from France in 1919, he moved to Cambridge and practiced for the next forty-five years.

He served his community as mayor for five terms; was Union Pacific Railroad physician for thirty years; deputy county physician; camp physician for the Civilian Conservation Corps in 1932; medical consultant for Morrison-Knudsen Construction Company during the building of the Brownlee-Oxbow Dam on the Snake River. He was a member of the Southwestern, Idaho, and American Medical associations.

Dr. and Mrs. Whiteman were parents of a daughter, Mrs. Donald Beckstead of Sacramento, California; two sons, Robert of Mesa and Donald of Riggins; and nine grandchildren.

Dr. Whiteman enjoyed writing memories of early days in medical school and problems met in practice, and overseas during World War I. The author has a fat file of letters received from him many years ago containing stories on everything from treating dope addicts, Rocky Mountain Spotted Fever, maggots in areas of bone decay, of diagnosing a breast cancer in its early stages but the patient saying, "Since it isn't bothering me, I won't bother it," and, of course, dying from it later.

DR. H. A. ANDERSON

A *cum laude* graduate of Harvard Medical College in 1896, Dr. Hyrum A. Anderson was instrumental in the creation of Idaho's Jefferson County in 1913. He moved to Rigby in 1908 and remained until his death in 1951.

An unusual man in life, he did an unusual thing in issuing a posthumous statement to the press, to be used at his death. The statement, of his life and times, includes:

> Hyrum A. Anderson was born August 20, 1868 at Lehi, Utah, the son of Mans W. and Christina Benson Anderson, early converts to the L.D.S. faith. His youth was spent in hard labor on the family acres.
>
> Early in life he showed an unusual desire for that time, for higher education. Supported by the products of the farm, and the fact that his mother kept a boarding house for students, he was enabled to take full courses at Brigham Young Academy at Provo. At twenty he was named faculty secretary and instructor in English and stenography.
>
> In 1892, he entered Harvard Medical College and was graduated *cum laude* in 1896. He earned maintenance by stenographically reporting lectures of professors.

During 1896 and 1897 he was house physician at Boston City Hospital, returning to Salt Lake City in the fall of 1897 to enter general practice. In 1898 and 1899 he was physician of Salt Lake County and in 1902–03 was co-owner of the Salt Lake Private Hospital. Early in 1908, Dr. Anderson came to Idaho, locating at Rigby early in its development. Until invalidism in 1938, he served continuously a large general practice. He was an associate member of the staff of the Idaho Falls L.D.S. Hospital. He helped create Jefferson County in 1913.

He was survived by two foster daughters, Mrs. Aldon Tall of Rigby and Mrs. Gene Evans of Los Angeles, and a nephew, Emery Anderson of Rexburg. His only son, Pharas, died two years before his father.

DR. CLIFFORD M. KALEY

Dr. Kaley's great-grandfather on his mother's side of the family was a first cousin of George Washington. He was born September 22, 1877, at Olney and graduated from high school in 1896. For the next three years he joined his father in the mercantile business, but yearned to be a doctor and when sixteen made the choice to do so.

At sixteen, Clifford M. Kaley began to read medicine with the family physician, Dr. William H. Thompson, as his tutor. He acquired a foundation for medical training at Northwest University in Chicago. He received his M.D. degree in 1904 and for the next two years served an internship in Olney, Illinois at the Sanitarium. He first located at Newton, Illinois, moving to Caldwell in October 1909.

While serving his internship, Dr. Kaley was married on August 16, 1905 to Henrietta Godeke. They had one child, Mary Elizabeth. Dr. and Mrs. Kaley became members of the Caldwell Presbyterian Church and he belonged to the Idaho and American Medical Associations, Masonic Lodge, Elks, Modern Woodmen, and Moose.

DR. CHARLES B. BEYMER

Oakley, Idaho was completely snowed in during the winter of 1928–29. There was no doctor in the town and a meningitis epidemic was in full swing. The daily train was the only transportation in or out, so, the arrival in Oakley of Dr. Charles Beymer was one of note. Members of the

Commercial Club had tried without success to obtain a resident doctor for the community. Finally, Art Solomon and Duane Cranney were sent to Salt Lake City with instructions to stay there until a doctor had been obtained.

After desperate and long discussions, they convinced Dr. Beymer, then not long out of the University of Nebraska Medical School and an internship in Council Bluffs, Iowa, that Oakley was a good place to practice. He and his wife and the first of four children, Charles III, arrived in February 1929 and had an immediate patient load.

Dr. Beymer had a guaranteed income, as Oakley families were assessed twenty dollars each and the funds administered by the local bank, which paid for the services when the doctor submitted notes, given by the patients in lieu of cash.

Mrs. Beymer reminisced that, "After the snowed-in period the O.B. business was phenomenal. Never had so many babies been born in Oakley! Why? Parents laughingly admitted there had been no trips nor entertainment and there had been nothing to do during that isolated period." When the Beymers left for Rupert in two years, Mrs. Beymer wrote, "We loved the happy little town of Oakley and left it with regret."

After two years practice in Burley, the Beymers moved to Twin Falls in April of 1934, and he became associated with Dr. D.L. Alexander. He remained there for the next thirty years but later accepted the challenge to work with the student health department at the University of Georgia. "I'll be kept plenty busy keeping 10,600 students in good shape," he said.

Dr. Beymer was a member of the U.S. Naval Reserve and was called to active duty in World War II, sailing to the island of Efate in New Hebrides. He was surgeon at the base hospital for nineteen months and then reassigned to Farragut Naval Base Hospital on the shores of Lake Pend Oreille for two years. He was sent to Guam in 1945, where he stayed until the war ended.

The doctor was president of the South Central Idaho Medical Society, Magic Valley Hospital staff, and of the Idaho Chapter of the American College of Surgeons, and member of the Western Association of Railway Surgeons.

DR. JOHN BOECK

Dr. John Boeck's steady climb to learn more, improve his finances, to study and practice medicine and do good for others displayed ambition, persistence and hard work. He was born September 15, 1861, at Neuendeich, Germany and came to the United States at nineteen. Hs father was a professor and judge. Years later there were to be many doctors in the Boeck family, most of them inspired by John.

In 1880 he attended the Gymnasium (classical preparatory) in Schleswig-Holstein, Germany. He came to this country and hired out as a clerk in a furniture store at Reinbeck, Iowa, where he learned to make burial caskets and furniture. His speaking ability in German, French, Greek, Latin, and Hebrew did not help him in English, so he went to night school. As soon as he had mastered English, he clerked in a drugstore, and later became a druggist.

He moved his family to Boulder, Colorado, and opened his own drugstore, which was a great success. The president of the medical school at the University of Colorado was impressed with John Boeck's knowledge and urged him to study medicine. Years later, he recalled the conversation, and said, "I was then thirty-seven years of age and objected to changing my profession. President Giffin refused to take my 'no' as an answer, so I sold my store, entered medical school, and spent all spare hours in Dr. Giffin's office."

He entered medical college in 1897 and was graduated in 1901. He and his family moved to Boise and he practiced until retirement in 1946. Upon retirement, he remarked, "When I stepped from the boat in New York at age nineteen, I had just five dollars, all of the money I possessed." Dr. Boeck bought one of the first cars in Boise and was given the courtesy of Ada County License No. 1 for several years. He helped to establish St. Lukes and Booth Memorial hospitals and delivered more babies than any other Idaho doctor of that time. Among those were several who became Boise doctors.

Dr. and Mrs. Boeck had three girls and one boy. Among the doctors in the family were son, Dr. A.B. Boeck, Boise; son-in-law, Dr. J.E. Naugle, Sterling, Colorado; grandsons,

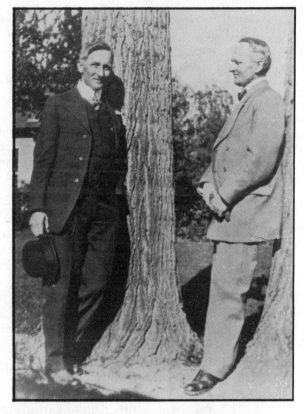

Doctors John B. Boeck and his son, Dr. A.B. Boeck, right, have an amazing story to tell of the difficulties which the father had in escaping from Germany. He arrived in this country in 1880 at age nineteen; he spoke German, French, Greek, Latin, and Hebrew. Dr. Boeck attended night classes to learn English. He aided in establishing both St. Luke's and Booth Memorial hospitals in Boise. The son became equally well-known.
(Courtesy Dorothy Korte)

Dr. J.E. Naugle Jr. and Dr. M.G. Nims in Colorado; Drs. F.E. and G.A. Mather of Boise; nephew, Dr. Cletus Schutte in Hamburg, Germany, and a niece, Dr. Elaine Allen in New York City.

DR. ALBERT B. BOECK

Albert Boeck had pioneer parents. He was the only son of Dr. and Mrs. John Boeck and came with his family to Boise in 1901. He was born February 13, 1888 in Nebraska, graduated from Boise High School in 1908, and received B.A. and M.D. degrees from the University of Colorado. He interned at St. Lukes Hospital, Denver, before moving back to Idaho. He practiced at Wilder from 1916–24 and in Boise from 1924–64. One year after retiring he died on May 14, 1965.

Albert Boeck and Armorel Nelson were married January 2, 1915 in Denver. They became the parents of three daughters, Dorothy Korte of Boise; Marjorie Keen, Illinois; and Patricia Eames, Connecticut.

He was active in civic affairs and received the Silver Beaver award for Scouting work. He was staff member of St. Lukes and St. Alphonsus hospitals and served as chairman of the advisory committee of Booth Memorial Hospital.

He enjoyed gardening, as did his father. He added a dimension in mechanical engineering and had a fully-equipped machine shop in which he turned out many works.

DR. GEORGE COLLISTER

The man for whom Collister, now part of Boise, was named was Dr. George Collister. He purchased 160 acres in the early 1880s, upon which he had a handsome home, and it was much of this acreage that became the Collister district.

George Collister was born October 16, 1856 in Willoughby, Ohio, to Thomas and Fannie (Young) Collister. His father, born on the Scottish Isle of Man, came to America as a young man and remained in Ohio until his death at ninety-six. He was the first person appointed by President Abraham Lincoln to a position in the Railroad Mail Service.

The future doctor attended grade and high schools in Willoughby and, for a short time, was a student at Ohio State University. He entered Heron Medical College at Cleveland and graduated as an M.D. in 1880. Before coming to Boise in June 1881, he practiced in Madison, Ohio. March 16, 1897 he married Mrs. Norden from Illinois. They had no children.

He enjoyed the practice of medicine so much that he rarely took a vacation. He was physician for Ada County, Boise city and the State Penitentiary. His memberships included: American, Idaho, Ada County, and Interstate Medical Societies; Masonic Blue Lodge, Elks, Knights of Pythias, Odd Fellows, and two years on the Boise City Council.

DR. HENRY C. WESCHE

He was a medical missionary in Taming, Hopei, China from 1926–41; practiced in Washburn, Wisconsin from December 1941–44; and at Nampa, Idaho from September 1944 until his retirement. He was Henry C. Wesche, born September 29, 1898, in Green, Iowa, and had a brother, Dr. Gerald Wesche, also of Nampa, and a son-in-law and two nephews who became doctors.

An Iowa farm boy, he learned to work and to study at an early age. Henry received his B.A. degree and did premedical study from 1920–21 at Asbury College in Wilmore, Kentucky. His M.D. was granted in 1925 from Northwestern University Medical School. His internship was at Ancon Hospital in the Panama Canal Zone, 1925–26, and residency in eye, ear, nose, and throat at Chicago's Passavant Hospital, 1932–33.

Dr. Wesche married a college graduate registered nurse and they had one daughter, who graduated from college and became a registered nurse. Dr. Wesche recalled home deliveries in China where the patient lay on a brick bed and was attended by a native midwife who made examinations with unwashed hands. Unusual means of travel for him included an ox cart, wheel barrow, bicycle, and motorcycle in China; a sled powered with a Ford motor, and using an airplane propeller on Lake Superior in Wisconsin. He remembered driving midway between rows of fence posts, unable to see the road, during a blizzard in Wisconsin. He had a private pilot's license.

He was a member of the China, American, Southwest Idaho, Idaho, Civil Aviation, Christian, Aero-Space, and Wisconsin Medical Associations. He was a member of the American Academy of General Practice.

DR. CASPER W. POND

Born October 16, 1882, to pioneer parents on the family homestead in the Gentile Valley near Thatcher, Casper Whittle Pond loved his family, medicine, and Idaho. His father organized the first cattle company in the Grays Lake area.

Through hard work on the homestead, Casper developed the strength that made him a fine athlete when he attended Utah State from 1900 to 1904. He often said, "A good athlete can also be a good student," and set out to prove it. Quarterback for the "Aggie" football teams, runner in the 100–yard dash, and relay races, he also posted high grades. He went on to secure his M.D. at Northwestern University in 1909, and interned in Chicago's Cook County Hospital 1910–11.

He opened offices in 1912 in Pocatello for one year before moving to Downey. He and a doctor at McCammon took care of the people in Marsh Valley. In 1919, he returned to Pocatello and practiced until retirement in 1960. He never regretted his decision to practice in Idaho.

It was on the homestead that, "I learned to stay with a job until I had finished it. I remember the long days of work, dust, and sweat, but I also remember that we didn't need to leave the homesite to fish in the Bear River, and could bag ducks and geese just by going out to the pasture. It was big fun to break wild horses, and I remember more of the fun than the work."

Being on twenty-four-hour call, traveling by horse and buggy through all kinds of weather, and emergency operations on kitchen tables helped Dr. Pond to notice changes were coming. Seven years after beginning general practice, he went to New York for two years of specialization in eye, ear, nose, and throat treatment. He returned to Pocatello and joined Doctors Frank and Charles Sprague and Tom Mullen. In 1931, he moved to the Spaulding Building and as his practice expanded, he brought in specialists Dr. E.V. Simonsen and Dr. J.B. Koehler. Other pioneers with whom he associated included Dr. W.W. Brothers and Dr. D.C. Ray.

Dr. Pond was convinced that Idaho was one of the healthiest states in the country and that medical research was paying off in a stronger race and increased years of good living. At age eighty, he was still promoting proper exercise, and light eating. "It is better to be slim and alive than fat and dead," he said. He had practiced during a time of many changes in treatment, the development of antibiotics, defeat of diphtheria and smallpox, elimination of crude pest houses, stemming of polio and the hope that greater numbers of doctors would appear.

He was a member of many medical societies and the Pocatello Elks. He died in January 1967, in a Boise nursing home. His wife, Nettie; a daughter, Genevieve Mahoney of Boise; son, Robert S. Pond of Silver Springs, Maryland, and six sisters survived. Two brothers preceded him in death.

DR. WILLIAM ROBERTSON KINNAIRD

The caliber of Dr. Kinnaird, who practiced in Idaho Falls for nearly forty years, is graphically stated in an article by his daughter, Kay Kinnaird Woolsey of Burbank, California, in early 1963.

Dad and his associates many times recounted experiences in early Idaho. One of the most harrowing was with his team of mustangs...half wild, tough, fast horses. Careening at breakneck speed across the prairies and along rough dirt roads, he many times raced The Stork or the Grim Reaper. One cold night, a man rode his horse into town to report a desperately sick child.

Donning a heavy, nearly ankle-length sheepskin-lined coat, Dad hitched up his mustangs. Suddenly, as he stood in front of them, fastening the last snap, something frightened them and they jumped forward, breaking into a dead run. With a hand desperately clinging to each horse's bit, Dad threw his feet up over the singletree (or whatever it is called). His long coat, dragging beneath him, was torn to shreds by the hooves of the frantic horses. It was nearly a mile before a horseback rider could catch and bring them to a halt. Dad, his coat in shreds, dropped to the ground, nearly exhausted, but he went on to call on his patient, and while I can't know for sure, I like to think he beat Death yet again.

Another time a miner from the Challis area rode in to report a seriously injured man, lying in a mountain cabin. Dad went alone, a two day trip one way. He found the cabin surrounded by a high fence. On opening the gate to approach the cabin, a Great Dane, the size of a colt, put a paw on each of Dad's shoulders and snarled in his face! Dad spoke quietly to the animal and was understandably relieved when the injured miner heard the commotion and called off the dog. Dad stayed several days and tended him until he could be moved and then took him back to Idaho Falls for further treatment.

When Dr. Kinnaird arrived in 1901 or 1902 (exact date not known), Idaho Falls boasted a general store, livery stable, saloon (over which he rented a room), a bank, and the Porter Hotel. Nearly every Saturday night there was a shooting. To the new doctor fell the task of patching up or pronouncing "dead."

He was born July 26, 1873, in Decorah, Iowa, and died in July 1950. His father was president and stockholder in the First National Bank, which had a branch in Idaho Falls (later the First Security Bank, but then the American National Bank of Idaho Falls). The family home was on the banks of the Mississippi River, where Will learned to love the outdoors and fishing.

Prior to entering medical college, he attended Rensselaer Polytechnic in Syracuse, New York and Purdue in Indiana. He was graduated in 1900 from Northwestern School of Medicine and served his internship at Jackson Memorial Hospital in South Chicago. When that was completed he started west, intending to go to Seattle, but stopped in Idaho Falls to visit his father's branch bank. He was fascinated with the countryside and the hunting and fishing. He decided to remain a year, but stayed until 1940, when he retired and moved to Los Angeles.

The Kinnairds had one daughter, Kay Kinnaird Woolsey, and a son, Robert, and six grandchildren.

DR. C. A. B. JENSEN

Driving a team of horses pulling his sleigh, Dr. Jensen was traveling at a fast clip from Mackay, Idaho, to the White Knob Copper Mine, where an injury had occurred, when the horses went around a bend and the sleigh tipped over. Doctor, medicine bags and all were sent down the mountainside. By the time the horses were stopped, the sleigh uprighted and belongings gathered, the doctor's hands were nearly frozen.

Dr. Jensen was spared none of the experiences of the pioneer doctor after he arrived in Mackay. There was no dentist in the village and he had to pull teeth of aching patients. He thought nothing of making house calls one hundred miles away. At one time it was necessary for him to remove a rock slide by hand before he was able to continue his journey. On several occasions he found it necessary to take patients 200 miles to a Salt Lake hospital. He traveled by sleigh, horse and buggy, a Model T Ford and when necessary, borrowed a railroad handcar.

Home surgeries were the order of the day. He performed two appendectomies, using the kitchen table for operating and kerosene lamps for lighting. One was done with the assistance of Dr. N.H. Farrell and the second with Dr. F.P. Richards. He went through a spinal meningitis epidemic and knew he had saved lives.

He was born May 13, 1891, in Baldwin, Wisconsin, attending school there and Valpraiso University, Indiana, 1908–12, graduating as a pharmaceutical chemist and pharmacist. He worked with his brother, August Jensen, for ten years before and after graduation in his drugstore in Butte, Montana. From 1910–20 he studied at Creighton University in Omaha, graduating as an honor student as he received his M.D. His internship was at Holy Cross Hospital in Salt Lake City, after which he moved to Mackay from 1921 until 1945. He was appointed as doctor at the State Hospital in Blackfoot, where he stayed for two years and then moved to Drummond, Montana.

During World War I, he was a second lieutenant in the Army. His recreation was playing several different musical instruments, writing and as a chef. He was a member of the Lutheran Church and a Master Mason.

DR. JOHN MONTFORT FINNEY

In the Idaho Panhandle the name of Dr. John Finney is recalled with a bit of awe for his accomplishments and confident attitude toward life. John Finney successfully used gasoline as an antiseptic in surgery. He formed a Citizens' Committee in the town of Harrison and rallied townspeople to force the city council to provide a pure water supply. Many had become ill from drinking contaminated water.

It was John Finney who came into Harrison in 1910, the year of the "Big Blowup," the worst fire to strike the west. The fire moved from Montana, jumping from one mountain range to another, blackening the town of Wallace, on through the St. Maries area and halfway down the rivers and lake toward Coeur d'Alene, with many losing their lives. John Finney battled back during the typhoid and influenza epidemics in 1918, saving the lives of many. He had the first automobile in Harrison, traveling before that with horse and buggy, horseback, walking, and motor boat.

He exchanged his car for horse each September until the next April, because of the deep snow in those years. He was in Harrison from 1914 to 1924, when he moved to Spokane and practiced until retiring in 1957.

He was born in Springfield, Ohio, March 14, 1881. His father was a farmer and a teacher. John and a younger brother joined forces to operate a hotel and restaurant to put themselves and two sisters through school. He was graduated from Cedarville College (Ohio) in 1903 with an A.B. degree; Medical School at Ohio University in 1910 with an M.D. degree. During World War II he served as medic.

The doctor enjoyed wood-working, masonry, boating, and fishing. He and Mrs. Finney became the parents of three sons, one a Methodist minister, one a physician, one an administrator; and a daughter, the wife of anthropologist Dr. William S. Laughlin. They had twelve grandchildren.

DR. RUSSELL TRUITT

Dr. Russell Truitt was born in Montgomery County, Illinois, May 2, 1852, and educated in the public schools. For three years he attended Hillsboro Academy; a year at McKendree; a year at Carthage College, and earned his degree from Eclectic Medical College, Cincinnati, in 1877.

He practiced in Illinois, visited the Willamette Valley, and in 1880, moved to Walla Walla and later to eastern Oregon until 1895. He then moved to Cottonwood, Idaho, as a pioneer physician. He was a member of the Idaho State Medical Society, of the State Board of Medical Examiners, for twelve years. He was a Republican, and belonged to the Masonic Lodge.

On August 1, 1878, Dr. Truitt married Louise A. Smith, of Albany, Oregon. They had two sons.

DR. RICHARD JACOB SUTTON

Dr. Richard J. Sutton practiced in Paris, Idaho from 1913 to 1922; Magna, Utah, 1922 to 1926; Idaho Falls, 1926 to 1936 and Oakley from 1936 until his death in 1951.

He was born in Paris, Idaho December 13, 1882. Much of

his youth was spent at the mine his father owned and in herding sheep for his father and uncle. He learned to shoe horses; hauled bricks and poles to the mill at Garfield; and helped build a large smokestack.

On October 5, 1904, he married Mabel Rich, daughter of William L. and Ella Amelia (Pomeroy) Rich. They settled in Pleasant Green where their first two children were born. He decided to become a doctor, moving his family to Salt Lake, to attend the University of Utah for one year. He attended Chicago College of Medicine and Surgery at Loyola University, graduating in 1913.

During early years in Paris he traveled long distances through cold and snow in the winter and deep mud in the spring. His Ford car, purchased in 1914 was stored in the fall, when a single buggy, cutter or small bob sleigh and team, depending on the severity of weather, were used. The sleigh had a canvas top for protection and the doctor donned fur coat, cap and gloves, with a robe of horsehide. He carried heated rocks for his feet, which his wife kept in the oven at all times during cold weather. For night calls he carried a spotlight attached to a car battery.

His hobbies included fishing, hunting, and horse racing. He had his own horses and raced a cutter on the ice in the winter, and did harness and quarter horse racing in the summer. He won many ribbons at county fairs.

The family lived on the ground floor of a three story house. The second story became a hospital, with operating room, patient rooms, and the third floor was living quarters for the nurses. Many deliveries and emergency surgery cases were performed in patients' homes, with makeshift equipment, kerosene lamps and mirrors. He labored long hours during the flu epidemic of 1918, two diphtheria epidemics and one of meningitis.

A son, Richard Pomeroy Sutton, also became a physician.

DR. HARMON TREMAINE

Dr. Tremaine was born June 16, 1881, Astoria, Iowa. His father was a physician. Through high school he studied in Ida Grove, Iowa. From 1902-05 he went to Armour Institute of Technology and graduated from Hahnemann School of Medicine, Chicago in 1915. Schooling was interrupted because of suspected tuberculosis, and he was advised to go west. He went to Colorado where he ran a small drug store and gave general medical and obstetrical service, there being no physician in the town.

From 1914 to 1915 he interned at Streeter Hospital, Chicago, returning to Colorado to practice from 1915 to 1924, when he moved to Boise. He practiced until his death in 1960.

He was on the staffs at St. Lukes and St. Alphonsus and from 1931–58 he was Idaho Chairman, American Academy of Pediatrics; charter member, Rocky Mountain Pediatric and North Pacific Pediatric Societies; director, Idaho Child Health Recovery Project in 1932.

He had a son and two daughters.

DR. JOHN MILLS MINTER

Dr. Minter was born in Madisonville, Kentucky, October 15, 1882. His father was a plantation owner.

He earned money for his schooling and was graduated from Northwestern Medical School. He interned for one year at the Deaconess Hospital in Milwaukee. He practiced in Burley from 1908 until his death, December 1916. His work was his hobby. The Minters had one son and one daughter.

DR. NEWELL JONATHAN BROWN

Dr. Brown was born in Stanstead, Canada, March 10, 1854. He was educated at McGill University, Montreal, and at Dartmouth College. He received his M.D. degree November 3, 1875, and began practice in Montreal. Three months later he moved to Red Oak, Iowa, and in 1977 moved to Grundy Center, Iowa.

October 19, 1878 Dr. Brown married Celia Frances Eastman. In December, 1878, they moved to Colorado because of his health. In April 1883, they moved to the two-year-old Idaho mining town of Hailey. He regained his health, opened a medical office and had a prosperous practice.

He was a member of the American Medical Association, and was local surgeon of the Union Pacific and the Oregon Short Line Railroad Companies. He was one of the highest ranking Masons in Idaho; member of the Ancient Order of United Workmen and the Modern Woodmen of America. The Browns had four sons.

DR. FREDERICK S. KOHLER

Dr. Kohler located in Nampa when the town was just beginning, and was its druggist and physician. He was born in Lewistown, Pennsylvania, December 18, 1838, the youngest of eight children.

He was educated at Dartmouth and Swarthmore Colleges, graduating in 1860. At the start of the Civil War, he became surgeon of the 21st Pennsylvania Cavalry, under General Sheridan. He remained at the front with the wounded, and was present at the surrender of General Lee.

When hostilities ceased the doctor returned to Lewistown, where he practiced for five years. He moved to Vevay, Indiana, for ten years. In 1882 he went to Denver, and from there to Morgan, Utah, until 1887, when he left for the new town of Nampa. He had a drug store along with his practice.

After the war, Dr. Kohler married Sallie Carson, who died four years later, leaving two sons. Both became physicians.

DR. RALPH FALK

Dr. Falk was born in Boise, August 6, 1884, son of the Nathan Falks, pioneer merchants, who came to Idaho in 1864. In 1868, with his brother, David, Nathan established the business that became known as Falks, one of Boise's leading mercantile stores.

Dr. Falk went through high school in Boise, and attended the Mount Tamalpais Military Academy, California, where he was graduated in 1900. He spent two years at the University of California, and in 1907 graduated from the Jefferson Medical College of Philadelphia. His first medical work came as assistant physician in St. Louis City Hospital, 1907-08.

In 1908 he opened medical and surgery practice in Boise. From May 1918 until January 1919, he served as first lieutenant in the Army; later as captain in the Medical Corps. He was secretary of the Idaho State Board of Health from 1910-17, and member of the Idaho and American Medical Societies.

He was married to Marian Citron and they had one son, Ralph Jr., and daughter, Carol.

DR. OSSIAN J. WEST

Dr. West was born in Oregon, August 24, 1866, son of the Reverend W.F. and Jane (Whipple) West. His father, born in England, was ordained minister in the Methodist Episcopal Church. The Wests crossed the plains to Oregon in 1851, and located near Salem. Of six children, all were farmers except Dr. West.

Dr. West was educated at the Willamette University and graduated with honors from the medical college in 1889. He practiced in the Portland hospital and spent two years at St. Helens. He was appointed government physician and surgeon at Idaho's Fort Lapwai Industrial School by President Benjamin Harrison, and named to succeed himself by both Presidents Cleveland and McKinley. Dr. West was with the agency for eight years. He was associated with General McConville, and when the General was called to the Spanish-American war, Dr. West had charge of the school. He became government physician and surgeon at the Nez Perce Indian Agency at Spalding.

He was a member of the Idaho State Medical Association, and prepared many papers of value to the medical fraternity. He was a Republican and a civic worker.

DR. SAMUEL M. C. REYNOLDS

Dr. Reynolds was born in Missouri, December 15, 1847, son of William and Didame (McClure) Reynolds. He had a somewhat limited education in Missouri. Despite his youth, he enlisted in the Civil War, and was with Sanborn's Brigade at Scofield. Later he became a member of the Sixth Missouri Cavalry and fought throughout the war. When it ended he returned home, and was editor and owner of a newspaper in Linn County. He wanted to be a doctor, sold his paper, entered Missouri Medical College, and received his M.D.

In 1881 he went to Boise and after practicing medicine for a brief time, went to work for the *Statesman* for a year. He moved to Weiser for five years and resumed his medical career. Then he moved to Salubria, Idaho, and practiced for ten years, when he was appointed Adjutant of the Soldiers' Home, and continued in that office until the administration of Governor Steunenberg. In 1896, he practiced in Meridian, where he was appointed postmaster, receiving successive appointments from Presidents Teddy Roosevelt and Taft. He was a staunch Republican. Dr. Reynolds was president of the Meridian Telephone Company; member of the Grand Army of the Republic; and the Odd Fellows.

DR. THOMAS AMMON ELLISON

Dr. Ellison was admitted to Idaho practice in 1918 and located at St. Anthony, where he owned St. Anthony General Hospital. His affiliations included: Latter Day Saints Church, Republican party, American, Idaho, and Upper Snake River Valley Medical associations and president of the latter in 1934.

He was born June 7, 1886 to Thomas and Annie Jane (Rowan) Ellison in Murray, Utah. He received his B.A. in 1912 from the University of Utah, and M.D. from Western Reserve in 1918. He married Addie Robison at Farmington, Utah in 1911.

DR. EDMUND EARL RIVERS

Dr. Rivers lived in Texas, Tennessee, Virginia, California, and Old Mexico, practiced medicine in all of them after finishing study in 1882. He came to Idaho in 1890 and practiced for a year before settling in Idaho Falls to share offices with his cousin, Dr. Wilson.

DR. EDWIN F. GUYON

Dr. Guyon spent much of his life working to stamp out tuberculosis. Born November 7, 1853 to Leon John and Emily Louise (Shattuck) Guyon in New Orleans, and when Edwin was a baby, his father disappeared and no trace of him could ever be found. When he was two, his mother took him and moved to California. She married again and the family lived in several places, including Portland, Oregon, where the doctor attended grade school.

His stepfather bought some Indian cattle and ranched at Pilot Rock, Oregon, where Edwin learned about the old west, the remuda, roundup, chuck wagon, branding, roping, and cutting out, until he was twenty-five. His mother died at that time, and Edwin decided to secure an education, graduating from Walla Walla College in 1875, and went on to study medicine at the University of Cincinnati. He received his M.D. degree in 1891, and studied further medicine before returning west. He practiced in Pendleton until February 28, 1896 and moved to Montpelier, Idaho, to open practice the next month.

In 1897, he was named assistant surgeon for the Diamond Coal Company in Wyoming and the Oregon Short Line, remaining for three years. He practiced in Montpelier and continued his interest in tuberculosis. In 1907, Governor Steunenberg appointed him to the Board of Medical Examiners where he helped author laws pertaining to medicine. In 1911, he was the sole Idaho doctor to attend the Denver national convention on tubercular diseases. In 1912, he was named one of five to the International Convention on Hygiene and Demography in Washington, D.C. The Grand Lodge of Odd Fellows was taking steps to provide a hospital where members suffering from tuberculosis could be treated. They asked Dr. Guyon to work with them.

Dr. Guyon had two children by his first marriage to Marguerite Jones at Pilot Rock, July 6, 1879; and three by his second marriage at Montpelier in 1903 to Effie Moore.

DR. HERMAN ZIPF

Herman Zipf was born and educated in Germany, coming to Idaho about 1865. His advertising card in the *Idaho World* stated that he was a surgeon and accoucher (child delivery). He lived in the Boise Basin and was one of the few physicians who wanted to remain there after the gold rush subsided. He had located a homestead adjoining a drugstore lot he purchased in 1874. Droves of people moved out of the basin and he finally moved to Boise and practiced until his death in 1890.

Dr. Zipf was especially successful in obstetrics and continued interest in the children he brought into the world as they grew to adulthood. He had great self-confidence and a Boise woman who knew him said, "He would attempt anything medically, and he always made a good job of it."

He was over six feet tall and weighed over two hundred pounds, but must have kept in good physical condition, as he had many rugged trips to take to care for patients. The late Mrs. Stella Graham, daughter of Mrs. Zipf, told of an unusually arduous trip that he took into the back country, above Idaho City. In a logging camp miles away, a man had a seriously infected leg from an imbedded iron splinter shot from a wedge he was using to fell a tree.

Realizing the terrain was rugged, Dr. Zipf hired a much younger and experienced woodsman, Barney Aveline, as guide. The route lay over high mountains, some heavily timbered, some with jagged lava rocks, frozen hard snow, or soft slush and mud. After miles of hard-going they reached a raging stream in full torrent with the spring thaw. There was no bridge, only a fallen pine tree spanning the stream. The tree still had its bark with sharp points of limbs that had been chopped off. Straddling the tree with their feet in the water, and the doctor holding his surgical kit in one hand, they hitched themselves across.

There were more miles of walking before they arrived at the logging camp and the patient. The doctor was exhausted from the trip and rested for a few hours. Then, in a crude cabin with a small kerosene lamp and simple medical instruments, no sterilization nor antiseptics, he amputated the man's leg at the hip. Dr. Zipf cared for the patient for several days and, feeling he would survive, left with Aveline on the same route back. Mrs. Graham said that the patient made a full recovery.

DR. I. H. HARRIS

An article in the *Portland Oregonian* of August 4, 1863, reported that: "Matt Bledsoe was killed in Placerville, Idaho, last week by Dr. I.H. Harris. Bledsoe shot at Harris, whereupon Harris stabbed him to the heart with a knife."

In *All Along the River*, author Nellie Ireton Mills, added, "Bledsoe was listed with a number of the most desperate outlaws of the Pierce City and Florence camps, and doubtless deserved his fate. Boone Helm, another well known criminal from the north, also was in the Basin and up and down the river."

No report was given on what happened to the doctor. Likely nothing, except congratulations for ridding the world of another outlaw.

DR. HARLAN PAGE USTICK

On Ustick Road in Boise is what was once the community of Ustick, with its own post office, store, church, bank, and fruit orchards. It was built by Dr. Ustick who arrived in Boise in late 1888 or early 1889, and was the twenty-seventh doctor to receive an Idaho medical license. He built the Boise-Nampa Railroad about 1912 and the Boise Gas Company about 1916. He purchased land and sold it in five or ten acre tracts.

Dr. Ustick was born November 26, 1848 in Fayette, Ohio, the youngest of thirteen children. His father was a farmer and also bought and sold wool on an extensive scale. An elder in the Presbyterian Church, he was uncompromisingly opposed to oppression of the Negroes. The Ustick home became a station on the famous underground railroad in ante-bellum days, aiding many Negroes on their way north to freedom.

Dr. Ustick graduated from Miami University in 1870, and from Hahnemann Medical College in Philadelphia in 1883. He practiced in Ohio, Chicago, and Portland, before arriving in Boise in 1892. He made a specialty of treating chronic diseases. He had a number of business interests. He was secretary of the Fruit Growers of Idaho, Knights of Pythias, Woodmen of the World, Pioneers of the Pacific, a leading member of the Presbyterian Church and Republican party.

Dr. Ustick and Mrs. Margaret Pittenger were married soon after his arrival in Boise. By her first marriage, she had a son, Fred, who was graduated from the Chicago Homeopathic Medical College in March 1899. The doctor had two sons and a daughter by his first marriage: Roy, Faye, and Clyde.

DR. GEORGE P. HALEY

Dr. George P. Haley, a Boise doctor, remembered the days of making calls by horse and buggy during most of the year, and replacing the buggy wheels with runners during the snowy season. He exchanged one potato state for another when he came to Idaho from Main in 1888 as a specialist in ear, nose, and throat ailments. Dr. Haley also made progress in the early-day study of cancer.

He was born April 24, 1854, to Benjamin and Mary Hunt Haley, East Corinth, Maine. Up to age twelve, George attended schools at Corinth and completed an academic course in New Jersey. He then went back to his father's farm and worked until he reached his legal majority. He began to fulfill his dream by entering Jefferson Medical College in Philadelphia, where he received his medical degree in 1879. Between Maine and Idaho, he practiced in Newport, New Jersey, until 1885 and at Laramie, Wyoming until 1888.

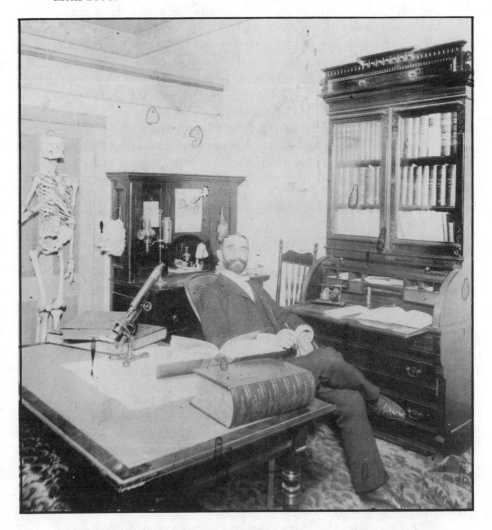

Dr. George P. Haley in his Boise office of medicine near the turn of the century. Note the skeleton which he used to point out "where it hurts" and why to the patient. Dr. Haley was born in Maine, educated in New Jersey, and arrived in Idaho in 1888. One of the early day doctors to take special study in cancer treatment, he became a well-known physician.
(Idaho Historical Society photo)

He watched Boise grow from a small village to a city. In 1903, he took a postgraduate course in the study of surface cancers at Chicago's Medical College. Dr. Haley was medical examiner for the United Artisans and Woodmen of the World. He was a delegate to the Pan-American Medical Society in St. Louis in 1889. Politically he was a Republican and fraternally a member of the Odd Fellows, which he joined in 1884. He held all of the chairs in the I.O.O.F. Dr. Haley was a member of the Methodist Church.

In 1881, Dr. Haley married Eliza J. Read of Vineland, New Jersey, and they had four children: George B., Marcus, Jennie, and Alice.

DR. SAMUEL A. SWAYNE

Samuel Swayne was born in Fort Wayne, Indiana, December 24, 1887. He went through high school there and received an A.B. degree from De Pauw University, Greencastle, Indiana. He attended Indiana University, College of Physicians and Surgeons, Columbia University.

His two year rotating internship at Kings County Hospital, Brooklyn was shortened to eighteen months by doubling the work, so he could serve in World War I. For one year he was at the hospital, U.S. Naval Academy. After the war he came to Idaho.

From 1920-61 he practiced in Nampa. He once did an appendectomy on the husband of a registered nurse in their home, as she was in a dispute with the hospital. The patient made an uneventful recovery. In the early years, the doctor carried a large shovel to dig out of snow drifts. One winter he treated two high school girls for severe frostbites on their lower thighs. They had walked to town through cold and snow in the days of above knee skirts and rolled stockings.

Dr. Swayne was on the staff at Mercy and Samaritan Hospitals. He belonged to Southwest Idaho, Idaho State and American Medical Associations.

He was interested in riding horses, hunting, camping, and ghost towns.

Three of Dr. and Mrs. Swayne's four daughters are still living. They are Rachel Schilde and Julia Hyslop of Nampa and Phyllis Thomas of Boise. A namesake nephew, attorney Sam Swayne, and his wife, Zoa, live at Orofino.

CHAPTER
3

"DON'T FORGET THE LADIES"

The man and woman on opposite ends of the venerable old Ford Theatre stage in Washington, D.C., were in the play, *John and Abigail*. They read from actual letters John Adams, second president of the United States, and his wife, Abigail, exchanged during their lifetime together. The letters were filled with happenings in the early days of our country, and very soon it seemed that the Adamses were standing before us, speaking to each other. June Duncan Hansen, British actress, who became the wife of Orval Hansen, Idaho Congressman, and this writer were at that play years ago. The quotations are as accurate as the memory.

In a time when women had been taught as little girls to obey and serve their husbands, Abigail and John Adams had based their successful marriage on equality. It was Abigail who had urged John and his countrymen in Philadelphia to declare independence for the colonies from the oppressive rule of Britain. With that accomplished, replying to his letter in which he told her of his labors in framing the laws by which America was to be governed, she urged the same men not to put unlimited power in the hands of husbands, as, "All men would be tyrants if they could." She ended her letter with, "Don't forget the ladies, John."

The women who doctored in Idaho cannot be forgotten because they cared. When examination finds nothing wrong with a patient, the medical folk use the word "unremarkable." This section is about a group of remarkable women, because there are so many things right with women who, in the early days of Idaho's history, chose to become doctors and gave extraordinary medical care.

While equality seemed to be a natural thing for John and Abigail Adams, it was not so with many in the eastern part of the country. Equality progressed at a much faster rate in the west. As the women of the frontier led rugged lives and worked by the sides of their husbands in building the homes, making the livings and lives of their own, western men were quicker to respond to the appeal of the suffragists who brought their message from the east. Idaho was among the first states to give the vote to women.

DR. MINNIE F. HOWARD

Few people living in Idaho during the first half of the 1900s had not heard of Dr. Minnie F. Howard of Pocatello and the good that she did for the state. She arrived in Idaho, along with her husband, Dr. William F. Howard, in 1902. It was only twelve years later that she was named as one of the "most energetic, active, and influential women in the state." There was hardly a facet of Idaho life in which she was not involved.

Born August 23, 1872, in Memphis, Missouri, Minnie Frances Hayden was a graduate of Central Normal College in Kansas and Cook County Normal School, Englewood, Illinois. In 1899, she received her M.D. degree from Kansas University Women's Medical School and took post graduate studies at New York University and in Vienna, Austria.

She married William F. Howard August 23, 1894 at Larned, Kansas, while both taught and worked toward medical degrees. She was constantly expanding her knowledge and took special training in both Chicago and New York, while practicing there. In 1902, the Doctors Howard moved to Pocatello and she was the 259th issued an Idaho medical license to practice on April 7, 1903. She and her husband had practiced together for twenty years when he died October 19, 1948.

The Howards had four sons, all becoming doctors: Dr. Richard P. Howard, Pocatello; Dr. Nelson Jr., San Francisco; Dr. Francis E., Redwood City; and Dr. Forrest H., Santa Ana, California. Dr. Minnie was a member of the Pocatello, Idaho, and American Medical societies.

Dr. Minnie was fascinated with the history of the old west and particularly Idaho. Fort Hall near Pocatello led to a study of all of the forts in Idaho. In a letter dated February 25, 1955, to Mrs. John Taylor, widow of Dr. Taylor of Boise, she wrote, "I always want to thank personally anyone who interests themselves in Idaho history." She became an early president of the Southeast Idaho Historical Society and an organizer and director of the Oregon Trail Memorial Association.

Two years after arriving in Pocatello, Dr. Minnie helped organize the Civic Club and was chairman of the committee to secure the Carnegie Library. The building now houses the Bannock County Historical Museum. She organized the Art and Travel Club, County Social Welfare Board, and was co-chairman of the first Red Cross chapters for Bannock and Caribou counties.

Dr. Howard seemed to have been born liberated. When her family was well-launched, she went alone to Italy and Austria for a year's study of the arts. When she returned, she "hit the ground running" and developed a traveling art exhibit for the Federated Women's Clubs. These exhibits traveled over Idaho, reaching twenty-six sites in two years. Dr. Howard met most of the expenses for the tour. She kept her family intact, cared for, and never neglected spiritual life as a member of the First Congregational Church. Friends marveled at her ability to handle so much. She died at age ninety-three in Pocatello, September 2, 1965.

DR. ELIZABETH L. MUNN

Where but in a western state, such as Idaho, would a woman doctor be bodily lifted from the saddle of her horse during a rodeo parade by a motorcycle policeman and rushed to the hospital for an obstetrics emergency? That and many other "typical Idaho" acts were experienced by Dr. Elizabeth Munn of Caldwell. She was born March 31, 1911, in Fairbury, Nebraska, and came to Caldwell before starting the eighth grade.

From the eighth grade through college, she attended Caldwell schools, receiving her Bachelor of Science degree, with a major in chemistry, from the College of Idaho in 1932. Her M.D. degree was earned at the University of Oregon Medical School in 1936, and followed by an internship at the Children's Hospital in San Francisco. She was granted a three year fellowship in obstetrics and gynecology, arriving back at Caldwell to open her practice in 1941.

She married Howard K. Eyestone in 1949, but retained her maiden name professionally.

Dr. Munn listed horseback riding as one of her interests and it follows that she was active with the Caldwell Night Rodeo and often rode in the parades and processions around the arena. On one occasion she rode her horse from the rodeo directly to the hospital. She said, "The horse was handy and the caller said, 'hurry'."

Home delivery of babies were still in vogue in the 1940s and the doctor remembers that she "was always called in the middle of the night." One delivery had seventeen spectators, all close relatives of the parents and baby.

In addition to practicing in two small private hospitals, the Sanitarium and the Memorial Park Hospital, she delivered the first baby born in the new Caldwell Memorial Community Hospital in 1951. Although she had no children, Dr. Munn felt like a grandmother when the first babies she delivered in the early 1940s came to her for care and delivery of their children.

She was a member and vice-president of the Southwest Idaho District Medical Association and delegate to the state meeting. She practiced as a member of the Caldwell Memorial Hospital staff and was chief of staff in the early 1950s.

DR. MARY ALLEN CALLOWAY

Mary Allen Calloway came with her family to Idaho when she was five years old and, with the exception of the time she was studying medicine, made it her home the rest of her life. She was the youngest of five children born to Dr. and Mrs. Thomas H. Calloway, pioneers of Caldwell. She was born December 29, 1878, at Decatur, Texas, and died at age seventy on October 15, 1948, in a Boise hospital.

Dr. Calloway was a descendant of an old Virginia family who had married into the Robert E. Lee and Jubal Early families. Her great-grandmother was an aunt of General Jubal Early, one of the distinguished officers of the Confederacy in the Civil War. (Interestingly, a Coeur d'Alene

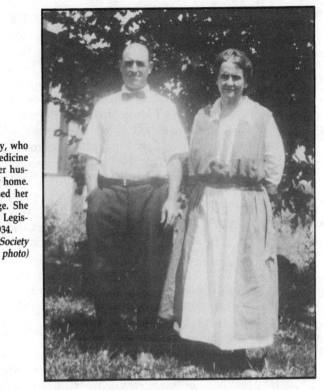

Dr. Mary Allen Calloway, who began the practice of medicine in Boise in 1902, with her husband, I.A. Joplin, at their home. Dr. Calloway always used her own name after marriage. She also served in the Idaho Legislatures of 1932 and 1934.
(Idaho Historical Society photo)

doctor, Robert M. McFarland, is the great-great-great nephew of General Early.)

Dr. Mary Allen Calloway received education in the Caldwell schools and graduated from the College of Idaho in 1897. She studied medicine at Texas Christian University, Fort Worth, graduating *cum laude* in 1902. She was licensed to practice in Idaho the same year and established offices in Boise.

Although married to Boise realtor I.B. Joplin, Dr. Calloway retained her maiden name in professional life. She was a member of Ada County, Idaho, and the American Medical associations. She served as Ada County physician. Elected as a Democrat, she served the 1932 and 1934 terms as a representative in the legislature. She was a member of the Christian Church, Women of Woodcraft, the Order of Yeoman, for which she was secretary; and the Rebekah Lodge.

DR. SUSAN E. BRUCE

Born in New Brunswick, Canada, located east of the state of Maine, Susan E. Bruce came to the United States with her parents in 1876 at age twenty-eight. She was born August 15, 1848. They located in Chicago, where she was graduated from the Homeopathic Medical School in 1880. She practiced in Chicago until 1905, when she came west. She was so impressed with the town of Lewiston, when visiting, she started making plans to move, and returned in 1906 to make Lewiston her home.

She was appointed by Governors of both political parties to serve on of the State Board of Health. Governor Frank Gooding, Republican, appointed her to a six year term in 1907. When Democrat Moses Alexander was elected governor, he named her to a two year term.

In 1911, she was named health officer for Lewiston, serving ten years. After a two year retirement, she was again appointed in 1923 and served until a short time before her death on December 24, 1934. She spent fifty years as a practicing physician.

During Dr. Bruce's administration, health affairs of the city were arduous and exacting. An epidemic of smallpox broke out in 1913, with ninety-five stricken. She enforced the health laws so stringently that the dread disease was prevented from spreading. At that time the jail was crowded and the epidemic spread there. Dr. Bruce took personal charge of the jail patients and held the outbreak in check. In 1927, she did notable work in a similar epidemic.

Dr. Bruce was representative of the business women in Lewiston during her day and maintained a vital interest in civic affairs. She participated in politics and was a delegate to the state convention of Democrats in 1920, and was sent as a delegate to the national convention in San Francisco.

DR. ALICE JEANNETTE TIPPETS

"Idaho had its share of great characters, and one of the most colorful was my grandmother Alice Jeannette Tippets, who was Bear Lake County's first and only woman doctor," are the words of Rhea Tippets Hall, with obvious pride in her ancestor. Writing memories of Dr. Tippets, Mrs. Hall referred to a journal kept by Dr. Tippets' husband, Joseph Mahroni Tippets, a distant cousin whom she married at age sixteen.

She had a soothing hand and a comforting word for the sick, and she was chosen to attend a school of medicine being opened in Salt Lake City after the Latter Day Saints Church leader Brigham Young had requested that Relief Society Presidents appoint three women from each ward to study hygiene and nursing. This was on July 15, 1873 and he proposed that the church Wards support those named.

A class in obstetrics was taught by Dr. Mary H. Barker. Private classes were given by Utah women physicians for about fifty years after 1877, during a shortage of male doctors. Professors included Doctors Romania B. Pratt Penrose, Dr. Ellis R. Shipp, and Dr. Margaret Rogers when Alice Jeannette was a trainee. She graduated from the School of Medicine and Surgery in 1884. Three years later she moved to Georgetown, Idaho, and for many years was the only doctor in Bear Lake County.

She told her grandchildren stories of coming west with the great band of Mormon pioneers. She was the oldest child of William Plummer Tippets and Sophia Burnham Mead Tippets. The family left Council Bluffs, Iowa (then called Kanesville), with Captain Hunt's company, on July 4, 1850 and arrived the middle of October. Alice Jeannette was six years of age and walked most of the way. She remembered wearing a dress, the skirt of which had been made from an umbrella. Those experiences taught her not to put importance on material things. Later in life she would smile and say, "You don't feel bad wearing old clothes, so long as you have better ones at home."

An incident that remained important happened one day when they stopped near a grove of trees for the noon meal. She was with her little sisters and other children playing under the largest tree when a sudden storm pelted them with rain and the wind was gusting. Suddenly, it seemed to her that a voice told her to take the children back to the wagon. She gave the signal and they made a dash. The instant they left, a dazzling flash of lightning struck the large tree under which they had been standing and slivered it to shreds.

Her medical training was a year, meager at best today.

Dr. Alice Jeannette, as she was most often called, took care of patients and healed many a broken bone. In one incident, William McCammon was thrown from his horse with his foot caught in the stirrup. He was dragged quite a distance before the horse could be stopped. His scalp was almost torn from his head. Dr. Tippets sewed it back on so well that no ill effects resulted.

She felt her greatest success was saving the life of her son, Joey, twenty, in August 1883, when he was shot in the chest while hunting. She had not finished her training, so sent a telegram to a doctor to come from Ogden. He arrived at ten that night, examined the boy, said nothing could be done and left one dose of morphine to ease him into death. So, Alice Jeannette began working, picking shot out of his back, closing the wound as much as she could, keeping it dressed. Many prayers were said and in a few days the fever left and he began to gain strength. Joey recovered. The wound never completely healed. His mother, however, had earned for him twenty-eight more years of life.

DR. ADELLA N. HOBART

At the time of death February 12, 1957, Dr. Hobart was one of the three oldest women physicians in the country. She was ninety-five, and born in 1861 during the Civil War. She graduated from Monmouth College in 1884 and from Northwestern Medical School in 1890. Internship was at Mary Thompson College in Chicago. The length of days was not all that marked her life, as she used her skill and training to heal many illnesses.

She practiced at Monmouth, Illinois (1891), Davenport, Iowa (1894), and Twin Falls, Idaho (1910). She married W.E. Hobart at Canon City, Colorado, the same year and continued to practice in Twin Falls through 1915. Mr. Hobart died in 1923. She was survived by a step-daughter, Phoebe Miller of Portland, Oregon, and nine nieces and nephews. She was a member of the Presbyterian Church.

DR. NINA H. MAYNARD

The spell of Africa, particularly the children, drew Dr. Maynard back three times in her life and later she returned there to die. She was born in 1879 and came to Idaho from Baltimore, Maryland. She had attended Barnes College in

St. Louis, Missouri, and arrived in Idaho Falls in 1908. She specialized in obstetrics.

In 1912, she left Idaho Falls as a Baptist missionary to a leper colony in Africa. She became so fond of the babies she delivered, calling them her "Black Diamonds," and felt the need for physicians in Africa so strongly that she kept returning there to do what she could. Her husband, Jay Maynard, remained in Idaho Falls where he was a book-keeper, until his death.

DR. CLARA M. HASTINGS

A North Dakota native, Clara Cummings Hastings was one of four in the Cummings family to become doctors. They were brothers Walter in Glendale, Arthur in Marysville, and John in Los Angeles. She opened an office in Los Angeles in the 1950s and moved to Nampa for a practice of seven years before joining the medical staff at the Veterans Administration Hospital in Boise.

She was graduated from Madison College, Tennessee in pre-med and received her M.D. from Loma Linda University. Her internship and residency in pediatrics were at Los Angeles White Memorial Hospital. She received her M.S. in public health from the University of Michigan. Dr. Hastings had two sons.

DR. MARY ELIZABETH DONALDSON

Dr. Mary Elizabeth Donaldson of Boise was a cousin once removed of the great English novelist Charles Dickens. Her father, Zachariah Craker of Sadsdam, Buckinghamshire, England, was his first cousin. Craker came to the United States in the early 1840s. Her mother, Elizabeth D. Brown, was from Spring Prairie, Wisconsin, where they were married. Mary Elizabeth was the eldest of nine, born January 12, 1851 at Reedsburg, Wisconsin. She completed her grade and high school and taught there. After four years of teaching she became the wife of a Mr. Hesford in 1871. They had one daughter, Zella, who died as a child, and the Hesfords were divorced.

Soon after the death of her daughter, Dr. Donaldson accompanied her brother, James, who was in frail health, to Idaho, where he hoped to recuperate. While caring for her brother, she taught school. James recovered his health, coming to weigh over 200 pounds! Mary Elizabeth met and married Thomas L. Johnston, an early resident of Idaho Territory, from Millersburg, Ohio in 1862. He was postmaster at Bellevue for several years and had mining ventures in the Wood River Valley. He died in Boise in 1898.

Johnston encouraged his wife to practice medicine and in 1889 she entered the Wooster University Medical School in Cleveland, Ohio. She was the only woman to receive the M.D. degree in the class of 1892. With her return to Boise she began opening a series of sanitariums. Once it was established, the doctor started medical practice in Milton, Oregon, where she opened another sanitarium. She headed the hospital four years before returning to Boise in 1898. That spring she and her husband built the Idaho Sanitarium Institute, at which she gave medical service without charge. Her private practice continued to grow.

Fourteen years after the death of Mr. Johnston, she became the wife of Captain Gilbert Donaldson, well-known Boise business man. Subsequent to the marriage, Dr. Donaldson was able to fulfill a hope she had entertained since 1881 when she first visited a home for the care of aged men and women in Philadelphia. Many Boiseans joined the Donaldsons in promoting such a home, and the Donaldson Home for the Aged was located on Donaldson Heights in Boise. Again, she offered free medical care to those at the home. During the years she took in five orphans and provided them a loving home.

Dr. Donaldson was a charter member of the American Woman's League and a contributor to its literature. In December 1903, she aided in founding the *Idaho Magazine* and published and edited the *Reform Appeal,* organized the Prohibition Alliance, and worked diligently to bring about the prohibition amendment.

DR. JESSIE K. CLARKE

When Dr. Jessie K. Clarke came to Grangeville in October 1898, to visit her mother and sister, who were ill, she liked the people and area so much that they found it easy to convince her she should open an office there. She made a specialty of diseases of eye, ear, nose, and throat.

Dr. Clarke was born in Circleville, Ohio, June 1, 1861, one of eight children. She was educated in the Normal School and Business Institute in Paola, Kansas, and Willamette University in Oregon, graduating from the latter in 1879. She pursued medical education at Edsworth Medical College, St. Joseph, Missouri, graduating with honors in 1896. She spent a year in specialized study at New York Polyclinic. She practiced for a year in Topeka, Kansas, before coming to Idaho.

JANE GABY, DOCTORESS

The first news that "Doctoress" Jane Gaby had arrived in Idaho City in 1864, was a notice in the *Idaho City News* on June 4, announcing that she had fitted up rooms and beds for accommodation of the sick. Particular attention would be paid to those having fevers. A year later, a notice appeared June 28, 1865 in the *World*: "Mrs. Jane Gaby, Doctoress. Inflammation of the brain, inflammation of the bowels, etc., cured in 24 hours. No cure, no pay."

The *World* on June 18, 1865, indicated she wanted boarders to supplement her income: "Gaby's Hotel. Mrs. Gaby informs the public that she is prepared to receive permanent or transient boarders."

DR. MARY JANE BEARBY

Dr. Bearby arrived in the Boise Valley in the early 1800s and practiced in Boise and Mountain Home. She moved to Mountain Home about 1884 and established a drugstore and opened a "tent" school in back of the building. It was the first subscription school in Mountain Home and one of the students was her daughter, Hope Pyburn.

When licensure became the law, Dr. Bearby was the 152nd doctor to apply, receiving that number on October 3, 1899. Her Medical Doctor degree came from the Homeopathic Medical College for Women, re-named the Cleveland University of Medicine and Surgery in 1894.

Our Heritage reported that "Mary Jane Bearby, druggist, received the Mountain Home Hospital contract, at a salary of $150. She built a large, two story residence located between the Christian Center and a small house adjacent to Humphrey's Funeral Chapel."

Dr. Bearby was last known to be in Albion and her license was cancelled in 1931, which usually indicates leaving the area.

DR. HELEN PETERSON

Many northern Idahoans think of Paul Croy of Hope as the Poet Laureate of the Selkirks. His homespun poems have touched hearts and funnybones for years. When Dr. Helen "Pete" Peterson retired in 1955, a party attended by hundreds, heard Paul Croy's poem called "Doc Pete."

> She posed to be no better than she was.
> No saving saint nor fashion plate,
> But like the "Country Docs" of bygone days
> She "tied her horse to our front gate."
> There was no fanfare when she came,
> No crowds along the street,
> For many years she eased our pain—
> Have fun now, "Dr. Pete."

And fun she had. She loves the great outdoors and when younger, rarely missed a chance at trout fishing trip. She caught her share of lunkers. She was proud of the first huge Mackinaw she caught in 1958. She took it to the hospital, put it on a gurney, draped a sheet around it, and wheeled it all around, showing it to patients and visitors.

Each year, Dr. Pete entertains nurses with whom she worked. They enjoy it so much they formed a club, "A Bunch of Old Nurses and One Old Doctor." Penny

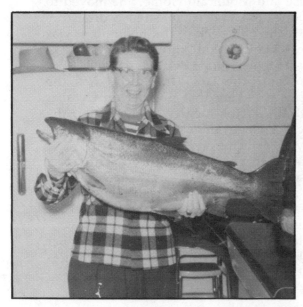

"Dr. Pete," as Helen Peterson, Sandpoint, M.D., was best known, happily displays the giant Mackinaw she caught in the waters of Lake Pend Oreille. The picture was taken in the kitchen of Dr. and Mrs. Malcolm McKennon before "Dr. Pete" took it to the hospital and showed in to workers and patients.
(Courtesy Penny Armstrong)

Armstrong belongs and, with her husband, prepared a special room in their home when the doctor had a stroke a few years ago, and she lives with them.

Dorothy "Brownie" Larson was the second nurse (June Dawson was the first) to work with Dr. Peterson and spent eighteen years with her. The hours were from 7 a.m. until 7 p.m. and she made fifty dollars a month. "I have great admiration for that woman," Dorothy said, "I went with her on house calls. Saturdays were rural calls, as far away as Clark Fork. It was good to watch her tending those she called 'the real people.' She was thoughtful of the patients and nurses, no matter how late she had to work."

Dr. William Tyler encouraged Dr. Peterson to go to medical school and later shared an office with her. Patients walked up many steps to get there. Dr. Tyler was something of a father figure to her. She says she couldn't have done it without him.

Mrs. Ted Navratil, nurse, said, "If patients came in feeling low, the doctor would tell a joke to make them laugh. . . ." She added, "I was working nights, and the phone rang about three in the morning, and it was Dr. Peterson, concerned about a patient. I told her the vital signs were good and she said, 'Good. Now I can get my sleep'.

"Another time, a patient had a bad reaction to a blood transfusion, so I called her office. She ordered medication to help with the allergy reaction and asked if I wanted her to come over. I said that I could handle it. Within a few minutes, she came in the door. 'I had to satisfy myself,' she said. The nurses could always depend upon Dr. Pete."

At the annual party, the nurses reminisce and Penny Armstrong usually has a poem saluting Dr. Pete. One included the stanzas:

> If you ask for advice at a party,
> As everybody knows . . .
> She will look straight in your eyes,
> And say, "Take off your clothes!"
> She's an unforgettable character
> It is really quite safe to say,
> The world is a little better,
> Because she passed our way.

DR. MARY JANE McGAHAN

Likely the most beautiful doctor (man or woman) to grace the medical profession in Idaho was Mary Jane McGahan, issued the 267th license to practice on April 7, 1903. It was at a pre-wedding barbecue at Redfish Lake in June, 1992, that Daphne Copenhaven (granddaughter of Dr. McGahan and medical writer in California), mentioned that her grandmother was an Idaho pioneer doctor.

Much was learned about the strong character and devotion of Dr. McGahan from conversations with Daphne.

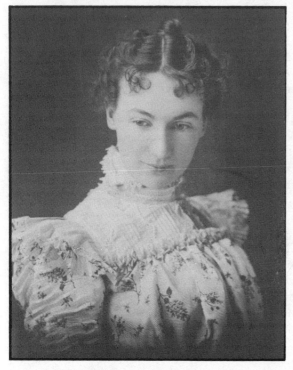

This beautiful doctor, Mary Jane McGahan, was the first woman to practice in Shoshone and Benewah counties. Her tragic death occurred about 1912, shortly after the Federal Narcotics Act was passed. She was murdered for the narcotics she was carrying in a "horse and buggy" call to a patient. The murderer was never found.

(Courtesy Daphne Copenhaven)

Dr. McGahan was the first woman physician to practice in two northern counties, Shoshone and Benewah. It is known that she had an office, along with her drugstore, in the bustling timber town of St. Joe on the river, and likely practiced for awhile in St. Maries.

Dr. McGahan was married to a "travelin' gold prospector and miner," who moved from one place to another. His daughter said that he had made and lost great sums of money. For sometime, Dr. McGahan followed him but the

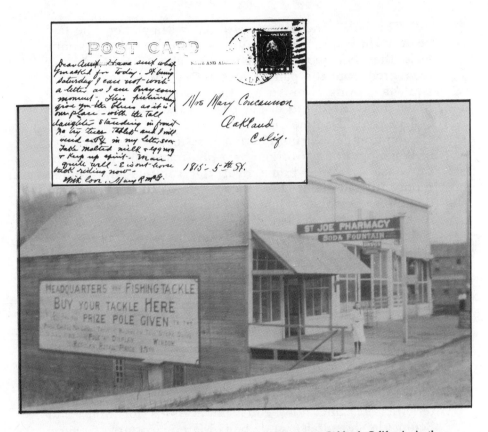

On the back of this postcard, sent to Mrs. Mary Concannon, Oakland, California, in the early 1900s her niece, Dr. Mary R. McGahan, then practicing in the timber town of S. Joe, Benewah County, wrote: "Dear Aunt . . . It being Saturday, I can not write a letter as I am busy every moment. This picture may give you the blues as it is our place—with the tall daughter—standing in the front . . . Take malted milk and egg nog and keep up spirit. We are quite well. E. is out horseback riding now. With love, Mary R."
(Courtesy Daphne Copenhaven)

marriage eventually ended in divorce. A nephew, Jack Lambrecht of San Jose, California, remembers her as a generous woman who loaned one of her brothers $500, so his family could buy a house.

Her granddaughter thinks she studied medicine in Minneapolis. Her only daughter, Ellen, was born in Mullan on January 11, 1901. Dr. McGahan suffered a tragic death about 1912. This was shortly after the federal Narcotics Act was passed. She took a horse and buggy to make a house call. The horse and buggy returned without her. She had been murdered for the narcotics she was carrying. Daphne feels that her mother, Ellen, then about twelve, never recovered from the pain of loss. She went to live with an aunt, a young woman in her twenties. "I can now understand the depth of her passion that narcotics should be legalized," Daphne said.

Ellen graduated from Pharmacy School at the University of Washington and worked as a pharmacist in Seattle. She purchased a large home near the campus and rented rooms to augment her income and to support her daughter, Daphne. When the daughter graduated from high school, her mother said, "I can't send you away to college, so I am leaving. You can have the house. Be selective to whom you rent the rooms, and you can have the twenty-five dollars a month support money your father sends." This all happened and the daughter received her education.

Ellen Berlin, who led the drive for generic drugs ahead of her time and worked for racial integration in the hospital and community, was chief pharmacist at Mills Memorial Hospital in San Mateo for many years. Her daughter, Daphne, began there thirty years ago as community relations director, editing the newsletter, annual reports, etc. She now edits publications for Mills and Peninsula hospitals, and San Mateo County General Hospital.

DR. MARY SHAW SHORB

Dr. Shorb, scientist, microbiologist, immunologist, bacteriologist, was an extraordinary woman by any measure. She was born January 11, 1907, to Ernest Leroy and Mary McKean Shaw. Her Bachelor of Science was earned at the College of Idaho in 1928, and Doctorate in Science at Johns Hopkins, 1933. She took time away from her studies on July 8, 1929, to marry Doys Andrew Shorb, parasitologist at the Ag Research Center, U.S.D.A., in Maryland. They had three children, Barbara Ann, Alan McKean, and Carole Elizabeth.

To list all her degrees, honors and titles would leave scant room for other doctors. Some of them are Immunologist, Abel Fund Research on common cold, Johns

Hopkins, 1929-32; Merck Post-Doctorate Fellow in nutrition, University of Maryland, 1946-49; Research and Emeritus Research Professor, Poultry Husbandry, Maryland; visiting scientist, National Institute of Health, 1960; Awards: Hematology Research Fund, 1948; co-recipient Mead-Johnson award for research on Vitamin B complex, 1949; Outstanding Woman of Maryland, Hood College, 1951; College of Idaho Alumnae, 1966; first Merck-Mary S. Shorb lecture, 1970.

Her publications include over sixty-five papers and abstracts on scientific experiments and developments.

DR. AMY ANNIE COHEN

From family papers of the late Judge Theron Ward of Twin Falls, came the historical note that Amy Annie Cohen was born on August 1, 1835 in Bethelgreen, London, England. She married William Sawyer Jr. She was graduated from the University of England with an M.D. Dr. Cohen-Sawyer practiced medicine in the towns of Malad, Samaria, and Arbon, Idaho. Her husband died March 7, 1876, and she raised her family alone. She died December 28, 1915, at Malad.

DR. MARY LOUISE HOLDREN

The *Idaho Sunday Statesman* saluted Dr. Mary Louise Hinson Holdren as an outstanding Idahoan for her medical and community service in the Boise Valley. She was born to farmer-rancher parents in Amarillo, Texas on June 3, 1923. She grew up in Texas and received a Bachelor of Science degree at Texas State College for Women in 1944 and a Master of Science degree from the University of Iowa, where she did an internship in dietetics. Her medical degree was earned at Tulane University in 1951.

From 1951-53, Dr. Holdren did an internship and residency in obstetrics and gynecology at the Women's and Children's Hospital in San Francisco. From 1953-55 she served another residency at Gorgas Hospital in the Panama Canal Zone. Her most interesting experience in the Canal Zone was delivering a baby on a chiva (bus).

Dr. Holdren was on the OB/GYN staff at the Madigan Army Hospital in Fort Lewis, Washington, 1955-57; School Health Service, Denver, 1957-59; and from 1959 until her untimely death from cancer, she shared an office with her husband, Dr. Robert Holdren, in a private practice in Boise. She was on the staffs of St. Luke's and St. Alphonsus hospitals and named a Fellow in the American College of Obstetrics and Gynecology in 1957. The Doctors Holdren became parents of a son, Glen, and daughter, Barbara.

OTHERS LICENSED

Women physicians and surgeons who were licensed to practice in Idaho included: Frances B. Delano, Carrie E. Lieberg, M. Addie and Effie Kester, Angeline G. Hamilton, Anna R. Steuernagle, all 1899; Mary E. Bates, Eva M. Gardner, Edna L. Cruzen, all 1901; Harriet N. Ballence, 1905; Sadie Lynch, 1907; Mary G. Loughlin, 1908; Gertrude W. Welton, 1911; Emily L. Mosage and Cora E. Alcorn, 1913; Lillian A. Arendall, 1916; Mabel Link, 1918; Dorothy Agee Rich, 1920; Ethel Page Westwood, 1921 (see Bonner County); Susie Vincent Standard, 1923; Emily F. Bolcum, 1928; Marjorie M. Heitman, 1930; Elizabeth Curtis French, 1933; Mary Frances Clark, 1935; June P. McBride, 1937; Evelyn M. Weissross, 1938; Ruth J. Raattma, 1941; Margaret M. Davis, 1946; Margaret Gerber and Helen Beeman, 1947; Madelene M. Donnelly, 1948; Lois Lemen Miller, Helen Frances Craig, Clara Cummings Hastings Baird, all 1950. The numbers have proliferated since that decade.

CHAPTER
4

THE DOCTOR-GOVERNOR

DR. CHARLES ARMINGTON ROBINS

Sammy Stewart, Twin Falls, young but seasoned legislative attache, was talking with new pages to the Idaho House and Senate. It was minutes after Governor C.A. Robins of St. Maries had given his inaugural address in January 1947. "I knew back in 1939 that 'Doc' could become Governor if he wanted to. It was his first term in the Senate and he was chairman of the committee that had to do with health institutions. With committee members, he left for St. Anthony, Blackfoot, and Orofino. When they came back he reported on horrible conditions that still existed. There wasn't a dry eye in that Senate." Improvement of the institutions began with the next budget.

To know what went in to the makeup of the doctor-turned-governor it is necessary to go back. Charles Armington Robins was born to Charles McAlester Robins and Rebecca Jane Burke Robins on December 8, 1884 in Rocky Ford, Colorado. As a small boy, Charles McAlester often rode on the horse in back of his circuit-riding, Baptist preaching, father through the Hartford, Connecticut area. The father was an adventuresome lad and went as a cabin boy on a sailing vessel which visited Rotterdam and Amsterdam. At age twenty-three, he moved west and purchased a mercantile store in Council Bluffs, Iowa. He was second lieutenant in the Civil War, at Antietam, Fredericksburg, Chancellorville, and Gettysburg. Out of the service as major, he married Rebecca Burke in 1870.

They moved to Rocky Ford, where daughter, Anna, and sons, Henry B., and Charles A. were born, and moved in 1887 to LaJunta (Spanish for The Junction) Colorado. Charles had summer jobs, played quarterback on the second string football squad, and graduated in 1912 from high school. He produced the high school paper at the town's newspaper and learned to hand set type. Perhaps it was there that he developed his interest in writing, which never left him.

His vacation employment was as varied as one summer on a ranch, to the Wells-Fargo express transfer and timekeeper for the Santa Fe Railroad, later as a "straw boss" and moving up to blacksmith's helper. He worked ten hours a day and earned $1.085 per day, scarcely more than ten cents an hour.

Charles' desire was to become a doctor, but there was no money. He entered William Jewell College and waited on table and washed dishes at a house to pay tuition and books. Still no money, so he taught history in the Springfield High School, Missouri, at seventy-five dollars per month. In 1908–09 he taught chemistry, physics and biology. At an education meeting in Denver in 1909, he was hired to teach science at the Billings, Montana, high school. In June 1910, he went to Laurel, Mississippi, to be secretary for an Industrial YMCA, and taught at the high school. He became a scoutmaster and established the first summer camp in Mississippi.

While singing in the choir at the Laurel Baptist Church he met Marguerite Granberry, the organist. They were later married in 1918. Mrs. Robins suffered from then-incurable chronic nephritis combined with hypertension most of their married life and began to fail in 1935, dying in the St. Maries Hospital on May 1, 1938.

All those years, he thought of medicine and when he went to Chicago in 1913 and entered the University of Chicago, he had, "far less funding than necessary for the first year. Only the first two years of a medical course were given on the university campus. My last two were at historic Rush Medical College in the west side of Chicago."

He shared a flat with three other Phi Gamma Deltas and took all the spare time jobs he could. For two summers he worked at the *Chicago Daily News* and as clerk for the Bureau of Indian Affairs. "Having been out of college for six years, I had to learn again how to study," he said. He attended a rush party with C.E. Watts, graduate of the University of Idaho from Juliaetta, Idaho, later a Seattle internist. He heard of the wonders of Idaho from young Watts.

The last two years, he paid tuition and lab fees by addressing letters to a large alumni list. One summer he earned a huge sum, seventy-five dollars per month, to operate a first aid room for a manufacturing plant. He interned at Cincinnati General, and was asked to work with prominent Dr. Bertram W. Shippy, who had a large practice in gastro-enterology. Dr. Shippy had also been one of Charles' professors at Rush, and Charles was his intern at Washington Boulevard Hospital.

In August 1918, Dr. Robins was commissioned a first lieutenant, U.S. Army Medical Corps, and sent to Medical Officers Training Camp, Fort Riley, Kansas, then on to Camp Sherman.

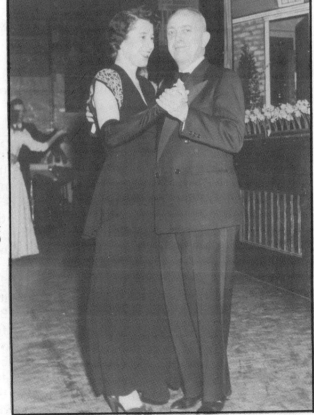

The new Governor and First Lady, Dr. C. A. and Mrs. Robins of St. Maries, pause for the photographer during the first dance at their Inaugural Ball in Boise in January 1947.
(Louise Shadduck photo file)

His father died while he was in the service. His mother lived to eighty-five and died in 1932. In writing to his daughters years later, he said of his mother, "She was gentle, firm, considerate, quiet and deliberate. Her sense of humor was keen but never in noisy evidence. Her Christian faith was deep and abiding and her chief ambition for her children was that they might develop into exemplary Christian members of the community." Such a description fitted him almost to a T.

How did this man, who had been asked to remain in practice with Dr. Shippy, get to St. Maries, Idaho, where he found deep satisfaction in caring for the lumberjacks, miners, farmers and their families? As discharging officer on December 15, 1918, at Camp Sherman, he made short work of it and left on December 16 to see Dr. Shippy about the invitation to practice with him. Dr. Bauffleur of Seattle, chief surgeon of the Chicago, Milwaukee, St. Paul, and Pacific Railroad was in Shippy's office and offered Dr. Robins a roundtrip to Seattle if he would look at two towns on their road needing doctors. He was interested in the west and agreed. The first was Three Forks, Montana, and the governor later said he "looked over" Three Forks from the vestibule of the Pullman.

Heavy snow and bitter cold caused the train to be twelve hours late as it reached the St. Paul Pass Tunnel at the summit of the Bitterroot Mountains and began the descent over many switchbacks and through numerous tunnels toward St. Maries. "I was so struck by the beauty of the snowy tree-covered mountains and finally the winding St. Joe River that I was sure that this was the place where I was meant to practice," the doctor said.

He got off the train in St. Maries on Christmas Eve 1918, walked the wooden sidewalks to the handsome old Kootenai Inn, where he registered for a room. He then crunched through the snow to the hospital to see Dr. D.E. Cornwall, who became a lifetime friend. Beginning January 1, 1919, Dr. Robins was an associate for four years, and in 1923 a partner until the death of Dr. Cornwall on July 5, 1939. He was then in full charge of St. Maries Hospital and district surgeon for the Milwaukee Railroad. Dr. Robins had been the local surgeon for more than twenty years.

He married Olive Patricia Simpson, nurse at the St.

Maries Hospital, November 15, 1939 in the Coeur d'Alene Episcopal Church. They became the parents of, Patty, Paula Jean, and Becky, and had two granddaughters. Just before they were married, he was joined in practice by Dr. E.G. Peacock.

They liked living in St. Maries and the practice of medicine in a small town which was a challenge. There were no surfaced roads, and very few graveled. He traveled by train, (doctor for the Milwaukee Railroad); handcar, boat, and sleigh or buggy. Dr. Robins was a charter member of the St. Maries Post, American Legion, 1919. He was commander during the building of the Legion Memorial Building. He and other Legion members invited Marshal Ferdinand Foch, Supreme Allied Commander in Europe during World War I, to stop in St. Maries during a visit through America. Foch accepted and poured the first shovel of cement to set the cornerstone November 29, 1921. Old-timers still tell of the more than one thousand people who turned out to welcome the Foch special train at the Milwaukee depot.

He became a Master Mason with the 33d degree, and he and Mrs. Robins were associate patron and matron of the Eastern Star. He was city physician for two years and county physician for ten; Selective Service medical examiner; member, St. Maries school board; director, chamber of commerce and president of the North Idaho chamber; an Elk and a Kiwanian.

He was elected as a Republican to the State Senate in 1938, 1940, 1942, and 1944, serving as assistant minority leader in 1943 and majority leader and chairman of the State Affairs committee in 1944. Recognition on a statewide basis came when he submitted his resignation during the 1945 session, because there was no other doctor in St. Maries and "the people of my county have been so good to me that I can not run out on them." Delegations of fellow legislators began to call upon him in St. Maries, urging him to run for governor. A statewide committee, composed of both Democrats and Republicans, was formed, pledging their support and he became the successful candidate. A large number of doctors were supporters and Dr. F.M. Cole of Caldwell was on the original committee. The campaign was on. Election day was

November 4, 1946 and when the doctor drove the north-south highway to St. Maries, he was met by a large Benewah County delegation at Plummer, forming a caravan to escort him home.

The good doctor had spent years in healing the people of the area and they responded, "almost to the voter" as one said, when he became a candidate and was later elected governor.

"Liked Lumberjacks"

Practice of medicine in the area in the early days, was a never ending challenge. Governor Robins found the lumberjacks the most picturesque and interesting group of people he served. He had a special place in his heart for them until the end. He told many stories of them and their lifestyle. He usually had a lumberjack visitor or two on Monday mornings, after a weekend in town and spending all their money, putting the hit on him for anything from two to ten dollars for coffee and commissary money until the next payday. It seemed to be a pleasure for the doctor to accede. He said that during the twenty-eight years there, he handed out an unknown amount of money and never kept books on it, but was firmly convinced that he was out only five dollars, and that "to a poor chap who had sustained a severe permanent disability in a logging accident."

"Two Old Coots"

Governor Robins told of becoming acquainted up and down the river in the St. Joe Valley and among them was an odd pair of "old coots," Montgomery and Monroe, who lived in the logging area of Herrick. One day he had a call to attend one of them who had been poisoned. He rode on a freight train to the nearest siding and was met by a buddy of the victim. He seemed a bit tipsy, but said he had a boat ready to cross "the Joe" and asked the doctor to follow him.

The friend could not light his pipe as they walked along, in no particular hurry, and stopped at the water's edge to complete the chore. As he stood with his back to a log, he teetered a time or two and, lighted match in hand, fell over backward, wedging his rear-end between two logs in a puddle of mud two inches deep. Doctor Robins had to bodily rescue him and was finding the prospect of even a short boat trip with him at the helm less than appealing. But they got there, went into an unfinished house and saw the victim lying on a cot.

He learned that the victim had been bothered by a cough in the night, got up and in the dark reached over the door and got what he thought was cough medicine. He put the bottle to his lips and took a healthy swig, suddenly realizing he had drunk from the bottle of carbolic acid, which they used in treating cuts on horses. The doctor asked either Montgomery or Monroe (the one who had not drunk carbolic acid) what had been done for the victim. He was told that he had eaten more than a half-pound of butter and had drunk at least a pint of straight moonshine whiskey. Upon examination the mucous membrane of the mouth and throat showed only slight evidence of corrosive action. "He was quite comfortable," the doctor said, and added, "and also quite tipsy." His pulse rate was normal, so continuation of the treatment, as needed, was advised and the doctor caught another freight back to St. Maries. "His recovery was complete," was the end of the story.

"Buried in Manure Pile"

That was not the end of experiences with the two old coots, and the doctor never knew which name to apply to which man. One of the old fellows had been missing for days. His cabin had been ransacked and possessions stolen. Eventually, someone's curiosity was aroused by a pile of manure beside an old stump. Examination revealed the body with a bullet hole in his head.

As the body was over the line in Shoshone County but closer to St. Maries, officials asked help from Benewah County coroner O.G. Merager, who exhumed the body, took it to St. Maries, and asked Dr. Robins to do the post mortem. He said that the wound of the bullet entrance was on the right side of the head, and he felt an indentation just back of the left ear, due to the final impact of the bullet against the skull. When the skull cap was removed the bullet was in that spot.

Soon the suspect was apprehended and a preliminary hearing set. It was at Wallace, and quite a group of St.

Maries people showed up. The trial took three days. Among the witnesses was Luke S. May, ballistics expert from Seattle, who gave evidence tying the bullet to the stolen gun found among the accused's possessions. When Doctor Robins had removed the bullet from the skull he carefully marked the butt end by scratching the Greek letter Phi. That caused an exchange between defense counsel and the doctor.

Defense counsel insisted that the doctor's mark would invalidate May's findings. Doctor Robins was equally insistent that it would not. The counsel finally asked, in a sarcastic tone, "Well now, why not?" The doctor slowly and carefully replied, "Because I was very careful to place it on the butt end of the bullet where it could not affect ballistics examination if any were made." Judge Albert H. Featherstone was presiding and the trial resulted in a conviction.

"Battling Polio Epidemic"

In many instances as governor, he found experience as a doctor helpful. The polio epidemic beginning in Caldwell and moving rapidly, caused the governor to speedily form a state committee to coordinate activities to meet the crisis. Members included Lieutenant Governor Donald S. Whitehead, Dr. Madeline Donnelly of the Idaho Public Health Department; Joe Imhoff, president of Elks Crippled Children's board; Mr. Belveal, March of Dimes; L.J. Peterson, director of Public Health, and his director of public information, Armand Bird; Doctors West of Idaho Falls, Hearne of Pocatello, Douglas of Lewiston; Helen Ross, St. Lukes superintendent; Sister Alma Dolores of St. Alphonsus; Colonel LeBrun, Bishop Rhea, Fred Graff, R. Kimbrough, American Red Cross representative; and Dr. F.B. Jeppesen, Idaho Medical Association president.

A rush was put on the opening of the new Elks Center and countless Elks, members of service clubs and their wives worked diligently so that cases at St. Al's and St. Lukes which were past the dangerous stage could move to the Elks and leave hospital space for the continuing parade of acute cases.

An advertised war surplus building from Gowen Field had been applied for and seemed so certain of being granted to the state, that L.J. Peterson and the governor, in their haste to make more room for the ill, had the building sawed in two, raised on dollies and ready to move. A man from Surplus Properties arrived to inspect the building. He either chose to ignore the sawing job or realized the necessity and the papers were signed.

"We had to have that building and almost overnight it was readied and just as soon filled. This sort of an epidemic is a terrible thing to have to meet," Doctor Robins solemnly said. His tone turned to joy and pride as he added, "but Idaho met it well."

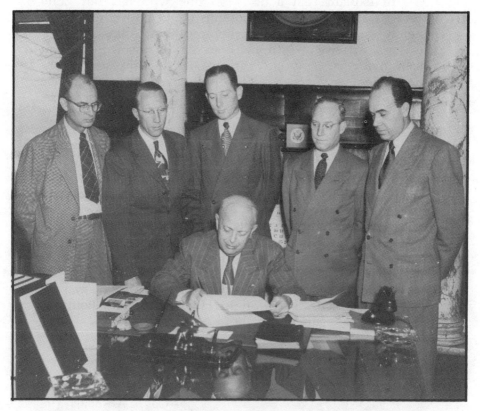

Medical history was made when Physician-Governor C.A. Robins of St. Maries, the first doctor to be elected Idaho Governor, signed the Medical Practice Act of 1949. Standing behind him are the five Idaho Medical Association physicians who worked on drafting the legislation. Left to right, are Doctors Robert S. McKean, Alfred M. Popma, Raymond L. White, S.M. Poindexter and F.M. Jeppesen.

(Idaho Medical Association photo)

The doctor-governor never lost his great pride in Idaho. Once, in telling of places he had lived, he said, "After having lived and labored in nine states, and having traveled in most of the others, I acknowledge that I found much of interest and made many friends. But having spent fifty years in Idaho, I must confess to a most ardent devotion to this, my adopted state.

"To few people have so many doors been opened as to me in Idaho. That after so many years of intensive application to my profession I should have chosen to give it up, in a measure, has been excuse for many questions . . . to explain that action. No one who has not gone through a four-year governorship could know how completely such an experience divorces him from any professional activity . . . tremendous strides in medicine had been made . . . myriad changes in therapy, new techniques in every area . . . I could not return to practice without an intensive refresher course of a year or more, and I was in my sixty-seventh year . . . again fortuitous circumstances moved in to help solve the problem . . ."

The circumstances included an invitation to become medical director of the North Idaho District Medical Service Bureau at Lewiston, which had grown to such a point that a medical director was needed and it would put the governor into "the most intricate relationship with my colleagues and the hospitals of the area." His wife, Pat, joined him in feeling it was a good move and they were to make Lewiston their home until his death on September 20, 1970.

Two days later the *Lewiston Morning Tribune* ran an editorial entitled, "He Brought Honor To Idaho Politics." The editorial began with a quote:

> I refuse to indulge in a party Donnybrook. I wouldn't call anybody names. Politics doesn't have to be dirty. It's as dirty as a man makes it. It can be an honorable calling.
>
> —Gov. C.A. Robins

A part of the editorial, signed with the intials B.H. (Bill Hall, still editorial page editor) follows:

> Gov. C.A. Robins, who died Sunday, had his moments as a state administrator, but he should be and will be remembered for the example in high-road politics he set for an entire generation of Idaho politicians.
>
> **Governor Robins was probably the most decent man ever to grace the Governorship of the state of Idaho.**
>
> That's saying quite a bit. The charlatans exist in politics as they do in any other profession, and so do moral giants . . . So Robins was not alone in the quest of high principle. But he alone was in large measure responsible for that trend in recent Gem State politics.
>
> . . . His accomplishment was extraordinary because of where it occurred. It would be one thing for a minister to succeed in the pursuit of morality. It is even almost expected that a man should serve so unselfishly in Governor Robins' first profession-medicine. But to provide decisive moral leadership in a profession where morality is supposed to be shunned . . . is a triumph for right and an affirmation of the propriety of principle.
>
> . . . The explanation is not very amazing. Governor Robins would have had the same effect on any profession he entered. He was, for all his many years, far ahead of his times. He had discovered many years ago the principle that the young people of today whom he understood and loved, sometimes in their innocence, think they invented . . . He was one of those rare and sanity-inspiring individuals who refused to think anything but the best of everyone.
>
> . . . The more he expected of those around him, the more they performed as he expected. Goodness does rub off, and he rubbed his state for the better for many long and fortunate years.

CHAPTER
5

DOCTORS IN UNIFORM

Doctors were always among the first to answer the call of the United States in wartime. Many Idaho doctors who saw war on the horizon, began to prepare for service before action began. Doctors and nurses served from the Revolutionary War on through the latest action in the Persian Gulf. In these profiles are a number of Idaho doctors whose ancestors fought in the Revolutionary War. The Idaho doctor was capable of great strength and bravery on the battlefield. The first of these did amazing things to save lives during the Civil War.

DR. MARSHALL W. WOOD

Highly respected and fondly called "Colonel" for his wartime service, Marshall W. Wood's medical career was as notable, if not more so, as his military. He arrived in Boise January, 1895.

Colonel Wood was a private in the Civil War and a medical officer during the Spanish-American. In a letter which the late Mrs. Alice (John) Taylor provided, someone had written: "He was a poor boy, his parents were exemplary, refined, intelligent persons. During the Civil War, his father and younger brother, Jason, had gone to the war when the government offered $1,000 bounty for additional men. Marshall, then a slender, undeveloped boy, went, giving the money to his mother. He had two wounds in battle."

He entered Rush Medical College, Chicago, after receiving an M.A. degree from Bowdin College. Marshall Wood was named an honorary member of the Chicago Society of Physicians and Surgeons while on duty on the frontier in 1876, because he had made the first successful transfusion of defibrinated human blood in a case of pulmonary tuberculosis. The soldier-patient was cured.

In 1889, while at Walla Walla, he was ordered to the middle west, but his transfer was postponed until a case of uterine cancer which he was then treating with electrolysis could be more definitely determined. He was made an honorary member of the Hawaiian Medical Society 1899, following his success in combatting a typhoid epidemic in Honolulu. A year later he was in Jefferson Barracks in St. Louis deeply interested in improvement of the untreated water supply, which was from "Chicago Sewage."

The colonel arrived in Boise after fifteen months at Harvard in bacteriology and pathological histology. One of the first things he did was to organize a class in bacteriology for local physicians. His influence helped to mold public opinion that led to the Idaho Bacteriological Laboratory.

Doctor Wood was credited with the first aseptic abdominal surgery in Boise. With Dr. Carol Sweet, he worked for the organization of the Idaho State Medical Society in 1883, and was instrumental in the passage of the Medical Practices Act in 1897, and when it was revised in 1899.

Although advanced in age, he answered the call to serve in World War I, after having served in both the Civil and Spanish-American wars. At eighty-seven years, he died in Boise, August 5, 1933.

DR. WILLIAM E. WALDROP

The first doctor to reach the bedside of Governor Frank Steunenberg after he had been fatally injured in a bombing at his front gate in Caldwell was Dr. William E. Waldrop, then living in that community. He also lived in Parma and Boise.

William Edgar Waldrop was born in Kentucky and spent much of his life in military action for his country. When he was eighteen, he enlisted in the U.S. Army and came west with a cavalry regiment seeing service in the cattle war in Wyoming. Despite the war, he loved the wide and wild country and knew his future would be spent in medicine in the west. To prepare, he studied pharmacy at the Ohio Normal School at Ada, and was acting steward in the

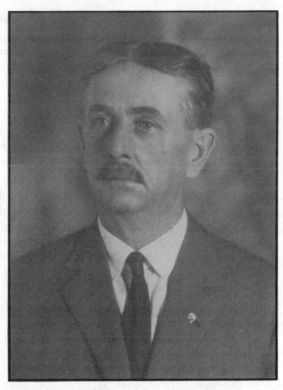

One of Canyon County's best-known pioneers was Dr. William E. Waldrop of Parma. He was born in 1873 in Kentucky, served his country in the military and medicine. He died at Boise in 1943.

hospital corps. Again, the Army called and he enlisted as hospital steward in the 28th Infantry. During the Cuban campaign he was cited for bravery for taking care of the wounded under fire. He contracted a tropical disease in Cuba from which he never completely recovered.

After that war, he studied medicine at Louisville Medical College and graduated in 1902. In April 1903, he arrived in Boise and after passing the state medical boards, located in Caldwell as an associate of Dr. Hamilton. In July, Dr. Waldrop opened an office in Parma, where he spent most of the rest of his life. Christmas Day, 1904, Dr. Waldrop married Lulu Stockton of a pioneer Parma family. They became the parents of three daughters, Mrs. Rex (Ila) Wendle, Spokane; Mrs. George (Alice) Cooke, Boise; and the late Mrs. Robert (Beth) Schroeder, Coeur d'Alene.

From 1905 until 1909, he was Canyon County physician and from 1932 until his death in February 1943, was Commandant of the Idaho Soldier's Home at Boise.

DR. LOY T. SWINEHART

Dr. Loy T. Swinehart was on active duty with the U.S. Naval Reserve in the Pacific theatre during World War II, and served from 1950–51 in Korea. As Lieutenant (MC) USNR, he was awarded the American Theatre medal; the Victory medal; the Asiatic-Pacific theatre, the China theatre, the Japanese Occupation, and the Korean War medals.

Born to a Lutheran minister and his wife on August 7, 1916, Dr. Swinehart attended the University of Washington, receiving a Bachelor of Science degree, 1940; Northwestern University Medical School granted his Doctor of Medicine in 1944; and served a pediatric residency in 1948–50 at the University of Colorado. He joined Alpha Kappa Kappa medical fraternity.

His naval internship was at Mare Island, California. From August 1946 until February 1947, he conducted a general practice in Spokane, and practiced in Boise from 1947–48, returning from his pediatric residency in Denver to resume practice in 1951.

Dr. Swinehart held staff appointments at St. Lukes, St. Alphonsus, and Booth Memorial hospitals; Elks Rehabilitation Center in Boise; consultant in pediatrics at Mountain Home Air Force Base; and the Idaho State Crippled Children's Service. He served as president of the Idaho State Pediatric Society; secretary-treasurer of the North Pacific Pediatric Society, and president of the Ada County Medical Society.

Dr. and Mrs. Swinehart have two daughters and three sons.

DR. MAX D. GUDMUNDSEN

Idaho born and educated until his college years, Max D. Gudmundsen came from the big potato country of Burley, where his father was a potato broker and gasoline consignee. After graduating from Burley High School, he received a degree from the University of Utah. He entered the University of Louisville Medical School and received an M.D. He joined Phi Chi medical fraternity.

He spent one year interning at Lucas County Hospital, Toledo, Ohio, and a second year residency in OB/GYN. 1941–42 he practiced in Boise. He entered the U.S. Army

Medical Corps with overseas duty in the Pacific, 1943–45. His rank was captain.

He returned to Boise and practiced at St. Lukes and St. Alphonsus hospitals and became chief of staff at the Booth Memorial Hospital. Dr. Gudmundsen was president of the Southwest Idaho and secretary-treasurer of the Idaho Medical associations.

He and his wife, Helen, became parents of two sons, Robert Max and Taylor; and two daughters, Elsie Lee and Jan.

DR. QUENTIN LORING QUICKSTAD

Quentin Quickstad spent 1953–55 in the U.S. Army, sixteen months of which was in Korea. He was a first lieutenant in the Medical Corps.

He was born at Toronto, South Dakota, December 5, 1926, and his early years were on the family farm. During high school he moved into Toronto. There were ten in his graduating class.

He attended the University of South Dakota, 1945–46. He received his Bachelor of Science degree from the University of Oregon in 1948, and Doctor of Medicine degree in 1952. He joined Sigma Alpha Epsilon. Dr. Quickstad took internship and residency at St. Vincent Hospital in Portland, July 1952 through October 1953.

He was with the Army Medical Corps in Korea, and upon return, he practiced general surgery, 1955–59, at St. Vincent. His certification by the American Board of Surgery was given in June 1960.

He moved to Boise, which remained his home. He practiced at both St. Alphonsus and St. Lukes hospitals, and in 1955, he married Barbara Gartrell, who describes herself as a "has-been" nurse. They have three children, Kent Loring, Karen Ann, and Kristie Ellen. Dr. Quickstad retired in 1933.

DR. GUSTAV V. ROSENHEIM

If laughter is as good as medicine, as it is said, Dr. Gus Rosenheim's patients must be the healthiest in Idaho. A man with a wry wit, he lists as his hobbies and interests, "Bird watching and beaver shooting!"

Born in Boise to Ed Rosenheim and his wife, he attended the University of Idaho and was awarded a Bachelor of

Science degree in 1941. He was a member of Beta Theta Pi. His Doctor of Medicine degree was received in 1945 from Jefferson Medical College.

Internship was at the Swedish Hospital in Seattle for one year. He served one year's residency at Kapiolami Maternity Hospital and one year at Queen's Hospital, Honolulu, Hawaii.

Dr. Rosenheim was a U.S. Air Force captain for one year, returning in 1952 to open a Boise practice. He has continued to practice since then. He and his wife, Alice, have a son, Gustav Alan, and a daughter, Leslie Maurine.

DR. VERNE JOHNSON REYNOLDS

Dr. Johnson and his wife, Agnes, have been active in Boise civic affairs. He was born January 14, 1907 in Elwood, Nebraska, where his father was an estimator and bidder for the Standard Bridge Company in Omaha.

At twelve, the family moved to Omaha, and he attended Central High School, playing four years on the basketball and baseball teams. From age seven until twelve, he herded cattle during the summer. In Omaha, he said that he ran an ice station and "scraped school desks and ground down school boards (slates) in the summer."

His premedical was at the University of Illinois, 1926-29, and at the University of Omaha in the summer of 1929. Medical study was at the University of Nebraska College of Medicine, 1930-33. At Illinois he joined Beta Theta Pi and Phi Eta Sigma honor society.

Dr. Reynolds' rotating internship was at St. Francis Hospital in Jersey City, New Jersey, 1933-34; residency in obstetrics and gynecology at Bellevue Hospital in New York City, 1934-35. A three months internship in 1935 was at Bellevue, and his residency was at Margaret Hague Maternity Hospital in Jersey City, 1935-37. He was chief resident at the same hospital for six months in 1937; practiced at Lincoln, 1937-42; and with the U.S. Air Force, 1942-46.

He was an Air Force captain in 1942 and advanced to major in regional hospitals doing OB/GYN, 1944. He was discharged in 1946 and moved to Boise to practice. When asked if he had done home surgeries, Dr. Reynolds replied, "The only dog obstetrics I ever performed ended in a caesarean section, with the mother dog and all the pups dying. I tried to perform the delivery with a sponge and a stick. It was unsuccessful." But he had unusual and successful experiences and in one case performed a caesarean to deliver a seven pound baby to a three-foot tall midget mother. Two mothers who would deliver triplets were conducted through pregnancy and delivery by Dr. Reynolds.

The doctor served on the staff of the Bryan Memorial, Lincoln General, and St. Elizabeth's hospitals in Lincoln; on staffs of St. Lukes and St. Alphonsus, Boise; was gynecology consultant at the Veterans Administration Hospital, Boise.

Positions held and association memberships include: American Board of Obstetrics and Gynecology; American, Idaho, and Ada County Medical societies; Idaho Obstetrics and Gynecological Society; Central Association of Obstetrics and Gynecology; Pacific Northwest OB/GYN Society, of which he was president in 1957; Founding Fellow of the American College of OB/GYN in 1951; and a Fellow of the American College of Surgeons.

His wife, Agnes, was graduated from New York's Bellevue Hospital School of Nursing. She is past president of the Ada County Medical Auxiliary, Women of Rotary, Hillcrest Women Golfers; Young Women's Christian Associations board; and an active golfer and bowler. They are the parents of a daughter, Sandra, and a son, Thomas G.

DR. WALLACE PIERCE

Wallace H. Pierce lived on a farm at Cottonwood in Idaho County, a part of the beautiful Camas prairie, and ancient home of the Nez Perce Indians. The starchy camas root provided food for tribe members for as far back as any of them could remember. There was good fishing in the rivers and creeks and fine hunting in the harvested fields and in the foothills and mountains—a boy's paradise.

When Wallace was grown, educated, studied, and degree granted to become a Doctor of Medicine, he served in five overseas countries during wartime, and came back a highly decorated major. He set up medical practice very near his boyhood home; he established a practice in Lewiston.

From 1928 through 1932, Dr. Pierce attended the

University of Idaho. He became a member of Sigma Chi and earned a Bachelor of Science degree. From 1932 until 1934 he attended the University of North Dakota Medical School; and Rush Medical College at the University of Chicago until 1936, when he was granted an M.D. He was a member of the OB/GYN Committee, and of the Academy.

His internship, from 1936–37, was at Ancker Hospital, St. Paul, where the future Mrs. Pierce was a nurse. They were married May 15, 1937. In 1946, he took a six months course in pediatrics at Harvard Medical School and three months in OB/GYN at the Poly-Clinic, New York.

In 1937, he returned to Cottonwood and associated in practice with Dr. Orr. During World War II, he distinguished himself with the 56th Medical Battalion in Africa, Sicily, Italy, France, and Germany. He returned with seven battle stars and a meritorious award, plus the rank of major.

He opened practice in 1945 in Lewiston, and remained. Dr. Pierce is a typical Idaho doctor with remaining boyhood interests in hunting and fishing. He added golf, boating, and ham radio operator.

Dr. and Mrs. Pierce became the parents of two sons and a daughter: Bob, Michelle Jean, and Dean Hamilton (Skip).

Dr. Pierce was chief of staff at St. Joseph's Hospital and chairman of the OB committee.

DR. WENDELL PETTY

It is a safe guess that the clear writing on information concerning Dr. Wendell Petty of Shelley, was done by his wife. Answering the question, "What do you do in your spare time?" were the words, "Fish, Fish, Fish."

Wendell Petty was reared in Salina, Utah, where he was born March 27, 1921. He worked his way through the University of Utah and taught for nearly a year before going into the U.S. Army. After three years in the military, during which he received a Bronze Star for bravery, his rank was sergeant major.

Upon graduation from Utah in 1942, he received a B.A. degree. He held membership in Phi Kappa Phi and was named to Phi Beta Kappa. He was the charter president of Alpha Omega Alpha, honorary medical society. In the manner of medical students and doctors, who like to play jokes, during his freshman year fellow students presented him an inscribed urinal as the top student in the class. At graduation, he received another for the top scholastic position throughout medical school.

His internship, from 1950–51, was at Wayne County Hospital, Eloise, Michigan, and surgical residency the following year at the Salt Lake Veterans Hospital. His general practice began in Shelley in 1951. He held positions as secretary, vice chief and chief of staff at Idaho Falls Hospital in 1957, 1958, and 1959.

An artist, Dr. Petty likes to paint in oils. He often performs on the piano with a humorous dialogue. He and Mrs. Petty have two sons, Wendell Eugene and Jerold Lee; and two daughters, Sandra Kay and Wendy Sue.

DR. ALLEN HUMPHREY TIGERT

Allen Tigert and his brother, Dr. Russell Tigert Jr., followed in the footsteps of their admired father, Dr. Russell Tigert Sr., and all practiced medicine in Soda Springs, Idaho. Allen was born February 24, 1914, at Dumas, Mississippi, and came to Soda Springs, where the brothers attended grade and high schools.

Four years of higher education were in Idaho: 1931–33, Idaho State College (now University), at Pocatello, and graduating with a Bachelor of Science degree from the University of Idaho in 1935. Allen entered Washington University's College of Medicine and received an M.D. in 1939. He was a member of Phi Beta Pi.

His internship and residency, all in St. Louis, were for six months at St. Louis Hospital; one year each at Depaul and Deaconess. He first practiced in Booneville, Kentucky (home of Daniel Boone of frontier fame), and in 1943 took two actions highly significant in his life. He married a registered nurse from the Lutheran Hospital in St. Louis, Alice Middelkamp, and joined the military service.

In the South Pacific he earned three campaign stars (in action in three battles), the Bronze Star for bravery, and a Presidential Unit Citation. Dr. Tigert was discharged in 1946, with the rank of captain. He was a major in the Reserves.

Dr. Tigert called himself "a football watcher," and enjoyed hunting and photography. He was active in community affairs and served as mayor of Soda Springs. The doctor and his wife became the parents of a son, Allen Ray, and two daughters, Alice Ann and Lynne Marie.

DR. JOHN R. NIELSEN

Winner of two Purple Heart medals for being wounded in action and two Bronze Stars for bravery under fire, Corporal John R. Nielsen, spent two and one-half years in the service during World War II.

Born in Norman, Oklahoma, May 29, 1925, to a medical doctor mother and a physics professor father, John received his Bachelor of Science at the University of Oklahoma. His M.D. was earned at Northwestern University Medical School where he joined Phi Beta Pi.

He had a rotating internship at Denver General and Denver Veterans Administration hospitals from 1953 through 1958, when he arrived in Caldwell, Idaho, to set up practice. He held staff appointments at Caldwell Memorial, Mercy in Nampa and Malheur Memorial in Nyssa.

The Nielsens became parents of Karen, Lisa, Marta, and Kristine and he was the stepfather of Stephen and Richard.

DR. PAUL F. MINER

Paul Miner had an aunt who practiced medicine in Macomb, Illinois, and served as vice-president of the Illinois Medical Association. He was born December 18, 1911 in Adair, Illinois, where his father was county agricultural agent and sold farm insurance.

Paul had elementary and high school educations in Mount Pleasant, Iowa, and pre-medical study at the University of Iowa. His Bachelor of Science and Medical Doctor degrees came from the Iowa College of Medicine in 1929 and 1935, and his Master of Medical Science degree from the University of Pennsylvania School of Medicine in 1953.

Internship and residencies were served from 1935–36, St. Lukes Hospital in Duluth, Minnesota, Cook County Graduate School of Medicine, 1939, Pennsylvania Graduate School of Medicine, 1946–47; and Harvard Medical School, 1947–48, and again in 1956.

Dr. Miner served with the famed Eighth Air Force, USA, in the European theatre during World War II. He was flight surgeon from 1942 until 1945, and awarded six battle stars and a Presidential Unit Citation. He left the Air Force as a lieutenant colonel with the inactive Army Reserve.

Dr. Miner practiced in Laramie, Wyoming; Denver, Colorado; and Boise, Idaho. His hospital staff appointments include St. Lukes and St. Alphonsus; staff president at St. Alphonsus; consultant at the Veterans Hospital and the Elks Rehabilitation Center in Boise.

He held positions in the American, Idaho, and Ada County Medical societies; Fellow in the American College of Physicians and American College of Cardiology, serving at different times as governor for Idaho in those colleges; Fellow in the American College of Chest Physicians, and of the Council of Clinical Cardiology of the American Heart Association; member of the Editorial Advisory board and a trustee of *Northwest Medicine*; member of North Pacific Society of Internal Medicine, American Therapeutic Society, American Society of Internal Medicine, and the International Society of Internal Medicine.

DR. RONALD P. RAWLINSON

Born a "Brit" in London, England on December 4, 1906, was Ronald Pinsent Rawlinson. He and his brother, Herbert, who also became a medical doctor were the sons of a British clergyman and his wife. Both brothers sailed for Canada when quite young, and Ronald taught in grade and high schools from 1924 until 1927 to secure funding to become a doctor.

With a 1926 degree from the Saskatoon Normal School, he earned a Bachelor of Science degree at the University of Alberta in 1930, and was graduated from that university's college of medicine in 1934. Internship and residency were taken from 1933-35 at the Misericardice Hospital in Edmonton, Alberta. At the end of that practice, Dr. Rawlinson moved to Emmett, Idaho, to practice. He became a captain in the Army Medical Services from 1942-46, and was a surgeon with the 110th Evacuation Hospital.

Dr. Rawlinson was chief of staff at Emmett Hospital and vice-president and president of the Southwest Idaho Medical Society. His greatest source of relaxation is in reading. The Rawlinsons had one daughter, Madelyn, who became a speech and hearing therapist.

DR. WARREN BELTRAN ROSS

Even though he received six battle stars for action in that many battles in the Asiatic theatre during World War II, Dr. Warren Ross' biography submitted to the Idaho Medical Auxiliary, contained less than one and one-half lines on his military service. He served as major in the U.S. Medical Corps from 1942–45.

Born January 10, 1912 in Muskegon, a port city on Lake Michigan, Warren Ross was graduated from the University of Iowa with a Bachelor of Science in 1931, and from the medical school there with an M.D. in 1935. He was affiliated with the medical fraternity Phi Rho Sigma.

One year's internship at the Akron, Ohio, City Hospital was followed by a year of residency in medicine and obstetrics. He and his wife came west to Nampa, where his late uncle, Dr. H.P. Ross had practiced. He was a member of the staffs at Mercy and Samaritan hospitals and chief at Mercy from 1955–58.

Dr. Ross was active in the medical community, serving as president of the Southwest Idaho Medical Society in 1952; secretary of the Idaho Medical Association, 1957; member, Idaho State Board of Medicine, 1947–61, and vice chairman from 1950–61. He was named a Fellow of the International College of Surgeons.

The Rosses are the parents of a daughter and son.

DR. THEODORE R. FLORENTZ

Dr. Florentz was another to give short shrift to his entire military biography, with, "Served four years during World War II as a flight surgeon in the United States and England."

He came to Boise from Detroit in 1948, after receiving an A.B. from Olivet College and M.D. degree from Wayne State University, both in Michigan. After military service, he completed his resident training in ophthalmology and was certified. He married and they had two children, Ted Jr. and Chrisanne.

DR. CLAYTON C. MORGAN

Born October 9, 1927 at Ontario, Oregon, Clayton Morgan had only to move over the state line to be an Idahoan. He attended grade and high school in Nyssa, Oregon, being active in football and basketball. His medical schooling was also in Oregon with pre-med from 1945–48 at the University of Oregon for his Bachelor of Science degree; then to the medical school in 1948–52 for his M.D. Dr. Morgan was a member of Delta Tau Delta at the University; Asklepiad Medical honorary; and Phi Beta Pi.

The doctor spent three years in the U.S. Air Force, one of which was with the rank of first lieutenant and did his internship at Madigan Army Hospital at Fort Lewis, Washington. The following two years he achieved the rank of captain and medical officer at Mather Air Force Base, Sacramento, and had two years of internal medicine residency. He practices in Boise.

In addition to flying his own plane for pleasure, he has flown it on medical calls. The Morgan children include one daughter, Cathy, and three sons, Mike, Frank, and Tom.

DR. RICHARD OTTO VYCITAL

Richard Vycital's interest in things to do, people to know, and goals to achieve, started early in life. The youngest of nine children, four brothers and four sisters, he was reared in a small resort town on a river fifty miles from Chicago. There were surrounding lakes where he enjoyed fishing, hunting, and trapping through his high school years. He earned the coveted Eagle Scout badge.

He was active in music and athletics, receiving an athletic scholarship to Lake Forest University. He put his talents to work in earning money for his medical education by selling live bait, caddying, driving a milk and a gas truck, working in hardware stores, mowing lawns, and pumping gas. He did not neglect his spiritual life, and attended the Methodist Church and Epworth League. With his brothers, he reconstructed an old Model-T Ford car and built a power-driven ice boat. He accomplished all of this in the few years since his birth on November 2, 1917 in McHenry, Illinois.

He attended the University of Lake Forest, becoming a member of Phi Pi Epsilon; Central YMCA College; University of Illinois College of Pharmacy, receiving his B.S. degree while being awarded the Kilmer research grant in pharmacognosy, August 1941; elected to Rho Chi, national honorary society in pharmacy; graduate fellow, University of Illinois College of Pharmacy, attending graduate school and teaching in the department of pharmacology. He was elected president of the senior class.

At the University of Illinois College of Medicine 1942-45, he received his B.S. in medicine in June 1943; M.D. degree, September 1945; M.S. degree in surgery, June 1951; and was certified by the American Board of General Surgery in January 1958. Active in class offices, he continued to work in a drugstore and the last two years of medical school joined the ASTP, and took honors. He was elected to the AOA fraternity and medical honoraries.

Internship was at the University of Illinois Research Hospital, October 1945 to July 1946. Residency with a fellowship was at the V.A. Hospital in Hines, Illinois, where he practiced general surgery 1948-51. He was able to continue his practice with the U.S. Air Force, with which he was a flight surgeon 1946-48; captain 1951-53, during which time he was chief of surgery at the V.A. Hospital in Grand Junction, Colorado, and advanced to flight surgeon and surgeon with the rank of major.

Dr. Vycital was ward surgeon at the V.A. Hospital in Boise 1953-56. He opened his private practice in Boise in June 1956. How he and his wife, Ann, a registered nurse, decided to live in Idaho is described by the doctor, "Ann and I met at the beginning of my internship at the University of Illinois and were married in June 1946. Daughter, Sherry Ann, was born November 5, 1948; and son, Richard Keith, on June 20, 1951. As do all young couples who are without outside funding for education, Ann and I worked during my residency.

"We were in charge of the first aid station at a Sulky racing track, although we had never seen a horse race before. We also rented a large home and sublet rooms to school teachers to help make expenses. I joined the National Guard during my residency and upon completion had to return to the service with the onset of the Korean War. I went to Europe and for more than a year we lived in France.

"Early one morning while on ship in the mid-Atlantic returning to the United States, we decided that we would move out west to raise our children. From new friends we had made in the military we had learned that Boise, Idaho,

was one of the nicest places to live. After residing here, we
so agree."

In Boise, Dr. Vycital has been active on the staffs of St.
Lukes and St. Alphonsus hospitals and the Elks Rehabilita-
tion Center. He has been a consultant in surgery at the
Veterans Administration Hospital, and held the positions
of treasurer, Southwestern Idaho Medical Society; chair-
man of various committees of both hospitals and Ada
County Medical Society; chairman of State of Idaho
Veteran Affairs; South Idaho Medical Survey Bureau;
American College of Surgeons Trauma Committee for
Idaho.

DR. J. WOODSON CREED

A reserve officer who returned to active duty and
assigned to the Civilian Conservation Corps, Dr. J.
Woodson Creed caught his first glimpse of Idaho from the
window of a narrow gauge troop train traveling from
Montana, over the high divide, down into Leadore and on
to Salmon. What he saw was fourteen inches of new snow
as they unloaded at Salmon, and he wondered what he
had done in requesting active duty.

He was born on a farm in Boone County, Missouri, July
26, 1907; graduated from Columbia High School, 1924;
received A.B. and B.S. degrees from the University of
Missouri and an M.D. from St. Louis School of Medicine,
the latter in 1933. It was in the depth of the depression
that he finished his internship. A return to active duty
seemed the only place to turn.

The following six months was spent at the laboratory at
Fort Riley, Kansas, and then assigned as doctor to take a
group of Kansas C.C.C. youth to the Black Hills for one
year before going on to Salmon.

He married Nona Milton on October 23, 1929. She was
driving west with their two sons, James, five, and Dudley,
one. In Wyoming, they ran into as much snow as the
doctor did in Salmon. Luckily, Mrs. Creed was able to
follow a large snowplow nearly all the way across
Wyoming, with the two small boys snuggled up beside
her. They stayed at Salmon while Dr. Creed took his C.C.C.
boys down the river to work. She began to wonder if they
hadn't made a terrible mistake.

The mood changed when they were transferred to a camp in the Stanley Basin, where the weather had improved and the beauty of the Sawtooth Mountains caused the Creeds to fall in love with Idaho. The C.C.C. boys felt the same way and later Dr. Creed said that more than one-third of them decided to make Idaho their permanent home. After his release as a first lieutenant from the C.C.C., he made a visit to Twin Falls and decided to locate in the county. He rented an old bank building in Filer and established offices in the front and family living quarters in the back.

In three years, the Creeds built a home on Yakima Street, with many patients aiding in the building as a way of paying their medical bills. Nearly all the babies he delivered were in the home, rather than the hospital. A third son, Robert, was born to the Creeds on January 26, 1939 at Filer. All three sons were graduated from Twin Falls High School.

As a reserve officer, Dr. Creed was put on alert when the Germans marched into the Polish Corridor. When Dr. Ivan Anderson moved into the community, Dr. Creed felt he was able to leave and secured a residency in pathology at Methodist Hospital, Indianapolis. July 26, 1941, he reported to Fort Ord, California for active duty. His family went with him and lived nearby.

Later he was assigned director of the second largest laboratory in the world at Fort Lewis, Washington. He was separated from the service in December 1945 after five years duty, with the rank of lieutenant colonel. He associated for several months with the department of pathology at Tufts Medical College in Boston.

He took the California board exams in both clinical pathology and pathologic anatomy and became a Fellow of the American Society of Clinical Pathologists and the College of American Pathology in July 1946. The Creeds spent a year in Salt Lake City, where he was associated with the pioneer pathologist Dr. Orin Ogilvie, and served at St. Benedict's Hospital in Ogden.

The family returned to Twin Falls and he set up a laboratory at the old Twin Falls Hospital. He organized the first community blood bank on a replacement basis. A summer training course for lab technicians which he set up at the hospital proved so popular that not all those who applied could be taken. Dr. Creed organized and was ready to start an intern program at the hospital when he became ill and was forced into retirement. In September of 1961 he suffered a stroke, the complications of which he later died.

Dr. Creed was as active in community affairs as in medical. He was president of the Filer Kiwanis Club and a member in Twin Falls. He belonged to the Filer Masonic Lodge and became a 32nd degree Mason in Salt Lake City. He belonged to Shrine El Korah Temple, Boise, and was past patron of the Magic Valley chapter, Order of Eastern Star; an elder, Sunday school teacher and president of the Men's Club in the Presbyterian Church; active in the Chamber of Commerce and Twin Falls Toastmasters Club.

For many years he served as county coroner and was often called upon to give expert testimony and perform autopsies in the Magic Valley. Once he was called from a formal dance and did an autopsy while dressed in his tuxedo.

DR. NEWELL HOWARD BATTLES

Dr. Battles saw much of the United States before deciding to settle in Idaho Falls in 1941. He was born in Central City, Nebraska in 1907 and attended public school in Genoa. His pre-med studies were at the University of Nebraska in Lincoln from 1925-29. He attended Northwestern University Medical School and received his M.D. in 1933. While at Northwestern University he was a member of Nu Signa Nu and Alpha Omega Alpha.

He interned at St. Louis City Hospital from 1932-33 and completed an eye, ear, nose, and throat residency at Barnes Hospital, 1933-35. He returned to St. Louis City Hospital as a resident intern, 1935-36. He completed an eye residency at Barnes Hospital in 1936-1937, after which he practiced in the Budge Clinic in Logan, Utah.

Dr. Battles was a captain in the Army, stationed at Letterman General Hospital, Hammond General Hospital, Modesto, California, and Fort Sill, Oklahoma, for a total of nearly four years, on eye, ear, nose, and throat. He was a member of the L.D.S. and Sacred Heart Hospital staffs, Idaho Falls; a Fellow of American College of Surgeons;

member, Academy of Otolaryngology and Ophthalmology; charter member, Centurion Club; member, West Coast Academy of Eye, Ear, Nose, and Throat; Utah Ophthalmological Society; American, Idaho State and Bonneville County Medical associations. He had three sons and one daughter.

DR. THOMAS WYNNE WATTS, JR

Dr. Watts was born December 28, 1920, at Portland, Oregon, where his father was a dermatologist. He went to grade and high schools in Portland; two years at the University of Oregon, and four years as U.S. Navy pilot; completed the University of Oregon and entered medical school. In June 1947 he received a B.S. degree from the University of Oregon, and in 1949 an M.D. from the University of Oregon Medical School. He had a rotating internship at Naval Hospital, Philadelphia, 1951–52; one year OB/GYN residency at Oregon Medical School Hospital and Clinics in 1953–54. He started general practice in Payette, Idaho in 1954.

Dr. Watts was on the Holy Rosary Hospital staff, Ontario, Oregon, and held all positions on the board and executive board.

For four years he was a Navy patrol bomber pilot, reaching rank of lieutenant senior grade. He was a physician in the medical corps for two years in Korea, and remained in active reserve with rank of commander M.C.

He had a ten acre horse and cattle ranch and enjoyed hunting, fishing, skiing, camping, and riding in the hills.

Dr. Watts was on the executive board of Ore-Ida Council of Boy Scouts; director, Treasure Valley Savings & Loan; lay advisory board, Holy Rosary Church. He married Dorothy Flanery of Springfield, Oregon, and they had two girls and one boy.

DR. LOUIS J. PERKINS

Dr. Louis J. Perkins was a veteran of the Spanish American War and World War I, serving overseas in both.

He was born near Utica, Iowa, March 12, 1866, and died June 1, 1923, at fifty-seven. He was educated in Iowa schools, and was graduated from the Normal School at Dexter, Iowa. He taught at the school for a few years, after which he entered the study of medicine. He was graduated

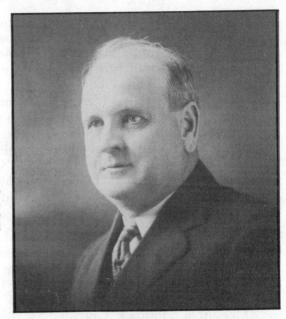

Dr. Louis Jay Perkins practiced in Lewiston. He was born in 1866 and died in 1923. He served as a medical officer in both the Spanish-American and World War I conflicts.

with honors from the Keokuk Medical College, March 8, 1892, and supplemented his education at Chicago and New York. He practiced for a time in Des Moines, Iowa.

In 1895 he went to Pendleton, Oregon to practice medicine and his family joined him later.

When the Spanish American War broke out, he enlisted and spent from 1900–01, with the Oregon Soldiery in the Philippine Islands. After the war he and his family remained for a short time in Des Moines, and then he took up his practice again at Pendleton. Later he went to Washington, D.C. to serve with the staff of the Pension Bureau.

From the capital city, he went to Lewiston in the fall of 1903, where he practiced for twenty years.

In all affairs of a civic nature, Dr. Perkins took interest, and this led his friends to nominate him for mayor of Lewiston in 1911. He was elected and served until June 1913. He was re-elected for the June 1915 to June 1917 term. He and those serving with him as commissioners made many city improvements. He was a member of the school board, and helped to establish a Home Economics Department at Lewiston High School.

Dr. Perkins answered the call to the colors in World War I, despite the fact that he had passed middle age. He served with the 80th and 88th divisions in France, from August 1918 until July 1919. When mustered out, he held the rank of captain.

He was married to Mamie E. Nelson, September 19, 1888. They had five children, Mrs. Ira Dole, Paul and Ralph Perkins, Lewiston, Dr. John N. Perkins, Helena, Montana, and a daughter who died at the age of four.

He was active in the Methodist Church and acted as trustee. He was a member of the Masonic Lodge, taking the Scottish Rite degree, and the Odd Fellows, Eagles, Elks, Spanish American War Veterans, and the American Legion.

DR. CHARLES E. MARSH

Dr. Charles E. Marsh graduated from Oklahoma University in 1954. He interned at Providence Hospital, Portland, Oregon, 1954–55. He entered the Air Force at Bryan, Texas, 1955–56, as flight surgeon, and was transferred to Marianna, Florida's Graham Air Force Base from 1956 through 1957. He was a major in the Idaho National Guard.

Dr. Marsh moved to Moscow to practice with Dr. J.G. Wilson for a year before moving to Buhl to open an office. He formed "The Nobles," a barbershop quartet that sang at towns in southern Idaho.

DR. ALBERT M. PETERSON

Dr. Peterson was born December 23, 1907, in Sawyer, North Dakota. Before medical school he was principal of Lawford School from 1933–35. From 1927–30 he attended Minot State Teachers College and received an A.B. degree. In 1938, he received a B.S. degree from the University of North Dakota. He received his M.D. from Temple in Philadelphia in 1940. To help pay for his education, he worked as seed salesman for Northrup King Company in the midwest during summers.

Dr. Peterson interned at Sacred Heart Hospital in Spokane, and for six months took a postgraduate course in obstetrics, gynecology, and general medicine at Polyclinic and Hospital in New York City.

In 1941–42 he practiced in Wallace and left to spend four years with the Air Force. He returned in 1946 and was staff chief at Providence Hospital, 1958-60. He was president of the Shoshone Medical Society and chairman of the county board of health.

During 1942-46 when he was flight surgeon with the Eighth Air Force's 388th Bomb group in the European theater, he received six battle stars and two Presidential citations. He left the service as a major.

DR. LEO F. QUIGLEY

As he sat in his home visiting with an old friend and Wallace attorney, J.L. Fitzgerald, on January 31, 1932, Dr. Quigley suddenly died. He was fifty-three and had resided in the Wallace district for twenty-nine years. He had first located in Wardner as an assistant to Dr. Hugh France at the hospitals. Three daughters and two brothers survived.

He was a colonel in the reserves at the time of death and during World War I was a major with the medical department. Military honors were accorded the funeral cortege while passing through Kellogg. A detachment of service men met the funeral procession at the city limits and with furled flags marched at the head of the column as it made its way through town. At the Idaho state line, officers from Fort George Wright met the procession and led the way to Spokane for burial.

DR. MAURICE M. BURKHOLDER

A native of Nampa, born April 6, 1915, Dr. Burkholder worked for the U.S. Forest Service before entering Northwestern University Medical School in 1943. In 1943-44 he was at Chicago Memorial Hospital. After completing college, he served from 1944-46 as a lieutenant in the Medical Corps of the U.S. Navy.

After leaving the service, he held a residency in internal medicine at Wesley Memorial Hospital until 1948. In July that year he relocated to Boise, where he practiced until retirement. He was chief of staff at St. Lukes and Elks Rehab Center and chairman of the department of medicine at both. He was a member of Ada County Medical Society and the American Medical Association Council on Mental Health.

Dr. and Mrs. Burkholder have been active members of Southminster Presbyterian Church for years. Both have worked in many community projects. In the fall of 1992 their children and grandchildren held an open house at the church to honor their golden wedding anniversary with a standing room only crowd in attendance.

DR. GEORGE EDWARD WEICK

From September 1942 until February 1946, Dr. Weick served as Army captain in the European theater. His father was a factory superintendent in Muskegan, Michigan, where Dr. Weick was born July 20, 1916. He received an A.B. in 1938 from the University of Michigan and an M.D. in 1941 from Michigan Medical School. Internship was at Westchester County Hospital in Valhalla, New York.

At the conclusion of World War II in Europe, where Dr. Weick was an anesthesiologist, he completed a two-year residency in pediatrics at the University of Michigan, 1946–48.

He moved to Boise in June 1948 and opened a practice. He and his wife, Catherine, have two sons and two daughters. In 1961, he was chief of staff at St. Luke's Hospital.

DR. ROY L. PETERSON

After completing his education at Creighton University and Medical School in 1933, Dr. Peterson entered the Air Force, serving as first lieutenant, 1933–34. He remained active in the USAF Reserve after discharge until 1940 when he established practice in Nebraska. He did post graduate work at Washington University in St. Louis, 1939–40.

Moving to Boise in 1940, he became an active staff member of St. Alphonsus Hospital until 1958, when he was named to the consulting staff as well as with the U.S. Veterans Hospital. He rejoined the Reserves as a lieutenant colonel from 1951–63 and in 1963 was promoted to full colonel.

Dr. Peterson was born in Chappell, Nebraska, July 22, 1908 where his father was a peace officer for the railroad. He married and had four sons and three daughters. Two of his daughters became registered nurses.

DR. GORDON WELD REYNOLDS

From Miles City, Montana where he was born December 2, 1918, Dr. Reynolds moved to Oshkosh, Wisconsin at seventeen. He worked to finance his education at the

University of Wisconsin. Graduating in 1940 with a B.S. he studied medical science at the University of Illinois, receiving an M.D. in 1943. A rotating residency in 1944 was at Cook County Hospital.

He joined the Army and spent two and half years at Deshon General Hospital, Butler, Pennsylvania as captain. Dr. Reynolds served as urology resident at Watts Hospital in Denham, North Carolina, 1946–49. He established practice in Idaho Falls, where he was on the staffs at L.D.S. and Sacred Heart hospitals.

He was regent for Idaho's International College of Surgeons; Diplomate, American Board of Urology; Fellow and Diplomate, International College of Surgeons; Fellow, American College of Surgeons; and member of the American and Western Urological Society. The Reynolds have one son and a daughter.

DR. WILLIAM SKELLENGER

Dr. William Skellenger of Coeur d'Alene, who flies his own Cessna 210, landing each week on the tiny runway alongside the St. Joe River to attend patients in St. Maries, flew during the Desert Storm War in the Persian Gulf. Although a resident of Idaho, he is a lieutenant colonel in the Washington National Air Guard.

Dr. Skellenger flew home with three decorations; the Air Medal, for having flown more than twenty missions in combat; the Air Force Achievement Medal; and the Liberation Kuwait Medal.

From December 29, 1990 to April, 1991, Lieutenant-colonel Skellenger (as flight surgeon) worked to maintain physical and emotional capabilities of the air crew through his medical services on wartime missions.

In the summer of 1992, Colonel Skellenger took about a dozen rides in the F-16 fighter plane, which operates by a "fly-by-wire" system run by computers. This was part of the Fighters Flight Surgeon School, known as "Top Knife", Air Force's Kingsley Field, Klamath Falls, Oregon. He enjoyed it, and remarked, "It's marvelous. I've never had more fun in my life. There aren't a thousand doctors in the world who get to ride in the back of an F-16." From there it was a short step to flying in the Gulf.

Dr. Skellenger's wife, Carol, was elected president of the Auxiliary to the Idaho Medical Association.

CHAPTER
6

MEDICINE — A FAMILY TRAIT

Bonds between parents and children are intricate and patterns of family life are extremely variable. "Depends upon the family," as the saying goes. Many children of doctors decide at an early age that they want a medical career. Doing research for this book and reading the material previously gathered by the late Irene Jones was, in many cases, like flipping through the pages of the family album. A few doctor mothers and children, many father and sons doctors, brothers, uncles, cousins, children and grandchildren fill the Idaho Medical Family album.

DRS. RALPH, EVERETT, and EVERETT, JR. JONES

For many years in the capitol city of Boise, the name of "Jones" meant one or more members of two unrelated, but of the same name, families practicing medicine.

Brothers Everett N. and Ralph Russell Jones were born into a farm family on Rural Route 1, Gervais, Marion County, Oregon. Everett was born February 19, 1904, and four years later Ralph was born on March 4, 1908. As the sons of a farmer, they learned to work hard, but enjoyed the horses, cows, pigs, sheep, chickens and, as Ralph said, "There was always a dog. And an occasional cat showed up."

Everett earned his B.A. from the University of Oregon, Eugene, in 1926; and his Doctor of Medicine two years later at the University's school in Portland. His internships and residency were taken at Ancker Hospital in St. Paul, 1928–29; U.S. Naval Hospital, Waukegan, Illinois, 1929–30; and Holy Rosary Hospital, Miles City, Montana, 1930–33. From 1933–37, he practiced in Wolf Point, Montana, and moved to Boise to practice with his brother and later with his son. He practiced in Boise from 1937–64.

"I did a home surgery, a resection of an *infarcted omentum* on a dining room table in a home south of Wolf Point, Montana. Getting there was as difficult as the operation. Crossing the Missouri River on ice in mid-winter when the temperature was sixty degrees below zero is what drove us to the Banana Belt of Boise," he said.

Dr. Everett was on the surgical staff at St. Lukes and St. Alphonsus hospitals from 1938 until 1964, and was chief of staff at St. Al's in 1951. He was president of the Southwest Idaho Medical Society in 1951 and councilor in 1952.

From 1942 to 1946, he served in the U.S. Naval Reserve and was presented a commendation by Admiral Wilkinson for action at Ronnell Island in the Solomons in January of 1943. He was promoted from lieutenant commander to captain (M.C.) U.S.N.R. On the homefront, Dr. Everett was honored by the Catholic Church with the *Pro Ecclesia Pontifice* Medal, which is bestowed to those eminent in their devotion toward church and community. Dr. Jones, who assisted in promoting the fund drive for the building of the new St. Alphonsus Hospital, was the first of ten Idaho Catholics to receive the award.

He and Mrs. Jones became parents of one daughter, Sister Mary Frances Dorothy, C.S.C.; and three sons, Everett Jr., surgeon; Harry E., electrical engineer; and John H., who earned his Bachelor of Science degree in political science at Idaho State College (now University) and worked as assistant commissioner of labor for Idaho.

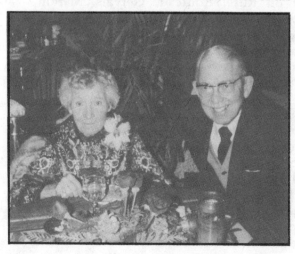

Dr. and Mrs. Everett (Dorothy) Jones Sr. lived in Boise, where he practiced with his brother, Dr. Ralph Jones, for more than fifty years, and later with his son, Dr. Everett, Jr. Dr. Everett was given the U.S. Navy citation for "Distinguished Service" for his efforts to evacuate his patients when his ship was torpedoed off the coast of Guadalcanal during World War II. In 1966, he received a medal from the Pope for his devotion to his church.
(Courtesy Dr. Ralph Jones)

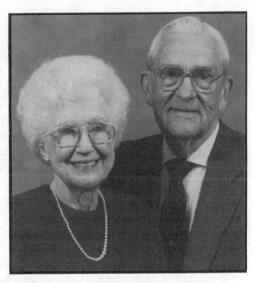

Dr. and Mrs. Ralph (Irene) Jones of Boise have played quiet and subdued, but very important roles in the development of Idaho medical history. Dr. Ralph and his brother, Dr. Everett Jones, opened a medical partnership in 1938 and have become among the most beloved and respected physicians in the area. Dr. Ralph is one of the few physicians to serve as president of the medical staffs of both St. Alphonsus and St. Luke's hospitals in Boise. He served during World War II aboard a destroyer in the South Pacific and at the Bremerton, Washington U.S. Naval Hospital.

Irene Jones was historian for the Idaho Medical Auxiliary and, for many years, had sought material for this book.

(Courtesy Dr. Ralph Jones)

Ralph Russell Jones received pre-medical education at Oregon State College, Corvallis, from which he was graduated in 1930 with a Bachelor of Science degree. His M.D. was granted on June 12, 1934, at the Washington University School of Medicine, St. Louis, Missouri. He interned at St. Vincent's Hospital, Portland, and was a surgical resident for two years at Holy Rosary Hospital in Miles City, Montana.

Dr. Jones received his Idaho license to practice medicine and surgery October 29, 1937. The following year he established a surgical practice with brother, Dr. Everett, in the Idaho First National Bank Building. During World War II, Dr. Ralph spent nearly four years in the U.S. Navy, twenty-two months of which were in the South Pacific and the remainder at the U.S. Naval Hospital in Bremerton. He was discharged as a lieutenant commander.

Following military duty, Dr. Jones took additional surgical training in St. Louis at the Washington University School of Medicine and at Bellevue Hospital in New York City. He is one of the few Boise physicians who served as president of the staff at both hospitals. He was president of St. Alphonsus medical staff in 1950-51 and at St. Lukes in 1967-69.

He has served as secretary-treasurer of the Southwestern Idaho Medical Society in 1950-51 and as president in

1958-59. He was a delegate from the society to the Idaho Medical Association on three different occasions for two-year terms; a member of the Ada County Medical Association, American College of Physicians and Surgeons, American College of Surgeons and president of the Boise Valley chapter in 1960-61.

Among the unusual happenings in his medical career, Dr. Ralph recalled that in June of 1938 he did emergency first-aid on a Milwaukee Railroad passenger car at Miles City, Montana, providing after-midnight emergency care and transportation of patients injured in a train wreck at the site of a washed-out bridge. Later he was in charge of transfer and admittance of fifty-three patients to the Holy Rosary Hospital twenty-five miles away. "The death rate at the site of the wreck and at the hospital was high," he reported, "and there were several fractures and surgeries."

He remembered when on board ship in Leyte Gulf of the Philippines during World War II, giving care to multiple casualties after the ship was dive-bombed by a Japanese Kamikaze (suicide) pilot in a plane which carried explosives. As first a lieutenant, senior grade, and later lieutenant commander, he was medical officer for twenty-two months on board a Navy ship in the South Pacific. From there he was assigned to the U.S. Navy Hospital in Seattle.

Dr. Jones and his late wife, Irene, had two daughters, Marcia Sands and Judy Combs, both in California. Each has a son and a daughter. The Joneses were active members of the Boise Methodist Church. An avid golfer, Dr. Jones is a member of the Hillcrest Country Club, Masonic Lodge, Scottish Rite Bodies and El Korah Shrine Temple.

Everett N. Jones Jr., was born May 6, 1932, in Miles City, Montana. He attended the University of Oregon for pre-medical education and received his M.D. degree in 1957 from Creighton University. He served an externship at Boys Town, Nebraska from 1955 to 1957; internship and residency at St. Joseph's Hospital in Denver, 1957-61; and was chief surgical resident at Denver General Hospital until 1963.

Dr. Everett Jr. says, "It was an inspiration to practice medicine with my father and my uncle." In addition to the three of them, another family member, Loy Cramer, is an orthopedic surgeon. He is a cousin to Everett Jr. While in medical school, Everett Jr. worked on two epidemics: newborn *staphylococcus* and pediatric *meningococcemia*.

Despite the fact that sometimes in winter weather he had to travel by snow van, Dr. Everett Jr. is proud of the fact that he was never late to do surgery in Boise, Mountain Home, or Emmett. He served on the active staffs at St. Alphonsus and St. Lukes and the consulting staff at Elmore Memorial Hospital in Mountain Home and Walter Knox Hospital in Emmett. He was president of the Idaho division of the American Cancer Society and remained a member of the active reserve of U.S.A.S. from 1959 until 1964.

Dr. and Mrs. Everett Jones, Jr., have five daughters, Kathy, Betsy, Ellen, Leslie, and Fay.

DRS. SAMUEL, RICHARD, and WILLIAM FORNEY

Dr. Samuel Wilcox Forney and his two sons, Richard A. and William D., established a reputation as being representative of what is best in the medical profession. They contributed much to the Boise area and to Idaho.

Samuel was born in Minonk, Illinois, December 29, 1883, to Mr. and Mrs. Henry Clay Forney. He attended grade and high schools in Minonk and entered Northwestern University, Evanston, for a three-year pre-med course before becoming a student at Rush Medical College, Chicago. He received his M.D. degree in 1908 and for the next year and one-half interned at Chicago Polyclinic Hospital and Postgraduate School and spent a part of his time at the Henrotin Hospital. He was associated in practice in Chicago for six months with Dr. Kleinspell.

Dr. Forney decided that the west was where he wanted to live and on March 30, 1911, arrived in Boise. He opened offices in the Overland Building and soon built a large practice. He never stopped studying and was actively interested in the Ada County, Idaho State, Tri-State, and American Medical associations. He was a member of the staff at St. Lukes Hospital. His memberships were in Alpha Kappa Kappa, the Masons, the University and Commercial clubs.

Richard A. Forney was born in Boise on April 8, 1914, to

Dr. and Mrs. Samuel Forney. He attended grade and high schools in Boise and his freshman year at the College of Idaho, Caldwell. His B.A. was from the University of California, Berkeley. In 1939, he received an M.D. from the University of Chicago, and in 1948, a Master of Science from the University of Minnesota. He interned at Ancker Hospital in St. Paul and was a resident Fellow in Surgery at the Mayo Foundation, Rochester, Minnesota, 1941-48. His fraternities are Alpha Omega Alpha, Nu Sigma Nu, and Phi Delta Theta.

From 1942 through 1945, he served as lieutenant colonel with the U.S. Air Force and was decorated with the Air Medal. He was staff surgeon at St. Lukes and St. Alphonsus hospitals and consulting cardiovascular surgeon with Veterans Administration Hospital. Dr. Forney was president of the Boise Valley Chapter, American College of Surgeons, 1958; Boise Rotary Club, 1960-61; and Idaho Heart Association, 1959-60.

He married Margaret Magel of Twin Falls and they have two boys and two girls.

William D. Forney was born July 12, 1918, in Boise, and followed his father and brother into the practice of medicine. He attended Boise schools; the College of Idaho from 1936-37; University of California at Berkeley, where he received his A.B. in 1940; University of Chicago School of Medicine to receive his M.D. in 1948; and received a Master of Science from the University of Minnesota.

Dr. William served his internship and residency in the city and county of San Francisco, 1949-50; the Mayo Foundation at the Mayo Clinic, 1950-53. He practiced at the Mayo Clinic and returned to Boise in November 1953 to practice. He served in the U.S. Army from 1942-45, as a "throttle jockey."

When asked if he had ever performed a home surgery, his response was, "Carpentry only." He has been on the active staff at both St. Lukes and St. Alphonsus, where he was chief of staff in 1965. He was on the active staff, and chief of staff, at the Elks Rehabilitation Center in 1959.

Dr. Forney was secretary-treasurer of the South Idaho Medical Service Bureau, past president of the Idaho Society of Internal Medicine and of the Idaho Heart Association; member of the American College of Physicians and

American College of Chest Physicians. He held membership in the American, Idaho, and Ada County Medical
associations.

On loan to the Air Force from 1942 to 1945 as squadron
commander of a B-17 group, Dr. Forney flew fifty-two
combat missions in the Mediterranean. He was decorated
with the Air Medal, Distinguished Flying Cross and
Presidential Group Citation and others.

He likes to hunt, fish, and is a fine enough carpenter
that he built his family lake home at McCall. He and his
late wife, Mae Shelton, had one son, Drew, and a daughter,
Lisa. Dr. William Forney and his wife, Mary, are living in
Boise.

DR. ROBERT L. NOURSE

The identification of Dr. Nourse with Boise began in
1897, but it was not until 1907 that he located there on a
permanent basis. He was involved with most of the
progress of medicine in Idaho from the time he arrived
until his death on June 25, 1949. He was secretary of the
first Idaho Medical Examiners Board, appointed by
Governor Steunenberg in 1899 and president, Idaho
Medical Examining Board in 1905.

Born September 27, 1864, at Cloverport, Kentucky, he
attended public schools and Columbus Academy.
Orphaned at fifteen, he left two years later to join his
uncle for several years in the hotel business at Stevens
Point, Wisconsin. He entered Rush Medical College,
receiving his M.D. in 1889. While a student and in practice
in Chicago, he served with the Illinois National Guard. He
married Marie Irvine Crawford of Chicago, daughter of
Samuel K. Crawford, surgeon of the Civil War period. Dr.
Nourse practiced at Chicago, Washburn, and Ashland,
Wisconsin where their two sons, Robert L. Jr., and Norman
C. were born.

With his family he moved to Hailey in 1897. From 1905
to 1907, he studied eye, ear, nose, and throat in New York
and in Europe. In late 1907, he opened practice in Boise.

His first wife died in 1921, and in 1923 he married Anna
Brakel of Portland, Oregon. They had one daughter,
Marianna (Mrs. George H. Lane of Boise).

In 1934 he became medical examiner for the Civil
Aeronautics Administration and in 1943 for United Air

Lines. He was a fellow of American College of Surgeons; member, American Medical Association, a licentiate of the American Board of Oto-Laryngology, both St. Alphonsus and St. Lukes medical staffs, as well as the Children's Home.

He was a lifelong Presbyterian and an elder since 1893. A director of the YMCA for twenty-five years, he was given a life membership. He was a 32nd degree Mason, member of the Scottish Rite Body, the Shrine, and was one of five honorary fifty-year life members of the Blue Lodge. He belonged to the Democrat party, but had no desire to hold political office.

DR. JOSEPH S. NUMBERS

A kindly physician who aided him in recovering his health was instrumental in Joseph S. Numbers becoming a doctor. Numbers, in turn, was the influence that caused his two sons, John and J. Reno, to obtain Medical Doctor degrees.

He was one of eight children born to Esau and Anna Smith Numbers on the family farm in Morrow County, Ohio, May 30, 1864. The numerous Numbers attended country schools. Joseph was thirteen when his mother died. He finished high school and entered Ohio Central College, Iberia. He then went to Paolo, Kansas, to teach, but became ill. During this illness, he was attended by Dr. Albert Reichard, and the two became fast friends.

Dr. Reichard persuaded Joseph to study medicine, and he read in the doctor's office before entering the Eclectic Medical Institute in Cincinnati, Ohio, graduating in 1885, and began his practice that summer. Soon he moved to Carbondale, Kansas, for a year. In the fall of 1886, he became assistant surgeon with the American Hospital Aid Association in Minneapolis. September 7, 1887, he married Mary B. Swartz, of Pennsylvania.

After two years in Minnesota, they wanted to move west, and in 1888 traveled to Weiser, where they spent the next twelve years. He was active in the community and was mayor from 1906–08. In 1910 they moved to Boise, and he continued extensive reading and research. He authored many articles for medical journals.

Dr. Numbers became president of the Idaho Medical Association, a member of the American Medical Association, and did post-graduate study at Rush Medical College, Chicago, in Baltimore, and New York City.

Dr. and Mrs. Numbers had three children. Their two sons became doctors. Donald, was graduated from the Barnes Medical College of St. Louis, Missouri, and was a captain and instructor in the Medical Reserve Corps of the U.S. Army. Joseph Reno was graduated from Rush Medical College. Their daughter, Josephine Letitia, married Buford E. Kuhn and died at an early age.

Dr. Numbers was a Republican, Knight Templar Mason, Mystic Shrine, and past master of his lodge.

DR. GEORGE HENRY WAHLE, SR.

The Wahle family could have staffed a hospital, with an adjoining clinic thrown in. Some kind of a record had to be set by George Henry Wahle, Sr., the son of a doctor, the father of two doctors, son-in-law of a doctor, brother-in-law of four doctors and one registered nurse! Dr. Wahle Sr., sixty-one, died June 20, 1955, in Boise.

Born February 7, 1894, at West Bend, Wisconsin, son of Dr. and Mrs. Henry Wahle of Marshfield, Wisconsin and Oakland, California, he lived in Rochester, Minnesota, before moving to Boise. He attended the University of Wisconsin Medical School for two years, receiving his B.A., and his M.D. in 1919 with honors from Washington University School of Medicine in St. Louis. He interned at Marshfield, and was granted a post graduate fellowship in surgery at Mayo Clinic from 1922 to 1924. He received a Master of Science degree in surgery in 1925 from Minnesota.

He was a fellow of the American College of Surgeons; American Medical Association; senior member, American Association for the study of goiter; member and later president, Southwest Idaho Medical Society; Mayo Foundation Alumni Association; member, Sigma Sigma, honorary medical fraternity; staff, St. Lukes and St. Alphonsus hospitals; and Knights of Columbus.

He and Mrs. Wahle, the former Elizabeth Mae Montgomery, had two sons, Dr. George Henry Wahle Jr., pathologist at King's Daughters Hospital, Temple, Texas; Dr. William Montgomery Wahle, pathologist, Fitzsimmons Hospital, Aurora, Colorado; two daughters, Betty Jane (Mrs. Peter Kalamarides), Anchorage, Alaska, and Joan Maurine

Wahle, Temple, Texas. Mrs. Wahle went to Texas to live with daughter, Joan, after the death of the doctor. She was the daughter of Dr. and Mrs. Alexander Montgomery Sr. of Wisconsin, and she had four doctor brothers and a registered nurse sister.

DR. EDWARD DEE PARKINSON

Edward Parkinson was born at Murray, Utah, December 1, 1903, and was a man of few words. He encased his entire life before entering medical school with, "The usual. Grade school, high school, university, working at odd jobs all the time when not in school."

He graduated from the University of Utah in 1929 and Northwestern University in Chicago, with an M.D. in 1932, going on to residency at Alameda County Hospital, Oakland. He practiced medicine in Emmett in 1934 and in Payette from 1935-41 when he moved to Boise. Dr. Parkinson was chief of staff at St. Lukes, 1950; president, Northwest Proctological Society, 1961; and was often invited to speak at medical meetings, including the American, Southern California, and Arizona Proctological Societies; Mexico City (where the paper was given in Spanish), Athens, Greece, and aboard the S.S. Monarch sailing to Bermuda.

The Parkinsons had three children, the oldest of whom, John, became a doctor of internal medicine. A second son is Edward James, and a daughter, Janeen, married Stan Daly.

DR. WESLEY E. LEVI

Wesley Levi was born and reared in Greenway, South Dakota, where his father owned farms and a grain elevator. He was another who described his youth as, "Nothing spectacular. Just hard work."

He graduated from the University of Idaho in 1941, with a B.S. degree; two years of medical school at the University of North Dakota; received his M.D. at Temple University in Philadelphia in 1945.

His internship was at the Great Lakes, Illinois, U.S. Naval Hospital, 1945-46; residency at the Bismarck, North Dakota, Hospital, 1956-59; and partial residencies at the University of Minnesota and the Children's Hospital in Cincinnati.

Dr. Levi practiced from 1950 until 1955 at Beulah, North Dakota; Veterans Administration Hospital in Sturgis, South Dakota, 1955-1956; Bismarck Hospital and Clinic, January 1959-June 1960; and arrived in Boise that same month to begin practice. He served in the U.S. Naval Reserve from 1943 until 1947.

A lasting memory of Dr. Levi's was of becoming lost in a North Dakota blizzard, with the temperature at twenty degrees below zero, and walking five miles to a town. He traveled by a ski-equipped plane to treat a patient at one time and by railroad handcar to another. Both cases were in North Dakota.

Relatives of the doctor, who also became physicians and surgeons were a brother, Dr. Donald Levi of St. Paul; a brother-in-law, Terry Havig of Kansas City; cousins, Dr. Harold Stokes of Sturgis, Dr. Kenneth Wilske and Dr. Jerry Minzel of Seattle. He and Mrs. Levi became the parents of three girls and one boy.

DR. HERBERT L. NEWCOMBE

Herbert Lewis Newcombe was born September 20, 1903, in Yarmouth Center, Ontario, Canada, where his father was a high school teacher. Through grade, high, and Normal schools, he was in Calgary, Alberta. He taught school in rural Alberta, and in Calgary for three and one-half years before entering the University of Alberta, from which he received his B.A. degree in 1928 and his M.D. in 1932. He was freshman class president, 1925, and of the University of Alberta Medical Club in 1931. His internship was at Royal Alexandria Hospital, Edmonton, 1931-32; one year residency at University of Alberta Hospital, 1932-33.

From 1933-36, he practiced at the Provincial Mental Institute, Edmonton, and was director of the Kootenai County Health Unit in Coeur d'Alene from 1938 until 1944, when he entered private practice for several months. He went to Emmett from 1944-51 and on to Boise to practice.

In 1938, Dr. Newcombe received a Medical Public Health degree from the Harvard School of Public Health; in 1941, a postgraduate course in pediatrics, University of California; in 1948, postgraduate course in cancer and in 1955 in surgery, University of Oregon; 1960, short course at Oregon in obstetrics and gynecology; study at New York

Postgraduate Medical School and Margaret Hague Maternity Hospital in 1947.

Dr. Newcombe remembered traveling in northern Alberta in 1935 by a home-made propeller driven snow-mobile in below zero weather as he traced a typhoid epidemic.

He was on the staffs of St. Alphonsus and St. Lukes hospitals and executive and credential coommittees of St. Lukes. Positions held include secretary, Kootenai County Medical Society, 1940–44; delegate, Idaho State Medical Association from the Southwestern Idaho and Ada County Medical societies for six years; member of the Idaho Medical Association Committee on Care of the Aged, 1959–61; president of the Idaho Tuberculosis Association, 1945–46.

Color photography and gardening were "relaxers" for Dr. Newcombe. He and Mrs. Newcombe had a daughter and a son. The son, Edward H., became a doctor, studying at Whitman College, Walla Walla, from which he received his B.A.; McGill University in Montreal for his M.D.; interned at Montreal General Hospital. Dr. Newcombe also had an uncle, E.P. Lewis of Toronto, who was a physician.

DR. TIUS W. McCOWIN

Earning a Bachelor of Science degree in industrial technology from Utah State University and working as an agent for New York Life Insurance Company was not enough for Tius McCowin. He returned to school and earned his M.D. from George Washington University Medical School in 1958 at the age of thirty-two. He became a member of Pi Kappa Alpha fraternity.

Dr. McCowin completed a one year internship at L.D.S. Hospital, Salt Lake City, Utah, 1958–59, and residency in general practice, Tulare County Hospital, California, where he was chief resident from 1959–60. During his internship he received the Mead Johnson Award for Outstanding General Practice residents. Dr. McCowin opened his practice in Shelley in 1960. He was on the staff at the L.D.S. and Sacred Heart hospitals in Idaho Falls.

Dr. McCowin served in the U.S. Coast Guard as a radar operator from 1943–45 and was a member of the U.S. Air Force Reserve for twelve years. He has three sons and one daughter.

DR. THOMAS CLAIR HORTON, JR.

A desire to enter medicine was fostered in Thomas C. Horton, Jr. by his physician father, who practiced in Colorado and Arizona before moving to Nampa. The younger Dr. Horton was born in Pueblo, Colorado in 1919, and attended school in Nampa.

Dr. Horton graduated from the College of Idaho with a B.A. in 1941. While there he was a member of Beta Chi fraternity. He joined Phi Beta Pi while at Northwestern Medical School from 1941-44. An internship at St. Joseph's Hospital, Chicago, from 1944-45 followed by a mixed residency at St. Mary's Mercy Hospital, Gary, Indiana, preceded his return to Nampa in 1947 to practice. Dr. Horton served in the U.S. Navy, as lieutenant (jg) 1945-46; and lieutenant commander, 1953-55. The Hortons had three children.

DR. ARTHUR C. JONES, SR.

Dr. Arthur C. Jones, Sr., liked to joke that the town of Shamrock, Nevada, where he was born June 26, 1887, disappeared from the maps after the Jones family left. He was the son of Marvin Preston and Kathleen Riley Jones. He credited his mother with a dogged insistence that he have the advantages of a good education. While being reared on a ranch out of Havre, Montana, he attended grade school and continued his schooling in Spokane, Washington, and then enrolled at Shattuck Military School, Faribault, Minnesota, graduating in 1909. He took his M.D. degree from the University of Michigan Medical School in 1912.

Drawn again to the west, Dr. Jones interned at Murray Hospital in Butte, Montana, and went east for residency with Dr. Henry Cunningham at Marquette, Michigan.

Before going abroad to study, he married Lois Caroline Gunn, daughter of Doctor and Mrs. J.W. Gunn of Butte on January 3, 1914. The years 1914-15 were replete with riches of travel and associating with learned medical people in London and Vienna, but war clouds were hovering and they left Europe just before the onset of the first World War.

Back in Butte, Arthur practiced his specialty of eye, ear, nose, and throat with Dr. Peter Potter. While awaiting call to the armed forces, he was requested by the governor to go to Whitehall, Montana, where a flu epidemic was raging. He remembered that, "The only medications available then were a gallon jug full of aspirin tablets and two cases of whiskey!"

He joined the Mayo Brothers Clinic in Rochester, Minnesota, in 1915, and spent the next two years studying plastic surgery under supervision of Dr. Gordon New. In 1918, he returned to Butte to practice until 1921, when he moved to Boise where he made his home for the rest of his life.

His mother's insistence on all the education he could get never left him, and he spent several months of late 1926 and in 1927 studying with Dr. Harris P. Moser in Boston. On June 4, 1927, he became a Diplomate of the American Board of Otolaryngology. He was a lecturer at meetings of the American Academy of Otolaryngology for several years. His course titled, "Helpful Hints in the Everyday Practice of Ear, Nose and Throat," was always popular.

He lectured at the Los Angeles Midwinter Course and at Gill Memorial Hospital. He was a Fellow of the American College of Surgeons since 1930, serving in 1953 as president of the Idaho chapter; member of the Board of Governors of the College 1951–57; first vice-president of the American Academy of Ophthalmology and Otolaryngology, 1947; vice-president, Triological Society, 1938; president, Idaho Medical Association, 1938, and of the Pacific Coast Oto-Opthalmalogical Society, 1929–30; member of the American Medical Association; American Association of Physicians and Surgeons; and the Pan-American Association of Opthamology and Phi Rho Sigma.

Long active in civic affairs, he was named consulting opthamologist by the Idaho Department of Public Assistance; consulting plastic surgeon to the Crippled Children's service, Idaho Department of Public Health; chief of staff as well as head of the eye, ear, nose, and throat department at St. Lukes Hospital; on the consulting staff at St. Alphonsus; and consulting physician for the Union Pacific Railway.

Known as "Artie," he was active in outdoor sports and for many years returned to Michigan in the fall to see football games with old friends. In June 1962, he returned for his fiftieth medical class reunion at Ann Arbor.

Dr. and Mrs. Jones were communicants at St. Michaels Episcopal Church. He was a charter member of the Arid Club; and held membership in Hillcrest Country Club, the Elks Lodge, a 32nd degree Mason, El Korah Shrine; Boise Rotary, for which he served as president. He also belonged to the Bohemian Club of San Francisco.

Dr. Jones enjoyed a full and enthusiastic life until the death of his beloved wife, "Mimi," April 15, 1962. He

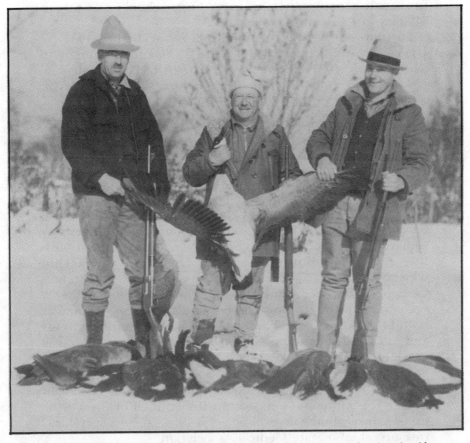

Dr. Arthur C. Jones, center, proudly shows his prize Canadian goose on a hunting trip with two "youngsters," Dr. William A. Koelsch and Dr. Jones' son, Dr. Winfield Jones. Doctors Koelsch and Winfield Jones are dentists. The successful shoot was near Lake Lowell and Caldwell.

(Courtesy Lodi Anderson)

continued an active office and surgical practice, but his children noticed that the spark was gone. He played golf with friends on September 1 and 2, but on the third said that he did not feel well. He refused to go to the hospital, but on the morning of September 4 he was admitted to St. Lukes, and died on September 6. The Jones had five children.

DR. A. CURTIS JONES, JR.

Born in Butte on April 5, 1916, Curtis moved with his parents to Boise in 1921. He attended Garfield and Roosevelt schools, then went to high school at Shattuck Military in Faribault, Minnesota.

Further study was at the College of Idaho, 1934-36; University of Michigan, 1936-37, 1938-39; and University of Washington, 1937-38 to earn a Bachelor of Science degree. He received an M.D. from the University of Michigan in 1949 where he joined Nu Sigma Nu and Phi Delta Theta.

Just before an internship at the University of Michigan Hospital, he married Martha Downs, a doctor in her own right, on June 4, 1942. An assistant residency and residency were taken at the same hospital, 1944-45; and he returned after a two-year military stint, to become an instructor in E.N.T. from 1947-48.

Dr. Jones was a first lieutenant stationed at Carlisle Barracks, Hiff General Hospital in Santa Barbara; Letterman General Hospital, San Francisco; advanced to captain with the A.U.S. at Border General Hospital, Chickashu, Oklahoma, 1946-47; thence to Army Aural Rehabilitation Center, Walter Reed General Hospital, Washington, D.C.

Upon returning to Boise he became a member of staffs at both St. Lukes Hospital and the Elks Rehabilitation Center and on the consulting staff at St. Alphonsus. He was president of St. Lukes staff, 1960; secretary-treasurer, Southwestern Idaho Medical Society, 1955; secretary-treasurer and president of Boise Valley Chapter, American College of Surgeons, 1954-58; on the council of the Pacific Coast Oto-Opthalmalogical Society, 1958-60; and secretary-treasurer, Idaho State Medical Association.

DR. MARTHA DOWNS JONES

Martha Downs was born October 23, 1917, in Highland Park, Michigan, where her father was superintendent of schools. Her girlhood was spent in Pleasant Ridge, a Detroit suburb, the youngest of three girls.

She joined Phi Mu sorority and received her Bachelor of Science degree at Duke University; became a member of Alpha Epsilon Iota and earned her M.D. degree at the University of Michigan in 1943. The year before graduation she married Arthur Curtis Jones Jr. Her internship and residency in ophthalmology were taken at the University of Michigan Hospital.

The Doctors Jones are the parents of three sons and one daughter: Arthur Curtis (Ace) III, Charles Downs (Chuck), Philip Armin, and Martha Merritt. Dr. Martha found occasions when she had the time to go hunting with her husband.

THE DOCTORS MAXEY

For more than one hundred years the distinguished medical family of Maxey ministered to Idaho and Idahoans. The first of them to come to Idaho was Dr. William Cannon Maxey. He was born New Year's Day in 1844 on a farm in Wayne County, Illinois. He arrived in Canyon

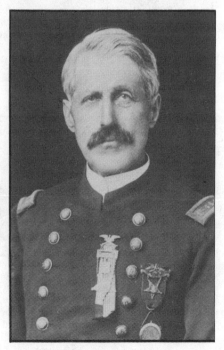

Dr. William Cannon Maxey arrived in Canyon County in 1887 to practice medicine and became favorably known in a short time. He was a member of the first Constitutional Convention on July 4, 1889. He is shown here in the uniform of the 1st Independent Regiment of the Illinois Cavalry in the Civil War. His son, Dr. Edward E., and son-in-law, Dr. Julius Wright, also practiced medicine.

(Courtesy Jeannie Reese)

County in 1887 and practiced medicine in and from there for the rest of his life. He died December 27, 1912, and is buried beside his wife in the Pioneer section of Morris Hill Cemetery, Boise.

Dr. William C.'s father, also a physician and surgeon, was Dr. William M.A. Maxey, native of Tennessee who settled in Illinois in 1818. It was in Illinois in 1861 that William C., imbued with patriotic fervor, joined the 1st Independent Regiment of the Illinois Cavalry. It was mustered out after a few months of service, and William C. re-enlisted in Company G of the 80th Illinois Volunteer Infantry. The excitement and hardships had just begun as he was captured by the Confederates and confined to Bell Island for several months.

At the close of the war he held the rank of second lieutenant. He went home and began the study of medicine until 1883, when he moved to Marcus, Iowa. Four years later he moved to Idaho.

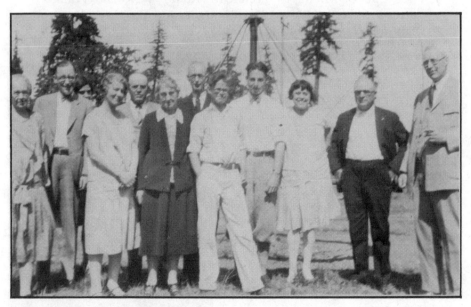

The remarkable family Maxey, left to right: Clara Kimble and Guy Maxey, daughter and son of William C.; Bess, wife of W. W. Maxey; Edna, wife of Dr. Edward; Mr. Kimble, husband of Clara; Jenny Wright and W. W. Maxey, daughter and son of William C.; Edward Maxey, son of Dr. Edward; Leonard, son of W.W. Maxey; Maude, wife of Guy Maxey; Dr. Junius Wright; and Dr. Edward E. Maxey, son of Dr. William C.

(Courtesy Jeannie Reese)

Dr. William C. became quickly known. He was a member of the first Constitutional Convention, held July 4, 1889 in Boise; and the first Commandant of the Soldier's Home. He became grand commander of the Grand Army of the Republic in Idaho. In 1886, he married Sarah Gertrude Lane and they became the parents of five children: Dr. Edward E. Maxey, Jenny (wife of Dr. Julius Wright of Caldwell), Clara of Caldwell, Woodruff William, and G.G., both located in Portland. Woodruff William was graduated from the first class at the College of Idaho.

When the Maxeys arrived in 1887, Caldwell had been a village for five years. Dr. Maxey was away from family and office two or three days at a time, attending to the sick in surrounding areas. At that time, all surgery was done in the homes as there were no hospitals. He worked equally hard in the development of Idaho. He was active in the Methodist Church, the Masonic Lodge, and a staunch Republican.

DR. EDWARD ERNEST MAXEY

Edward Maxey completed high school in Marcus, Iowa, engaged in farming and teaching school, before coming with his parents to Caldwell in 1887. The trip west was made in a box-car, with his father's three work horses and household goods to be used in reclaiming government land. Edward spent much of that first summer hauling lumber from the Emmett sawmill, twenty-six miles away, to erect the family's buildings.

The next fall, he went to Chicago to study medicine at the College of Physicians and Surgeons, and graduated with honors in 1891. That July he located at Walla Walla, but after two months returned to Caldwell and associated with his father until February 1902. He then moved to Boise to join Dr. L.P. McCalla in general practice.

On December 20, 1900, Dr. Maxey married Edna Horn, daughter of the Jacob Horns of Caldwell. A daughter, Marie Elizabeth, was born February 13, 1907, and a son, Edward, April 21, 1913.

He went to Europe in 1908 to study eye, ear, nose, and throat in Vienna, Berlin, and London. He practiced in Boise from 1909 until July 1917, when he received a commission as captain in the Army Medical Corps. Within six months he was promoted to major. After a month at Boise Barracks recruiting, he went to Fort D.A. Russell, Wyoming, for training before going to Camp Sherman, Ohio, to be chief of the eye service in the base hospital. He was discharged in April 1919, and practiced in Boise with Dr. R.L. Nourse until 1924. He then moved to Aberdeen, Washington to practice.

Dr. Edward was a charter member of the Idaho State Medical Society, organized in 1893; secretary from 1897 to 1917, with the exception of 1901, when he was president; member of American Medical Association, Academy of Ophthalmology and Oto Laryngology, and the Pacific Coast Oto-Ophthalmology Society; Fellow of the American Institute of Medicine and American College of Surgeons; a 32nd degree Scottish Rite Mason, Shriner, Republican, and an Elk.

In 1898, Dr. Maxey published the first extensive description of the disease now known as Rocky Mountain Spotted (Tic) Fever, and continued to publish articles on the subject. For this work he was awarded a place in *Who's Who in America*. He worked for better medical organization, higher standards of education and licensure, health legislation, and enforcement of medical laws. When the Idaho League for the Preservation of Public Health was organized in 1922, he was asked to be a council member and secretary.

Dr. Maxey was the first coroner of Canyon County and was Surgeon General of Idaho with the rank of colonel on the staff of Governor John M. Haines. He died suddenly of a coronary attack on August 31, 1934, at age sixty-seven.

DR. ORVID RAY CUTLER

Orvid Cutler had a father, brothers and a son, who were doctors. It was the natural thing to do to join them. He was born July 21, 1903 in Preston, Idaho, where he received his grade and high school educations and graduated from the Oneida Stake Academy in 1922. He received an A.B. degree and medical certificate from the University of Utah after five years study. His M.D. was in 1929 from Northwestern University in Chicago.

Dr. Cutler did his internship and residency at Staten Island Hospital, returning to Preston in October 1930 to begin a practice of many years. He held many offices in medical societies. Dr. and Mrs. Cutler had two sons and one daughter. One son, Clair Riley Culter, became a doctor with an M.D. from Northwestern University in Chicago, and practiced in Preston.

DR. ELVIN JAMES CUTLER, JR.

Elvin James was known as "Jim" from childhood, and was born in Burley, where his father was a school teacher. Jim received his B.S. degree at Idaho State College at Pocatello in 1953 and went east to George Washington University in Washington, D.C. for his M.D. in 1957. His internship and residency were at Fresno County Hospital in California and he began his practice in Burley in 1961.

Three uncles, Orvid W., Morton and Royal Cutler; two cousins, Clair Cutler and Gordon Daines were all medical doctors.

DR. WARREN DAVID SPRINGER

Dr. Springer, chief surgeon at St. Luke's Hospital in Boise from its founding until his death, was considered one of the most eminent physicians and surgeons in the northwest. He was born March 30, 1864 in Nelson, Ontario, Canada, to David Warren and Elizabeth (Ghent) Springer. There were eight sons and six daughters. A brother, Dr. John Springer, also lived in Boise. Dr. Warren graduated from Trinity College, Toronto, in 1889 and the College of Physicians, Ontario, in 1890. He opened an office in Toronto for one year before moving to Ogden, Utah. Soon afterward he moved to Boise to practice with Doctors Fairchild and Springer.

His focus was on surgical work and at the time of his death he was one of the foremost surgeons in Idaho. When the call for volunteers was made in 1898 for service in the Spanish-American War, Dr. Springer went to the Philippines as regimental surgeon with the rank of major.

Dr. Springer was married to Lulu Eymann in Warsaw, Illinois in 1894. The Springers had two sons, Eugene and Warren David, the latter born a month after his father's death.

DR. JOHN SCOTT SPRINGER

John S. Springer, one of fourteen children, was born and raised in Ontario, Canada. He graduated from high school in 1898 and began a career in teaching which lasted for three years. To study medicine and surgery he entered Toronto Medical College, graduating in 1905.

Attracted by the growing west, he made his way to Emmett, Idaho, where he practiced for a year after which he spent eight months in post-graduate work in Chicago. Upon his return, he opened an office in Boise and entered active practice with his elder brother, Dr. Warren D., that lasted until his brother's death in 1909. Dr. John Springer remained alone in the practice and served as surgeon for Idaho and Oregon Railroad and for all the electric inter-urban railway lines entering the city. In addition, he had a large private practice.

In September 1909, Dr. Springer was married to Neva Rice, daughter of one of the pioneer settlers, Frederick G. Rice.

DR. W. DAVID SPRINGER

The third member of the Springer family to practice medicine in Idaho, W. David Springer was the son of Dr. and Mrs. Warren David Springer and nephew of Dr. John Scott Springer. After attending the College of Idaho, he graduated as an honor student from the University of Oregon Medical College in 1936, as an honor student. He completed an internship at Orange County Hospital in Santa Ana, California, and began practice in Boise in 1937 where he remained except for military service. He was a flight surgeon and lieutenant colonel, 1942–46. Dr. Springer served as secretary and treasurer for St. Lukes Hospital staff; secretary and treasurer for Southwest District Medical Society. By presidential appointment in 1949, Dr. Springer was on the Idaho State Board of Appeals for Selective Service.

During his years in practice, Dr. Springer stitched two completely severed noses. One was a middle aged man who drove himself fifty miles for treatment; and, twenty years later he did the same surgery for a seven year old boy. Both operations were successful.

DR. WALTER RAYMOND WEST

Dr. West, brother of Dr. Jabez West, was born in Salt Lake City, Utah, February 7, 1897. Before entering medicine he served a Latter Day Saints mission and taught school.

Dr. West attended the University of Utah from 1919–23; University of Cincinnati, 1923–25; interned at Dee Hospital in Ogden; four two-week courses at Cook County, Chicago. Throughout his life he took numerous short courses to be aware of changes. Dr. West practiced in Rigby from June 1926 to August 1935. He moved to Idaho Falls, and practiced from August 1935 to January 2, 1958.

He was president of the Snake River and Idaho Falls Medical societies; president of the Idaho State Medical Society in 1950; Fellow, International College of Surgeons; member, Board of Trustees of Northwest Medicine.

In the first World War he was in the field artillery, and won the Selective Service Award in the second World War.

Flowers and shrubs (especially French lilacs), golf, Red Cross, and his family were outside interests. The Wests had one son and four daughters.

DR. JABEZ WILLIAM WEST
Jabez West was born in Salt Lake City, January, 20, 1885. His brother Walter R. West was also a physician.

He served an L.D.S. mission, and taught in high school before becoming a doctor. He graduated from the University of Utah in 1915. He went to Western Reserve, Cleveland, Ohio, and interned in Cleveland. Dr. West went to Idaho Falls in 1919 to practice medicine.

He and his wife, June, had two boys and two girls.

DR. JESSE CHARLES WOODWARD
Jesse Woodward, who practiced in Payette, graduated from the University of Colorado in 1900. In 1904 he married Elizabeth Margaret Morgan. October 29, 1910, a son, Jesse Charles Woodward, Jr., was born.

Dr. Woodward was vice-president of the Idaho Medical Society; president of the South Idaho District Medical Society; member of the American Medical Association, the Clinical Congress of Surgeons of North America, and the Ancient and Free Masons. He studied in New York Post-Graduate Medical School and Hospital and Cornell University Medical College.

In 1904 he joined his brother in partnership. Their practice became so large, and the necessity for a hospital so apparent, that within a few years they built a modern private hospital for medical and surgical treatment.

They were the local surgeons for the Oregon Short Line; chief surgeons, Payette Valley Railroad; local surgeons, Mountain States Telephone and Telegraph Company, Idaho-Oregon Light and Power Company; and the Michigan-Idaho Lumber Company. In addition to their hospital building, they owned other real estate and a modern building in which their own offices were located.

DR. IRA R. WOODWARD

Payette claimed as one of its leading citizens Ira Richard Woodward, M.D. He was not only a physician and surgeon, but a leader in civic, social and economic lines. Dr. Woodward practiced with his brother, Dr. J.C. Woodward. Their father, Israel Woodward, was a native of New York, and a contractor and builder. In the late fifties he moved to Colorado, by the overland route. He married Jennie Bell in Illinois in 1863. They had three children, Burton, Jesse Charles, and Ira Richard, born in West DePere, Wisconsin. Israel Woodward died in Denver in 1902 at the age of sixty-nine.

Dr. Woodward received early education in Denver, graduating from East Denver High School, and then entered the University of Denver, where he studied medicine. He graduated in 1897. He began his practice in Mercury, Utah, remaining there for two years. In 1899 he located in Payette. He became the oldest doctor in length of service.

Dr. Woodward was past master of the Ancient Free and Accepted Masons, a Knight Templar, and Noble of the Mystic Shrine. He was a member of the South Idaho District and Idaho State Medical societies; president of the Idaho State Board of Medical Examiners, president of the Payette Valley Building and Loan Association, secretary-treasurer of the Peoples Irrigation Company; and city president.

In Boise, December 4, 1907, he married Anna Josephine Hastings, daughter of Mr. and Mrs. William Hastings. She was a graduate of St. Mark's Hospital Training School of Salt Lake City. They had two children, Jean Elizabeth and Ira Richard Woodward Jr.

DR. C. L. DUTTON

Dr. C.L. Dutton of Meridian was born at Eldorado, Kansas, September 8, 1874, a son of Dr. Sherrod W. and Susie A (Lawrence) Dutton. His father was born and educated in Kentucky. Outbreak of the Civil War found him joining the Confederacy. For three years he served with the rank of major. On the close of hostilities in 1865, Dr. Sherrod Dutton moved to Kansas to practice in Eldorado. Dr. C. L. Dutton was the first of five children. His early education was in Kansas, following which he graduated from South Denver High School. Inheriting his father's inclination to the medical profession, he entered the University of Colorado, receiving his M.D. degree. He started practice at McKracken, Kansas. In two years he decided there was a wider field in the west, and moved to Meridian.

In 1910 he was elected president of the Southern Idaho Medical Society; belonged to American and Idaho State Medical societies, Meridian Blue Lodge No. 47, and Woodmen of the World. In political matters Dr. Dutton was a Democrat.

June 8, 1904, Dr. Dutton was married to Alice A. Ackerman, Grand Junction, Colorado, a graduate of the State University of Colorado, and daughter of J. Harvey and Ella Bell (Brown) Ackerman. Dr. and Mrs. Dutton had one son, Robert Roosevelt, born at Meridian, May 5, 1907.

DR. RUSSELL T. SCOTT

Russell T. Scott came to Idaho with his parents at age twelve. His father was a doctor, and moved from Watertown, Ohio, to Rupert to practice. Russell was born April 18, 1898, and graduated from the University of Idaho in 1921 with a B.S. degree. From 1921-23 he was an assistant in the bacteriology department at the University. In 1928 he was graduated from Northwestern University Medical School. He was a Beta Theta Pi, and a Phi Beta Pi in the medical fraternity.

He interned at Seattle General Hospital, assistant to Dr. A.B. Hepler, urologist, 1930-33, and an urologist on the active staff at St. Joseph's Hospital, Lewiston. In 1951 he was president of the Idaho State Medical Society. Dr. Scott was a member of the American Medical Association;

American Urological Association; Fellow of American College of Surgeons; Diplomate, American Board of Urology.

He was a lieutenant colonel in the Medical Corps, and assistant chief, Surgical Service, 50th General Hospital, 1942–45, and was in the European theater for two years.

Dr. and Mrs. Scott had two daughters and one son.

DR. WILLIAM L. FRAZIER

Dr. William L. Frazier, Boise physician and surgeon, was born on a farm in Randolph County, Missouri, May 4, 1877, son of Dr. Joseph H. and Deniza E. (Epperly) Frazier. The father was born in Virginia and was a physician and farmer. He was graduated from a medical college at Keokuk, Iowa, and practiced for a third of a century in Missouri. Dr. William Frazier was the only member of the family living in Idaho, but one of his four brothers, Dr. Leland Frazier, was a surgeon in the United States Army.

Dr. William was reared on a Missouri farm and his early education was in a country school. He was fourteen years of age when his father died, after which he assumed the responsibility of operating the home farm, until he reached the age of twenty. He assisted in caring for his mother and the younger children of the family. He earned the money to pay for medical college. After reaching twenty, he taught school for three years, and at twenty-four, entered the Missouri Valley College, a Presbyterian institution, where he took a two year academic course.

When twenty-six, he entered the medical department of the Missouri State University at Columbia, and was graduated in 1908 with an M.D. degree at thirty. He practiced medicine at Warren, Texas, from 1908 until 1910, and in the latter year came to Idaho, settling at Mountain Home, where he followed his profession until December, 1917. In 1915, he had taken a post graduate course in surgery under the Mayo Brothers.

Moving from Mountain Home to Boise in 1917, he continued in the general practice of medicine, and was particularly skilled in surgery. He did much research work as to the cause of diabetes, and kept in touch with the latest scientific discoveries and frequently contributed to medical publications. One of his treatises on typhoid fever was published as a book. His chief interest and recreation was in research. On June 23, 1908, Dr. Frazier was married to Mary S. Walsh, of Miami, Missouri, a former teacher. They became parents of three sons, William Lawrence, Jr., Edward Leland, and Virgil Lowry.

Dr. Frazier was a Presbyterian and in early manhood ordained to the ministry. He was a Master Mason and a Knight of Pythias.

DR. LOUIS A. HARRIS

Dr. Louis A. Harris was a popular physician in New Meadows. His father was Aaron Harris, noted physician of Boston, where he died in 1906 at the age of eighty-four. His mother was Jerusha Sherwood, native of Massachusetts, and of English parentage. She died in Boston in the same year as her husband, at the age of eighty-two.

Louis was born in Melrose, Massachusetts, October 25, 1872. He attended public schools and Boston Latin School, then to the School of Pharmacy, from which he graduated in 1894. He entered Harvard University from which he was graduated in literature. He then went to the University of Kansas for his professional work, graduating in 1900.

He began medical practice at Sheridan, Wyoming, and in 1903 came to Idaho, for a time. He went to San Francisco, where he practiced until the earthquake. He returned to Idaho and located in New Meadows. He was in practice there for many years.

Dr. Harris' sole efforts in politics was as president of the Board of Pension Examiners and county coroner. He was a member of the Ancient Free and Accepted Masons, belonging to the Blue Lodge, the Independent Order of Odd Fellows, and of the Knights of Pythias. In professional circles he held membership in all of the medical societies.

Dr. Harris married Fannie T. Levy, of Chicago in 1907. Mrs. Harris was a daughter of Jonas and Theresa Levy. They had no children.

DR. JOSEPH FREMSTAD

The first permanent drug store in southern Idaho's new town of Burley, was the enterprise of Dr. Joseph Fremstad. As druggist, physician, and surgeon, he became a leader in business and his profession.

The doctor's father was also a physician, a graduate of

one of the best schools in Sweden and later of the College of Physicians and Surgeons at Chicago. For many years he practiced in Minneapolis, where he died in 1896. His wife died in Grantsburg, Wisconsin, in 1906, a graduate of the University of Stockholm and a woman of strong character and mentality.

A sister of the doctor was Olive Fremstad, a noted opera singer. In Wagnerian and other heavy roles she sang with the Metropolitan Opera Company of New York for many seasons. She had the distinction of being the originator of the role of Salome when that Strauss opera was given its premier performance in America.

Of the six children, Joseph was the second and the oldest son, born at Fredericksald, Norway, November 5, 1872. At the age of four he came with his parents to America, spending two years in Chicago and then moving to Minneapolis. As a boy he attended Minneapolis schools, and at an early age began earning his own way. When fifteen, he worked at a drug store for one dollar a week. That experience gave him the practical direction for a business career. In 1897, leaving Minneapolis, he went by boat to New Orleans, and a short time later he and his wife embarked on a schooner bound for Tampa. A hurricane drove the boat across the gulf to Yucatan, and it was only after a long and dangerous voyage that he arrived in Tampa.

Though successful as a druggist Mr. Fremstad had for some time thought of studying medicine. In 1901 he entered the College of Physicians and Surgeons at St. Louis, from which he received his M.D. degree in 1906. He paid his way through college. In the clinics and other work he came into association with many of the most eminent men of medicine.

Dr. Fremstad came to Burley in 1907, and established a drug store and medical practice. The doctor owned a fine farm four miles from town. He was married at Minneapolis on January 1, 1893, to Mabel Brusven, daughter of Mr. and Mrs. Abe Brusven. He was a thirty-second degree Mason. Hunting, fishing, and outdoor sports were his favorite recreation. He enjoyed scientific literature, general reading, and music.

DR. FRANCIS EMERSON BOUCHER

Dr. Boucher, physician and surgeon in St. Anthony, was born April 19, 1885, in Marshalltown, Iowa, where his father was a physician for thirty-six years. Dr. Boucher represented the third successive generation to have at least one member in the medical profession. His paternal grandfather was a surgeon on the staff of General Grant throughout the Civil War, and later became first professor of anatomy in the University of Iowa. Both father and grandfather were graduates of Jefferson Medical College, Philadelphia.

Dr. Boucher graduated from high school in 1904 at Marshalltown, and graduated from the medical school at the University of St. Louis in 1909. During his last half year in college he was resident physician of the German Evangelical Deaconess' Hospital of St. Louis. After his graduation he became resident staff physician and assistant surgeon of St. Mary's Hospital for a year. After the death of his mother in Marshalltown in 1910, Dr. Boucher practiced at home with his father. After a year he moved to Utah where he was employed by the Utah Copper Company as surgeon at Bingham Canyon. He remained there until October 1912, when he moved to St. Anthony.

Dr. Boucher was a Republican and a member of Modern Woodmen of America, Mystic Workers, Ancient Order of United Workmen, the Odd Fellows and local examining surgeon for all four. He was a member of Bingham Commercial Club, the Episcopal Church, National Guard of Missouri, and part owner of the Yerington Malachite Mine.

DR. CRISPIN WRIGHT

Dr. Wright came to Fruitland from Virginia, one of four sons who took up professions, three in medicine. Crispin was born July 16, 1882, at Chatham, Virginia, to Mr. and Mrs. Dryden Wright. His father was a Confederate veteran of the Civil War. He was a loyal supporter of the southern cause, and went into the Confederate Army under Captain Henry A. Wise, later a brigadier general. Mr. Wright served in both the infantry and artillery, and during four years at the front was not wounded nor taken prisoner. He was a farmer and planter. Octavia Clement Wright, mother of Dr. Wright, was born in the same Virginia county as her husband and son.

Dr. Wright was next to the youngest of eight children. His early education was in public and private schools, and later at Virginia Military Institute at Lexington. He entered the University College of Medicine, Richmond, for two years and completed two years in the University of Denver, Colorado. In 1910 he received the M.D. degree. Dr. Wright became an intern in St. Luke's Hospital in Denver and in June, 1911, he located at Fruitland.

He was deputy and local health officer of then-Canyon County, and was medical examiner for several life insurance companies. He was licensed to practice in Colorado, Oregon, and Idaho, and was a member of A.K.K. medical fraternity. He was a Democrat and a member of the Methodist Episcopal Church.

One of his brothers, Joseph, was a civil engineer in the U.S. Reclamation Service. Another brother was a physician in Virginia. Dr. F. J. Wright, the third brother, practiced at Fork Union, Virginia. Dr. Wright had three sisters, and another brother who died at the age of eight.

At Colorado Springs, Dr. Wright was married on June 30, 1910, to Emma Lane, daughter of George H. Lane, of Chicago. They had one son, George Dryden, born April 16, 1911.

DR. ALEXANDER AYER HIGGS

In 1919 Dr. Higgs was the only representative of the medical profession in Boise devoted exclusively to surgery. He was born in Owensboro, Kentucky, August 4, 1870, the eldest of the eleven sons of DeWitt G. and Rachel (Baird) Higgs. His father served as a commissioned officer in the Confederate Army.

Five of the brothers lived in Idaho. Two were physicians, Alexander A. and Dr. DeWitt P. Higgs of Gooding. Although his father was not a doctor, he came from a long line of physicians and surgeons in North Carolina. Dr. Higgs went to public schools of Owensboro, and also to a private tutor. He entered Cincinnati Medical College at twenty, and graduated in 1896. He began practice in Kentucky, and in 1898 was appointed to a professorship in a medical college at Atlanta for two years.

In 1901 he came to Idaho and practiced on the Camas prairie for the next eighteen years. In January 1919, he moved to Boise to practice only surgery. He did much postgraduate work in eastern clinics. He was a Fellow of the American Medical Association and a member of the Idaho State Medical Society.

On February 20, 1898, Dr. Higgs married Blanche King, also a native of Kentucky. They became parents of three sons and three daughters.

They belonged to the Roman Catholic Church, and Dr. Higgs was a member of the Knights of Columbus.

DR. JOHN H. SPICKARD

Dr. John H. Spickard of Idaho Falls followed in his father's steps when he became a doctor. His father was in medical research and development in Los Angeles. An uncle was a practicing physician in Seattle.

Dr. Spickard was born March 21, 1929, in Seattle. He went to Santa Monica City College, 1946-48; U.C.L.A. 1948-50, and was graduated with a B.A. degree. In 1957 he received his medical degree from Northwestern University. He interned in Los Angeles County from 1957-58. In 1958-59 he had a residency at Tulare County Hospital and practiced in Torrance from July 1959 to April 1960. He moved to Idaho Falls in 1960. The Spickards have a son and a daughter.

DR. DONALD MERRILL MACK

Born July 10, 1925, Donald Mack attended Columbia Academy before entering Walla Walla College in 1947. He worked his way through college by logging during the summer months and graduated with a B.A. in 1952. He completed his medical degree from Loma Linda University in 1956, and interned at Portland Sanitorium for one year. He began his practice in Boise in 1957.

Dr. Mack was on the active staff at both St. Lukes and St. Alphonsus. He was a member of the Ada County, Idaho State and American Medical associations. Dr. Mack had four cousins in the medical profession.

DR. LEON W. NOWIERSKI

Leon Nowierski had every opportunity to know the pros and cons of medicine before he decided to become a doctor. Both his father and grandfather practiced in Yorktown, Texas, where he was born on January 4, 1921. He received his B.A. and M.D. from the University of

Texas, graduating in 1944. He was a member of Phi Rho Sigma Medical fraternity and Osteon Intermedical fraternity. His internship was at the U.S. Naval Hospital in Acia Heights, Hawaii, from 1944–45 and his residency fellowship at Ochsner Clinic in New Orleans, from 1947–50. He began practice in Boise in 1950 and was on the active staff of St. Lukes and St. Alphonsus hospitals.

DR. FRED O. GRAEBER

Born sons of a minister in Aberdeen, South Dakota, brothers Fred and Mark Graeber became physicians. Fred played high school football and basketball and participated in boxing at the University of Iowa. He studied pre-law at Iowa from 1930–32, received his M.D. from the University of Minnesota in 1937. He completed a one year internship at Kansas City General Hospital and a one year residency at Broadlawn General Hospital in Des Moines, Iowa. He attended Johns Hopkins Medical School and received a Master in Public Health in 1941.

Dr. Graeber spent four years as lieutenant commander in the Navy, two of those in Australia. He practiced in Aberdeen, South Dakota from 1945–47, Eureka from 1947–49; Vale, Oregon, 1949–50, and came to Boise in 1950. Dr. Graeber served as the Director of Health for the State of Idaho.

DR. JOHN HAROLD CROMWELL

Since the time of the first Oliver down to the present day, the name of Cromwell has been associated with the sturdy virtues of that great leader of English Puritanism. Mixture with other blood has softened some of the harsher outlines of the old stock. One of the members who attained the high regard of the community where he lived was Dr. John Harold Cromwell of Gooding.

Dr. Cromwell was born in Pike County, Illinois, on Christmas day, 1876, and his father and grandfather were doctors. Dr. Cromwell grew up in Pike County, attending the Nebo grade and high schools, and graduated from Northern Illinois Normal School. He taught for four years in Pike County. He began the study of medicine in the College of Physicians and Surgeons at St. Louis in 1899, and was graduated in 1903 with an M.D. For the next five years he practiced in Nebo with his father. He located at

Altona, Illinois, for three years. In 1911 he came to Idaho, and settled in Gooding. He owned his own home and considerable real estate, having faith that Gooding had a great future.

Dr. Cromwell was married on November 1, 1904, to Willie E. Barry. Mrs. Cromwell was a graduate of the Illinois State Normal School, and taught for five years at Mackinaw, Illinois. The Cromwells had two sons, Frederick and James.

The doctor was a Mason, member of the Order of Foresters, member of the Knox County Medical Society, Idaho State and American Medical associations.

DR. ERWIN C. SAGE

Even though he left general practice because of the severity of winters in northern Iowa, Dr. Sage continued in the medical field in the Nampa area. Erwin Sage, born January 28, 1896, was the son of a physician. He received a B.A. degree in education from Iowa State Teachers' College, a B.S. and M.D. in 1924 from the University of Iowa, and a M.P.H. from Johns Hopkins Hospital in 1937. He was a member of Sigma Phi Epsilon fraternity. His internship was completed at University of Iowa Hospital in Iowa City.

Dr. Sage served for one and one-half years in World War I and during World War II was at the Naval Hospital in Shoemaker, California. He saw active duty as chief medical officer on an attack transport in the battles of Saipan, Iwo Jima, and Okinawa. Dr. Sage had a general practice in Eagle Grove, Iowa, was director of the health department in Burlington, Iowa, and assistant director of health for the city of San Francisco for twelve years.

Dr. and Mrs. Sage had two sons, one a doctor and the other with a Master's degree in hospital administration.

DR. JOHN B. COOPER

Dr. John B. Cooper was the oldest practitioner in Blackfoot, where he had followed his profession since 1895, and one of the leading physicians of Bingham County.

He was born near New Castle, England, on March 24, 1839, a son of Thomas and Ann (Bell) Cooper. His father was a successful boat builder at Blythe, England. Dr. John was the oldest of five boys and three girls. He studied in private schools in England until he was sixteen. At nineteen he entered the Medical College at Newcastle-upon-Tyne, from which he was graduated in 1860, with a degree of Doctor of Medicine.

For twelve years after his graduation, the doctor practiced in Pennsylvania, then moved to Virginia for three years. He moved west, and for eight years practiced in Weir City, Kansas, then moved to Ogden, Utah, for a brief time before moving to American Fork, where he practiced for eight years.

The new state of Idaho attracted him, and in August 1896 he established his home at Rexburg, later moved to Pocatello, and in February 1897, he located in Blackfoot.

May 3, 1877 he married Elizabeth Mary Richards of Hazelton, Pennsylvania. She was born in Cornwall, England, on January 11, 1839, the daughter of William and Phyllis Richards. Dr. and Mrs. Cooper had two children, the youngest, Dr. George Cooper.

DR. GEORGE H. COOPER

One of the most progressive physicians and surgeons in eastern Idaho was Dr. G.H. Cooper, son of Dr. and Mrs. John Bell Cooper of Blackfoot. He was born August 22, 1880, the younger of two children, at Meyersdale, Pennsylvania.

He attended schools in Blackfoot and Pocatello. He enrolled at Central Medical College at St. Joseph, Missouri, where, in 1905, he was graduated with honors, receiving his Doctor of Medicine degree. Returning to Idaho, Dr. Cooper established himself for his initial practice at American Falls. He remained there for one year, during which he was married. His next location was McCammon, where he settled in 1906.

In November, 1912, Dr. Cooper conceived the idea of establishing a private general hospital at McCammon. He leased large apartments over the McCammon Investment Company's store, and installed modern medical appliances. So great was his success in this hospital that he built a hospital of his own. The institution received, among other patients, all the cases of which he had charge for the Oregon Short Line Railway. He was physician for Bannock County. He belonged to the Elks Lodge, was a Republican and member of the Episcopal Church.

Mrs. Cooper was Ilene Cottrel of American Falls. She was a daughter of Samuel and Harriet (Lish) Cottrel. They were married February 17, 1906. The Coopers had two children, Caroline and John.

DR. ROBERT FRAZIER

Dr. Frazier was born August 31, 1915. His father was a tailor. There were two other Drs. Frazier in Idaho. Dr. William Lawrence Frazier began practicing in Boise in 1911. He passed away at age eighty-four. Dr. Leland Frazier practiced in Rupert, and died in the 1930s.

Robert lived and attended school in Pocatello, and in 1937 was graduated with a degree in pharmacy from the University of Idaho, Southern branch. In 1938 he managed a drug store in Evanston, Wyoming until 1947. He went to Utah Medical School and was graduated in 1950. From 1950–51 he interned at St. Mark's Hospital in Salt Lake City.

He moved to Boise in July 1951 and was on the staffs of St. Alphonsus, St. Lukes, and Booth Memorial.

His wife, Vera Redfield Frazier, was born and raised in Idaho. They were married in 1937 and had two boys and a girl. After her death, he married Loyce Young Mixon in 1973.

DR. THOMAS E. MANGUM, SR.

Dr. Thomas Mangum was born August 11, 1884, in Voca, Texas. Two of his sons are doctors, Dr. T. E. Mangum, Jr. and Dr. J. Robert Mangum, located in Nampa.

He was graduated from the University of Texas in 1910 with his medical degree. In 1919 he received his O.B. degree from Northwest Nazarene College. He interned at St. Mary's Infirmary, Galveston, Texas 1910–11. From 1911–16 he practiced in Ballinger, Texas; 1916–18 Hamlin, Texas, and moved to Nampa in 1918.

In 1913, in Ballinger, Texas, he did bone surgery in a home because the hospital refused a colored patient.

In 1919 he founded the Samaritan Hospital and in 1922 the Samaritan Hospital School of Nursing, both in Nampa. He was physician for Canyon County several times.

He was an ordained minister in the Church of the Nazarene. He raised Tennessee Walking horses and was an accomplished rider. He enjoyed fishing, golfing, and family.

Dr. and Mrs Mangum had six children, three daughters and three sons.

He had a fellowship in the American College of Surgeons, and was a member of F.I.C.S.

DR. JOHN ROBERT MANGUM

Dr. John Mangum was born in Ballinger, Texas, November 5, 1913. His brother and his father were physicians who practiced in Nampa.

He attended grade and high schools associated with Northwest Nazarene College. In high school he was active in music, forensic and athletics. From 1930–32 he went to Northwest Nazarene College; 1930–31 summer school at the College of Idaho, and University of Idaho 1932–34. Granted a B.S. in pre-med in 1937 following the first two years of medical school, he went to Washington University School of Medicine, St. Louis, Missouri from 1934–38, where he got his M.D. He had a rotating internship at St. Louis County Hospital, from 1938–39; in 1939–40, assistant residency in surgery at St. Louis County Hospital; 1949–50 Basic Sciences in Surgery, Washington University School of Medicine.

He moved to Nampa in 1940 and practiced until 1942. He was in the Army Medical Corps from 1942–46, being associated with the Air Force as a flight surgeon from 1943 until discharged in 1946. He then returned to Nampa.

He encountered unusual epidemics associated with extreme food poisoning twice while in the service. On one occasion lye was used in pancake batter, causing extreme toxic gastro-intestinal reactions in the entire bomb squadron.

He was chief of staff as well as chief of surgery at Samaritan Community Hospital on two occasions. The Mangums had two boys and two girls.

DR. HARRY L. WILLSON

Dr. Harry l. Willson, physician and surgeon of Idaho Falls, was born at Clarksville, Virginia, October 25, 1889, to Dr. Thomas C. and Adelaide (Shangle) Willson. The father was a physician, who practiced in Virginia, Pennsylvania, and Missouri, before moving to Idaho Falls about 1890.

Dr. Willson was reared and educated in Idaho Falls. He became a student at Whitman College in Walla Walla, graduating in 1910. He received his M.D. from the University of Pennsylvania in 1914. He practiced in the University Hospital until March 1917, when he returned to Idaho Falls and opened an office.

The Willsons belonged to the Methodist Episcopal Church, and he was a member of the Elks.

DR. JUDSON BENTON MORRIS

Judson Morris was born in Fort Atkinson, Wisconsin, where his father was a physician. He went to grade and high school in Fort Atkinson, and graduated in 1928. From 1928-30 he attended Lawrence College, Appleton, Wisconsin, received his A.B. degree from University of Michigan, Ann Arbor in 1932. He was graduated from the University of Michigan Medical School, 1936, with an M.D. In 1940 he received a degree in radiology from University of Pennsylvania Graduate School.

From 1937-41 he practiced in Hammond, Indiana. He was in the U.S.N.R. from 1942-46. The doctor moved to Boise in 1946, and was on the staff at St. Alphonsus Hospital (radiologist).

The Morrises had two boys and two girls.

DR. HENRY RAY HATCH

Dr. Henry Ray Hatch, the son of a lawyer, was born on April 20, 1886 in Ashley, Utah. His own four sons, Steven, John, Harvey, and Joe, became doctors. His life before becoming a doctor included working with livestock, prospect mining, hunting, and fishing. An injury (fractured femur) started the idea of becoming a doctor.

He earned his B.A. at the University of Utah and completed two years of medical school by 1908. He attended Rush Medical College to obtain his M.D. in August of 1910. At Brigham Young University he earned an M.A. in 1923, and did postgraduate study in Europe until 1926. He became a Fellow, American College of Surgeons, in 1929, and served as a governor of the College for Idaho in 1950. He served two terms as president of the Idaho Medical Society.

He began practicing in Heber, Utah in 1910 and stayed until 1919 with a brief interruption to serve in the U.S. Army Medical Corps as a first lieutenant in 1918. He began his practice in 1920 in Idaho Falls. He did a number of major operations in private homes while in Heber, and major surgery in Shelley in the 1920s until the L.D.S. Hospital opened in Idaho Falls in 1923.

He used several forms of transportation including horseback, buggies, carts, and cutters. In 1912 he had the only automobile in the county, but for summer use only. Winters were impossible for anything but sleighs. He was a physician during the deadly Spanish Influenza Epidemic in 1918-19 that filled the cemeteries of the nation. The harsh weather required the use of fur coats, caps, gloves, muffler, and mittens during below zero temperatures.

While practicing in Heber he took surgical patients to the old General Hospital and to the L.D.S. and Holy Cross hospitals in Salt Lake City and later to the General Hospital and Spencer Hospital in Idaho Falls. He was attending surgeon and member of the Board of Trustees of the L.D.S. Hospital and president of staff two terms. He was a member of the original building committee. He and Mrs. Hatch had five sons, four becoming doctors and one an Agricultural Attache to the U.S. Embassy in Ireland.

DR. CHARLES STEVEN HATCH
One of the sons of Dr. Henry Ray Hatch, Charles, was born March 30, 1919, while his father was a physician in Utah. He moved to Idaho Falls with his family at the age of one and continued to live there throughout his school years. He then filled his mission for the L.D.S. Church in France, Belgium, and Switzerland. He took summer courses at Ricks College, Brigham Young University, and Utah State College as well as the University of Paris. He graduated from the University of Utah with a B.A. and attended the University of Utah Medical School for one year. He then went to Johns Hopkins Medical School for the last three years to earn his M.D. He was a member of several medical fraternities and served as the bishop of the Baltimore Ward, L.D.S. Church during his medical school and residency. His internship was at Johns Hopkins Hospital in surgery, Church Home Hospital as assistant resident and resident in surgery in Baltimore. He completed his residency in surgery at the Salt Lake General Hospital from 1956-59.

He began practicing in Idaho Falls at the Hatch Clinic in

1949 and narrowed his specialty to urology in 1962 when he went to U.C.L.A. Harbor Hospital for further study and in 1962 to Palos Verdes, California to study. He returned to Idaho Falls to continue as a member of the Hatch Clinic.

He performed a number of firsts in surgical procedures in the Idaho Falls area. He did the first esophagectomy, first aortic embolectomy, first radical total cystectomy, first Whipple Operation (pancreatectomy), first successful open chest cardiac massage. He served as the chief of surgery, infection and record committees. Dr. Hatch was active in numerous professional civic and church organizations and family activities. He and Mrs. Hatch had five girls and three boys.

DR. HARVEY ALLAN HATCH

Dr. Harvey Hatch was born in Heber, Utah, October 5, 1914, to Dr. and Mrs. Henry Ray Hatch. He not only had four brothers and a father but also an aunt, Dr. Lorene Miles, and uncle, Dr. Leonard Southerland, and four cousins who were doctors. He lived in Idaho Falls from 1919, except for a brief period while on mission for the L.D.S. Church in Germany, and in 1943–46 while in the Army as a captain and flight surgeon in Scotland, England, and Germany. He was educated at Brigham Young University during summer sessions and graduated from the University of Utah in 1936 with a B.A. He went to Johns Hopkins at Baltimore from 1937 until 1940. He also obtained an L.L.B. degree through correspondence, an extension of School of Law, during his Army years. His internship and residency were at the University hospitals in Minneapolis from 1940–42 and postgraduate work at the University of Utah Medical School from 1946–47. He practiced in Idaho Falls from 1942–43 before entering the Army and then returned in 1947 to stay.

He rode often during winter months with Dr. Joe Hatch and Dr. Milt Rees and remembers the snow being so high on the Ammon Road that patients had to be brought by sled to the hospital. He faced considerable opposition by other doctors when he began getting his OB patients up after delivery without the two weeks in bed others were requiring.

He held the chief of staff position at the L.D.S. Hospital

in Idaho Falls and was certified by the Board of Internal Medicine in 1949, the Board of Pediatrics in 1947, and became a fellow of the American College of Physicians in 1959. He enjoys reading, hunting, fishing, astronomy, skiing, and swimming. He and his wife had two boys and four girls (one set of twins, a boy and girl).

DR. PRESTON MERRILL PACKER

Dr. Packer went to Ricks College, and to the University of Utah, where he received a B.A. degree in 1943. In 1946 he got his M.D. degree at the University of Utah Medical School. From 1947–48 he interned at Norfolk General Hospital. He started practicing in Blackfoot on New Year's Day in 1948.

During the snow problems of the 1949 winter, he made house visits by various means: airplane landing at the side of the house in a pasture; by horse; and by people meeting him at the highway with their horse-drawn sleighs. He was on the staff at L.D.S. Hospital, Idaho Falls, and chief of staff several times at Bingham Memorial Hospital.

For twenty-seven months he was in the A.S.T.P. program, and twenty-four months as a captain in the Air Force Medical Corps with a flight surgeon rating. The Packers had four boys and three girls.

DR. C. DEAN PACKER

Dr. Packer had two brothers, P. Merrill of Blackfoot and Alden M. of Idaho Falls, who were also doctors. He was born March 11, 1916 at Salt Lake City and raised in Rexburg through grade, high and two years of college at Ricks. He spent two years at the University of Utah and then entered the medical school there. He was active in acting and operatic singing in both high school and college and won the All-Around Athletic Award at Ricks for football, basketball, and tennis.

He worked his way through college with an athletic scholarship helping him through medical school. He received his B.S. in 1939 at the University of Utah and his M.D. in 1942 from the University of Colorado Medical School. He interned at Swedish Hospital in Seattle, 1942–43, and was in the Army 1943–46, discharged as a captain. His residency was at Swedish Hospital, Firland Thoracic Hospital and King County Hospital, 1946–49.

In 1950, he went to Blackfoot to open his practice and was chief of staff several times at the hospital; thoracic and general surgical consultant to the Idaho Tuberculosis Hospital at Gooding; original president of Idaho Thoracic Society, the medical arm of the State Tuberculosis Association.

He is active in the L.D.S. Church and has served in the presidency of the Blackfoot Stake. He enjoyed athletics and farming. He raised Black Angus cattle.

Dr. and Mrs. Packer had two daughters, Michaelene and Deanne; and four sons, Allan, Richard, Kelly, and Norris.

DR. ALDEN M. PACKER

Two brother doctors of Dr. Alden Packer are C. Dean and P. Merrill, both of Blackfoot. Alden was born at Rexburg, March 2, 1929 and attended schools there while he worked for his father on a dry farm during the summers. He attended Ricks College four quarters; married in 1948; filled an L.D.S. mission for two years; finished a pre-med course at the University of Utah and studied medicine there.

Dr. Packer's internship and residency were at Harbor General Hospital in Torrance, California, through July 1957, and he spent three years as a captain in the Air Force at Cambridge, England. When he returned to the United States in 1960, he opened a medical practice in Idaho Falls. He has held staff appointments at the Idaho Falls and Sacred Heart hospitals. He and Mrs. Packer have three girls and two boys.

DR. MILTON THOMAS REES

A father, two uncles and seven cousins who were medical doctors couldn't help but influence Milton Thomas Rees to study medicine. He was born to Dr. and Mrs. Thomas David Rees in Salt Lake City on April 1, 1910. He was raised in Nephi, Utah, where he attended grade school. He attended high school and the University of Utah in Salt Lake, and drove bus for the Union Pacific during the summer to help pay for his education. From 1931 until 1934, he filled an L.D.S. mission in Germany.

Dr. Rees attended the University of Utah from 1928–31 and again from 1936–38 for the last year of pre-med and two years of medicine. He transferred to the University of

Colorado Medical School where he was graduated with an A.B. and M.D. He belonged to Sigma Pi and Phi Beta Phi. While he was interning, sulfa drugs were introduced to the medical profession. His internship was at Colorado General Hospital in Denver, 1940–41. He started practice in September 1941 in Idaho Falls.

He had several firsts to enjoy, including the first four-wheel drive army surplus vehicle to make house calls in winter and the first Volkswagon in Idaho. He gave the first sodium pentothal anesthetic in Idaho and assisted the first commissurotomy (heart) operation in the state. He held many positions in local, state, and national medical organizations and enjoyed river running and exploring. Dr. and Mrs. Rees have two daughters and two sons.

His father, Dr. Thomas David Rees, was born September 11, 1877, and died November 3, 1952. Funeral services were at the North Idaho Falls Stake Tabernacle and honorary pallbearers were the forty-six doctor members of the Idaho Falls Medical Association, with whom he had practiced many years.

DR. ROBERT SYDNEY SMITH

Boise's well known Dr. Robert S. Smith was born September 19, 1906, the second of five sons of a physician and his wife in East St. Louis, Illinois. Two brothers who also became physicians are Harvey S. and Carl W. Smith. Robert was editor of his high school paper, won prizes in oratory, and was valedictorian and president of the senior class. High scholastic records won for him a full tuition scholarship to Washington University, St. Louis. He worked during the summers in Yellowstone Park.

He earned a B.A. at Washington University in 1927, and attended the School of Medicine until 1930, when he won a Rhodes Scholarship to Christ Church College, Oxford University, England, 1930–32; bachelor of science in bacteriology in 1932; and his M.D. granted *summa cum laude* at Washington University School of Medicine in 1933. He belonged to Pi Kappa Alpha, Nu Sigma Nu, Phi Beta Kappa, Sigma Xi, Alpha Omega Alpha. He was a member of the championship LaCrosse team at Oxford, and became first lieutenant in the Army Medical Reserve Corps upon graduation in 1933.

Dr. Smith did his internship and residency in surgical service at Barnes Hospital, Washington University School of Medicine, 1933–36. In Boise he became associated with Dr. Ralph Falk, member of the pioneer Falk family, until Dr. Falk's retirement in 1941. He practiced at Boise from June 14, 1936, with the exception of three years when on active World War II duty in the Army Medical Corps, until he suffered a severe stroke in 1971. His practice was taken over by Dr. Dean Sorenson and Dr. John Lung.

Dr. Smith was the first Idaho surgeon to become a Diplomate of the American Board of Surgery by examination. He was chief of staff at St. Lukes Hospital in 1958, and chief of surgery several years; on the staff at St. Alphonsus and Veterans hospitals, and surgical consultant at the latter, as well as to the Crippled Children's Bureau of Idaho.

In 1933 at St. Louis, Missouri, Dr. Smith and a medical secretary of the Department of Medicine, Washington University, Helen Ona Kempster, were married. They have three children: Robert S. Jr., Kathleen Anne, and Michael Ernest.

Dr. Smith has made emergency flights in light planes to Council and Twin Falls. From Twin Falls he flew a critically injured patient back to Boise and recovery. During a raging blizzard in January 1949, the Smiths were snowed in at Sun Valley and forced to telephone cancellation of surgery for two or three days. The trains were snowbound in Wyoming.

The doctor remembered an anecdote from an early hospital experience: "I was assisting Dr. Ernest Sachs, world-famous neurosurgeon, also famous for his temperament, during that particular operation a 'bleeder' was giving difficulty. A fuming Dr. Sachs said, 'Dr. Smith! If you don't help me stop this bleeding the patient will die!' From under the sterile drapes weakly came the voice of the locally-anesthetized patient: 'Dr. Smith *please* help Dr. Sachs!'" The patient survived.

DR. JOSEPH E. BALDECK

Dr. Joseph Baldeck of Lewiston has one brother, Eugene, and a son, Eugene M., who are both physicians. Dr. Baldeck was born and reared in Lewiston, attended St.

Stanislaus grade and Lewiston high schools. His pre-med study was at Gonzaga University in Spokane and he earned his Medical Doctor degree at Creighton University. He is a member of Phi Chi medical fraternity.

His internship was at the U.S. Marine Hospital and residency at St. Francis Hospital in Grand Island, Nebraska. He was captain and flight surgeon in the Air Force during World War II. Dr. Baldeck has served as hospital chief of staff and on all committees; as president of the North Idaho District Medical Society and two-term member of the Idaho Board of Medical Examiners.

In addition to the doctor son, Dr. and Mrs. Baldeck have a daughter, Joan Elizabeth, who married dentist John Lynn Hogan.

DR. HOYT B. WOOLLEY

Dr. Woolley was born May 7, 1903 in Pocatello. His father, brother, three uncles, and four cousins were doctors. His father practiced in Pocatello.

He was graduated from Pocatello High School in 1920, and Northwestern University Dental School in 1925. For four and a half years he practiced dentistry in Salt Lake City and Pocatello. In 1934 he received his M.D. degree from Northwestern University Medical School. From 1932–34 he interned at Illinois Masonic Hospital.

In 1934 he moved to Idaho Falls. He was on the staff at L.D.S. Hospital, and belonged to the Idaho Falls, Idaho State, and American Medical associations.

The Woolleys had a son and a daughter.

DR. HIRAM S. WOOLLEY, JR.

Dr. Woolley was born August 6, 1874 in the Hawaiian Islands, the eldest of eight children. His father was in business there. When he was a baby the family moved to Paris, Idaho, where he grew up. He went through high school in Paris and Fielding Academy in the same town. He was graduated from the University of Utah in 1893. As a boy he followed ranching and stock work, and in this way paid his way through school.

He went to Pocatello in 1896, and for seven years was in the Internal Revenue Service. He then went to the Northwestern University Medical School, Chicago, and was graduated in 1909. He interned at St. Mark's Hospital, Salt

Lake City. In 1910 he started his practice in Pocatello. He was physician of Bannock County; member of the Bannock County, Southern Idaho, and American Medical associations. His fraternal associations were Elks, Eagles, Modern Woodmen of America, and Woodmen of the World. He was a Republican and a member of the Latter Day Saints Church.

On June 21, 1896 he married Mary Budge, daughter of Mr. and Mrs. William Budge of Bear Lake. They had two sons and a daughter.

DR. ELWOOD T. REES

Dr. Rees was born August 7, 1907, at Scipio, Utah. His father, Nephi J. Rees, was a doctor in Nephi and Salt Lake City. His three brothers, G.S. Rees, Gunnison, Utah; David S. Rees, Provo, Utah; Robert L. Rees, Salt Lake City, were also doctors. His son, Jerome R. Rees, became a doctor.

He went to school through high school in Nephi, and in 1928 was graduated from the University of Utah, with a B.A. degree. From 1927-28 he attended the University of Utah Medical School, and the University of Pennsylvania Medical School from 1929-31. He interned at Northeastern Hospital, Philadelphia 1930-31, and Highland Hospital, Oakland, California, 1931-32.

The doctor practiced in Rains, Utah, 1932-34; Jerome, Idaho 1934-37. He did postgraduate in surgery, Cook County Hospital, Chicago in 1937. In 1939 he moved to Twin Falls. He was on the executive staff, Magic Valley Memorial Hospital; chief of staff, Valley Memorial Hospital, 1953, and was one of the founders of the Twin Falls Clinic in 1947. In 1942 he enlisted in the U.S. Navy Reserve, and was on active duty 1942-46 in the South Pacific, holding the rank of lieutenant commander M.C.

In 1932 he and Thelma Frances Jensen were married in Salt Lake City. They had three sons and a daughter.

DR. RICHARD DeWEESE SIMONTON

Dr. Simonton was born March 19, 1905, Wamego, Kansas. His father was a physician in Wamego, and later in Wendell, Idaho. His brother was a physician with Mayo Clinic, Rochester, New York.

He went through high school in Wendell. In 1927 he received his B.S. degree from the University of Oregon, and his M.D. from the University of Oregon Medical School in 1930. In 1935 he did postgraduate work at Mayo Clinic in surgery, and at John Hopkins University Medical School from 1936–37.

From 1931–33, Dr. Simonton practiced in Twin Falls with Dr. D. L. Alexander, and with Dr. Ralph Falk, Boise, 1933–35. In 1937 he began private practice in Boise. He was on the staff at St. Luke's Hospital. He belonged to the American Medical Association, and was a charter member of the Boise Valley Chapter of American College of Surgery.

The Simontons had one daughter.

DR. HYRUM J. HARTVIGSEN

So dedicated was Hyrum Hartvigsen to his studies, and so quiet about what he was planning to become, it was just before he entered Columbia University to study medicine, that a neighbor asked his father, "When is that boy going to get his education and start teaching school?"

Dr. Hartvigsen's medical successes as a rural doctor helps us to realize what miracles the early-day doctors accomplished with almost primitive equipment and surroundings. He was named Hyrum for the place in Utah where he was born March 20, 1885. The son of an immigrant father from Norway, who had a sawmill at Hyrum before homesteading near Downey, Idaho, young Hyrum received his schooling in a one-room schoolhouse, where he "became inspired," as he wrote, "to be a doctor." Still on the homestead, he studied correspondence courses that enabled him to pass entrance exams for college.

After two years at Utah State Agricultural College, he received his bachelor of science degree, and moved on to the University of Utah for two years of medicine. He was granted his doctor of medicine degree from the College of Physicians and Surgeons, Columbia University, New York, in 1916. Internship was not required as extensively as later, but the students trained at City Hospital, where he had the unusual experience of traveling by ferry to Blackwell or Welfare Island, where he helped treat "whole wards of blue babies, as well as a colony of lepers."

His first practice was at McCammon, Idaho, from 1917 to 1920, when he moved to Downey from 1920–34. He opened an office in Pocatello in 1934, remaining for the rest of his life. During his early practice there were no lab facilities available and diagnosis was strictly dependent upon his clinical judgement and experience. One winter he sutured a young girl who had her face slashed through her nose and ear in a sleigh-riding accident. Dr. Hartvigsen could not keep the happiness from his voice, when he said, "She grew to a beautiful woman with no disfigurement." He performed an operation in a Japanese home, where no one spoke English, on a man whose testicle had been torn out and was hanging by a cord. The operation was so successful that the man recovered and produced children.

He traveled by Model T as far as the road went, then by horseback to isolated homes to deliver babies or for emergency care. As a railroad doctor, he delivered a baby on a train, between stations. He experienced two epidemics in Marsh Valley, one for smallpox in 1920, when he vaccinated nearly 100 percent of the residents. About 1925–26, there was an outbreak of pneumonia when, after the first two patients treated, he decided to use numoquine (optochin base), and the following forty-two patients recovered. The first two, who did not receive the numoquine, died. The doctor told others about it, and they began its use.

Dr. and Mrs. Hartvigsen had three sons, of whom Dean, became a doctor; and Boyd a dentist; one daughter, Lila, married Keith Pearson, who became a Salt Lake doctor. Son, Vaughn, became an outstanding musician and accountant for Idaho Highway Department. Dr. Hartvigsen was a member (president) of the Pocatello, Southeast Idaho, Idaho State, and American Medical associations.

DR. HAZEN B. DAINES

Dr. Daines was born in Hyde Park, Utah, February 14, 1899. His father was a farmer, and two of his relatives were Utah doctors, Clyde J. Daines (Logan), and Orson Daines (Ogden). In 1926 he received a B.S. degree from the University of Utah, and M.D. degree from Columbia University College of Physicians and Surgeons, 1929.

He interned at the Thomas D. Dee Memorial Hospital, Ogden for one year, and had a two year residency at Newark Eye and Ear Infirmary Newark, New Jersey. From

1930 to 1939 he practiced in Preston, Idaho, and moved to Nampa in 1946. He spent four years in the Army during WWII as a lieutenant colonel.

Often during the deep snows of winter, his patients would meet him with one or two horses hitched to a log, he would balance on the log over the snow and drifts. He was on the staff at Preston Memorial Hospital, Mercy Hospital, and Samaritan Hospital, Nampa.

The Daines had two daughters.

DR. JACOB E. WYATT JR.

Jacob E. Wyatt Jr., who practiced medicine in Weiser from 1951-53; Pocatello, 1954-58; and became medical director of the City-County Health Unit in Boise in 1958, was born November 6, 1919 in Kansas City, Missouri. His brother, William M., became a doctor in pathology and practiced in Macon, Georgia.

Jacob received his B.S. degree in chemical engineering at the University of Kansas in 1940; worked for the explosives division of the Hercules Powder Company, in Delaware and New Jersey; was with the submarine service, U.S. Navy, at Radford, Virginia, 1943-46. His medical degree was granted by Creighton Medical School in 1950; and his master of public health from the University of California, Berkeley in 1954. He was named Diplomate of the American Board of Preventive Medicine in public health in 1960.

Dr. Wyatt married Margaret Ann Miller of Billings, Montana in 1949, and they had two boys and one girl.

In Boise, he became medical director of School Health Services, and later, administrative director of the Ada County Health Center. He worked to help handle a syphilis epidemic on the Fort Hall Indian Reservation from 1954-56. When the defective Cutter vaccine resulted in an epidemic of poliomyelitis in 1955, Dr. Wyatt aided in organizing polio clinics.

He was president of the staff at Weiser Memorial Hospital in 1953, and practiced at Bannock Memorial Hospital in Pocatello. He belonged to the Southeastern Idaho Medical Society, was alternate delegate to Idaho Medical Association, president of the Idaho Public Health Association, and chairman of the Idaho Conference of District Health Department directors.

DR. JOHN OLIVER MELLOR

Born July 17, 1881 in Fayette, Utah, John Mellor helped with the family livestock operations while a boy. He attended Brigham Young University at Provo, getting his bachelor's degree in 1903. The next month he was called to a mission by the Church of Jesus Christ of Latter-Day Saints and spent the next two and one-half years in Great Britain. He married Effie Barney Howe on September 5, 1906, and they went to Philadelphia, where he attended Jefferson Medical College. He received his doctor of medicine degree in 1910.

Dr. Mellor interned at the out-patient department of Jefferson and took a six-months postgraduate course at New York Post Graduate Medical College and Hospital. He spent two months at the clinic of Dr. Andrews, then a noted specialist in Chicago. He started practice in Idaho Falls in 1910, a practice which went well beyond fifty years.

He set up "The People's Hospital" of thirteen beds in 1918, and maintained it with two graduate nurses and student nurses. He and Dr. David L. McDonald operated the hospital until 1923, when the L.D.S. Hospital was opened. For many years, Dr. Mellor drove a team and carriage in the summer and a cutter in the winter. He was kept unusually busy during the 1918–19 influenza epidemic and at other times during epidemics of smallpox, typhoid, diphtheria, and scarlet fever.

Dr. and Mrs. Mellor had two sons, both of whom became doctors. Wendell John was born in Philadelphia on June 24, 1907, while his father was studying medicine, and after graduating from the University of Utah he entered Jefferson Medical College in 1936. His M.D. degree was received in 1940, and he practiced in Hollywood, California.

Joel Kimball Mellor was born December 5, 1926, in Idaho Falls and attended schools there. In September 1944, he enrolled at the University of Idaho, and during that winter entered the U.S. Navy, where he was assigned to the Medical Corps. During the following two and one-half years, he received much practical medical experience. Released from the Navy, he spent three years at U.C.L.A. in medical preparatory courses, before being called on a mission to the Netherlands by the L.D.S. Church. Upon return he entered Brigham Young University and graduated with a B.A. degree. He was graduated from the University of Washington with the degree of doctor of dental science in 1958. He married Mary Lou, the daughter of William and Beulah Hatch of Idaho Falls, and they moved to Spokane to practice. They became the parents of two boys and two girls.

DR. DALE BURNETT PATTERSON

Born December 19, 1916 in Arthur, Iowa, Dale Patterson moved with his parents to Idaho at age two. His early years were spent at Mackay and then Idaho Falls, where he attended high school. He attended the Southern Branch, University of Idaho, Pocatello, from 1934–37; the University of Utah, 1937–39; and received his medical degree from Louisiana State Medical School in 1942. He followed the footsteps of three doctor uncles, James and Beam Patterson and Frank Richards. The latter practiced at Mackay.

His internship was at the U.S. Naval Hospital in San Diego in 1942–43 and he served from then until 1947 in the Navy, when he was discharged with the rank of lieutenant. He had served aboard the U.S.S. Gallatin in the Pacific. Dr. Patterson died in 1955, at the age of thirty-nine, but accomplished much in the few years that he had left to him.

He and Mrs. Patterson had two boys and a girl. They lived at Cascade from 1947 until 1954, and he established the Valley County Hospital there. He made numerous trips into the back country to attend patients, using planes, horseback and snowshoes. He belonged to the Idaho and American Medical associations and the American Association of General Practitioners. He practiced in Boise for one year before his death.

DR. HAMILTON HILL GREENWOOD

Dr. Greenwood was born May 29, 1904 in Candler, North Carolina. His father was a physician in Waynesville, North Carolina, and one of his sons, William H., practices in Grangeville.

He went to grade school in Waynesville and high school in Mansfield, Washington. He was graduated with honors in pre-med, from Washington State College, Pullman. He received his M.D. from Rush Medical College in 1931. From

1931–32 he had a teaching fellowship. He interned for eighteen months at Presbyterian Hospital, Chicago. He moved to Coeur d'Alene in 1933, and practiced until his death.

He and his wife Mary had two sons.

DR. WILLIAM HAMILTON GREENWOOD

Dr. Greenwood was born March 28, 1932, in Chicago. His father was a physician, and the family moved to Coeur d'Alene when William was two. He lived there until he was nineteen. He attended North Idaho Junior College from September 1950 to June 1951. From September 1951 to June 1953 he attended Washington State College and in 1954 received a B.S. in zoology. He was graduated from the Chicago Medical School in October 1957, with his M.D. For one year he interned at Blodgett Memorial Hospital in Grand Rapids.

From January 1959 to December 1960 he was a captain in the U.S.A.F., spending most of that time in Japan. While in Japan he practiced at the 600th U.S.A.F. Dispensary, Tokyo, and the U.S.A.F. Hospital, Tachikawa, Japan. He practiced at State Hospital South, Blackfoot, April 1961–October 1961. He then moved and set up his practice in Grangeville.

The Greenwoods have one daughter.

DR. LOWELL B. PRIVETT

Dr. Privett was born December 3, 1900 in Woonsocket, South Dakota, and died in Boise, Idaho, June 13, 1960. He was the son of Mr. and Mrs. John Privett and received his early schooling in Woonsocket and Mitchell, South Dakota. His medical degree was granted from Creighton in Omaha, Nebraska in 1929. He took a basic course in ophthalmology at Washington University in St. Louis, Missouri, 1945–46. His internship was at Creighton Hospital in Omaha.

Dr. Privett married Agnes Marie Folda on July 3, 1930 in Howells, Nebraska, and they had two daughters and two sons: Geraldine Marie, John Rupert, who became a doctor; Robert Michael and Margaret Ann.

From 1930 until 1936, Dr. Privett maintained an office and hospital at Geddes, South Dakota, and then entered the Civilian Conservation Corps, practicing at Bend, Oregon, and McCall, Idaho for a year each. He started general practice in Boise in 1938 and remained until World

War II began. He was a major in the Army Medical Corps and commanding officer of the 45th Station Hospital. Dr. Privett was chief of the E.E.N.T. Service at the 220th General Hospital in Fort Smith, Northwest Territory, in Canada until 1945.

He returned to Boise and an ophthalmology practice from 1947 until his death in 1960. He was active in and president of the Southwest Idaho Medical Association and member of the American Medical Association.

DR. JOHN W. SMITH

Uncles, cousins, and three brothers as doctors convinced John Smith that he should join the group. He was born December 15, 1917 in Lincoln, Nebraska. From 1939 through 1945 he attended Atlantic Union College, where he was president of Phi Delta Chi; University of Southern California; and La Sierra College. From 1946 to 1950 he was at Loma Linda University, from which he received his medical degree. His internship was at Los Angeles County General Hospital, 1950–51. He practiced from July 1951 until January 1952 at Ukiah, California, and for the following ten years in Sandpoint.

From 1945 until 1946, he was a laboratory technician with the Army Medical Corps. He became president of the Bonner-Boundary District Medical Society and president of the Sandpoint Chapter of the American Red Cross for several years. Dr. Smith owned and operated the sixty-four bed Sandpoint Manor nursing home. He and his wife had three children, Jack, Nancy, and Charles.

CHAPTER

7

DR. C. K. AH FONG

The young Chinese doctor was broad-browed with black hair and intelligent, bright, black eyes, which shone with curiosity and anticipation. Dr. Ah Fong Chuck (soon to be officially renamed Chuck Ah Fong by an American immigration officer who understood virtually nothing of the Chinese language) was aboard a ship sailing from the Chinese mainland to the western United States. Even though there was sadness in his heart at leaving his baby son behind, Dr. Ah Fong was already making plans for the day when his son, Herbert, would be able to join him in the new world and life toward which he was sailing.

The doctor was to become one of the most colorful characters in the gold boom areas of southeastern Idaho. This was no easy feat, as colorful characters abounded in the Idaho of that day. He was also to cause some dramatic changes in the awarding of licenses to practice medicine in the state. Ah Fong had been born in Canton Province, China, which edges the southeastern shoreline facing the South China Sea. The city of Hong Sing (now known as Chun Sin) was the place of his birth and youthful days. After the birth of his son, Herbert, his young wife died and Ah Fong set sail for America. He left the baby with relatives with instructions that he, too, was to be trained in the ancient and classical art of Chinese and herbal medicine.

Two dates are given by separate sources for his arrival in Idaho—1865 and 1869. It could be that both are correct in the minds of those who cited the dates, as one source has him at Rocky Bar in Elmore County in 1865, and his great-grandson, Richard Ah Fong of Boise, has placed him at nearby Atlanta in 1869. Whichever the date, it was upon his arrival in California that the family surname of Chuck was switched to his first name, from which he later took the initials C.K., and Ah Fong was placed as his last name. Immigration authorities suffered an inability to comprehend the Chinese custom of giving the family surname first. The name stuck to him and his descendants. The grandson wrote, "My birth certificate still reads Richard James Chuck, not Ah Fong. I probably need to do something about that someday."

Hundreds of Chinese were pouring into that mountainous land of Elmore County which had become internationally famous for the production of gold and silver. The Ida Elmore mine, from which the county was named, was the greatest producer of gold in the late 60s. The year before Dr. Ah Fong arrived, the first quartz mill was built at Rocky Bar.

Dr. Ah Fong found a ready and willing clientele among both Chinese and Caucasians in the mining towns. The Chinese had often been denied medical attention by white "doctors," many of questionable training and whose prescribed treatment could be worse than the disease. The white miners and their families were also anxious to find someone who could make them well. Dr. Ah Fong's knowledge of health-giving herbs became well-known as far away as Boise. He became heralded as one who kept his patients well and strong. The Caucasians also looked forward to the Chinese celebration of the New Year, with parades, costumes, and fireworks, a program in which Dr. Ah Fong was a leader.

He was a born and trained leader and the Chinese were drawn to him as a source of learning and assistance. He was described as 'feisty' by his great-grandson, who told of the doctor's being schooled in the martial arts and accustomed to defending himself and the Chinese community.

The gold mines started playing out in the late 1880s and miners and their families began to migrate to Boise, which had by that time grown to the size of a handful of buildings. Dr. Ah Fong had joined the move in 1889 and established an office on Idaho Street, where the well-known Basque restaurant, the Valencia Club, later stood. As the town grew the Chinese population increased to

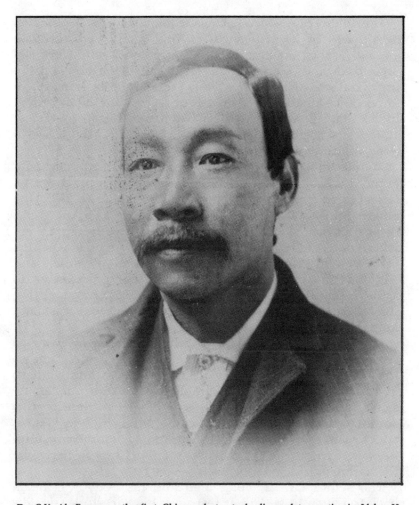

Dr. C.K. Ah Fong was the first Chinese doctor to be licensed to practice in Idaho. He practiced in the mining district of Boise County and later moved to Boise City. This photo was taken in 1890. He and his family became well-known in Boise and a son, Herbert, and grandson, Gerald, both practiced with the senior Ah Fong.

(Idaho Historical Society photo)

about 400, and the doctor moved into an office at 210 North Seventh Street, with Fong's Tea Garden nearby. His practice continued to grow.

Dr. Ah Fong married again and adopted two daughters. Amy eventually moved to California; Lena for years operated the popular Hong Kong Cafe in downtown Boise.

The Idaho State Medical Association had its beginnings in a series of letters, meetings, and many conversations among Idaho doctors in the year 1892, and formally organized and elected officers in 1893. History of the organization will follow, but the organization is of importance in the Ah Fong story. When the later-formed Idaho State Board of Medical Examiners began to review and grant licenses to practicing physicians, Dr. C.K. Ah Fong was among the first to apply.

"While most longtime physicians were automatically granted a license," Dick Ah Fong wrote, "this practice was not applied equally to Chinese physicians." In 1899, the board refused to grant C.K. Ah Fong a license. His response was to challenge the board in court. In an era when non-whites had little success in American courts, C.K. won his right to be a fully licensed physician and surgeon, making him the only Chinese practitioner to achieve that distinction in the history of Idaho and, at that time, it is believed in the United States. He was the 106th Idaho doctor to be licensed.

In 1917, the son, Herbert, who had been left in China to secure a classical education in Chinese medicine, came to the United States and to Idaho to join his father. Herbert, in turn, had left his son, Gerald, in China to pursue the same type education. Herbert's wife never came to this country, but the son, Gerald, came when he was sixteen and became an apprentice in the family apothecary until he had learned the proper uses of the Chinese herbs for the various medicinal purposes.

The senior Dr. Ah Fong died and his body was taken back to China to be laid at rest with his ancestors. Gerald's marriage was arranged in China and his bride, Sarah, who spoke both Cantonese and Mandarin, came to this country. In 1964, Dr. Herbert moved to San Carlos, California, where he purchased a home and small cafe. Gerald continued practice at the 611 Idaho Street office he had shared with his father.

Gerald and Sarah's five daughters and two sons thrived and were educated in Boise. Dick says that "To be graduated from high school was equivalent to a declaration of independence," and one by one the daughters moved to the San Francisco Bay area. Son Bill is in the computer business in San Jose and Dick wanted to remain in Idaho. He teaches English in Boise.

Dick started the study of pre-medicine to follow in the Ah Fong medical footsteps but found that modern medicine had so far surpassed that which his father and grandfathers had practiced that he gave it up to teach English. "When the Communists took over in mainland China, it became very difficult, and then impossible, to get herbs shipped out," Dick said, "and we were unable to serve the very faithful clientele who kept coming to my father." Now, herbal medicine is again being preached and practiced in many quarters.

The *Idaho Statesman* noted that "Mrs. Gerald Ah Fong, 423 Ada Street, was received into the First Presbyterian Church on Easter Sunday, April 19, 1950. The Ah Fongs children are in the Sunday School there."

Dr. Gerald died in 1968 in a tragic accident in California, where they were visiting a daughter and her family. She had left the baby in the car as she rushed into the house for something. The baby managed to take the car out of gear. As it began to roll, grandfather Gerald attempted to stop the car and was run over.

CHAPTER
8

FIRST IDAHO ALIENIST

Ask almost anyone today, "Who or what is an alienist?" and the answers will vary from "Someone from a foreign country," to "An extra-terrestial, like E.T. in the movie."

Dr. John W. Givens was neither a foreigner nor an extra-terrestial. He was Idaho's first psychiatrist, then known as an alienist. He was also a builder of hospitals. And, for the mid-1900s, he was well traveled, crossing the country several times.

He was born December 28, 1854, at Placerville, California, the son of Mary Russell and Thomas Jefferson Givens, who had crossed the plains from Illinois in 1849. His father died soon after his birth and, with his mother and three sisters, traveled to Illinois by the way of the Isthmus of Panama. His mother re-married in Illinois and, once again, the family crossed the plains in 1862, this time to Oregon. The family lived in Forest Grove and Hillsborough, where he he attended grade school. His high schooling was in Portland, where his interest in medicine was whetted by working in a drugstore owned by a Dr. Bailey, who also taught him medicine.

He received his M.D. degree from the University of Willamette on June 22, 1875, and began practice in Union, Oregon. The U.S. Indian Service soon hired him as physician for the Snohomish Indian Reservation at Puget Sound, where he remained until 1882. He then crossed the country again to take a post-graduate course at New York's Bellevue Medical College, receiving a second M.D. degree March 14, 1883. He was named the first assistant medical superintendent of the Oregon State Insane Asylum at Salem, where he remained from September 1, 1883, until December 1887.

Dr. Givens was hired by the State of Idaho in 1887 to become medical superintendent of the state asylum at Blackfoot. He had been married ten years earlier, April 10, 1877, at Hillsborough to Ellen E. Luelling. Two of their four children, Mary and Wallace, died in infancy. One son, John A., became an accountant in Portland, and the other, Raymond L., an attorney and member of the Idaho Supreme Court, in Boise.

Dr. Givens was admitted to medical practice in the states of California, Oregon and Idaho, receiving the 73d license to practice in Idaho shortly after the legislative creation of the Idaho State Board of Medicine in 1899. He served as president of the Idaho Medical Society and was a member of the American Psychiatric Association.

In 1891, the main building of the Blackfoot asylum burned and Dr. Givens was in charge of construction of a new brick central building and two wings. The brick was manufactured by the patients. He remained as superintendent until 1896, when he left for Baltimore to take a post-graduate course in nerve and mental diseases at Johns Hopkins Medical College. He practiced as a specialist in Los Angeles until returning to Blackfoot in 1898, remaining as superintendent until 1905.

He accepted the challenge of building the newly created North Idaho Insane Asylum at Orofino, which was built almost entirely by the patients under his direction. His reputation as a builder and superintendent of such institutions grew, and he was named by Governor James H. Hawley to the committee to locate and build a home for the feeble minded. Nampa was chosen as the site.

Dr. Givens prepared many medical papers on technical subjects for meetings all over Idaho and was frequently called upon to testify as an expert alienist in Idaho, Utah, and Washington.

Dr. Givens remained at Orofino until 1925, when he retired and moved to Boise, where he died on June 23, 1928. He took part in civic and business affairs wherever he lived, was a member of the Congregational Church and the Masonic lodge. Ellen Givens was equally interested in the development of Idaho and served as president of both the southeastern and northern districts of the Idaho

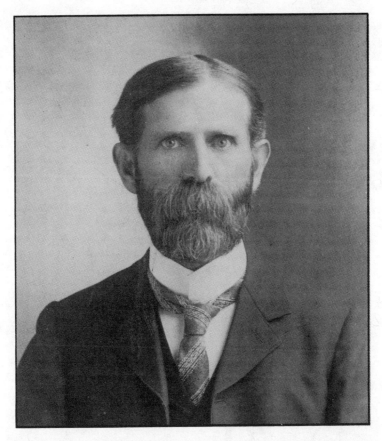

The first Alienist to practice in Idaho, Dr. John W. Givens, was the 73rd doctor to be issued a license to practice in the State. He was in charge of re-building the mental hospital at Blackfoot, which had burned in 1891. Dr. Givens also built the new North Idaho Insane Asylum at Orofino. He was on the committee to choose a site for the new home for the feeble-minded. Nampa was chosen. One son, Raymond L. Givens, was an attorney and a Justice of the Idaho Supreme Court.

(Courtesy Allee Givens)

Federation of Women's Clubs, and as vice-president of the state federation.

At different times, Dr. Givens was stockholder and director in the Standrod and Company Bank, Blackfoot; D.L. Evans and Company, Albion; W.G. Jenkins and Company, Mackay; Bank of Nampa, Lewiston and Nampa; but had severed connections with all but D.L. Evans and Company, prior to his death.

CHAPTER
9

"THEY WERE FIRST"

DR. C. W. SPRAGUE

How did a boy who thought he didn't like school, who ran away from home, "eloped school," as he described it, become an outstanding physician and psychiatrist?

The life and times of Dr. Charles H. Sprague, Pocatello, is a fascinating story. He was born to livestock-owning parents October 13, 1882, in Morrill, Kansas, attended country school, where he studied much Latin, and played in a country band. He "eloped school" and became a "boxcar pullman bum," riding all over Kansas until retrieved by his family and sent into the Army, 20th U.S. Infantry, December 15, 1898, at age sixteen. "I was sent to Fort Leavenworth as a trumpeter, and became so homesick I was in the hospital until the regiment was ordered to the Philippines in January 1899. We arrived at Manila (Corregidor) on February 22, 1899, and it was some sight from thirty miles away to see the fire that the insurgents had started to burn Manila. We landed at Manila and I was wearing winter clothes. We were sent direct to the firing lines at Guadalupe Church, Pasig City (later Fort McKinley). As the smallest, I was hoisted over the church door, where several 'insurrectos' were exterminated."

March 13, 1899, his battalion was ambushed with the heaviest loss of men during the insurrection. For the next two years, he played funeral marches with two to eight deaths a day from malaria, dengue fever, and dysentery. The band went on military campaigns to Loag and Batangas. They shipped home, arriving December 20, 1901, and celebrated New Year's Eve in Pocatello with his brothers. His brother, Frank M., was a pediatrician in Pocatello from 1909 until 1949.

He contracted malaria in the Philippines and was forced to quit high school. In 1902 he took a stenography course at Salt Lake Business College and was named an "expert stenographer." He worked at stenography until February 1907, when he returned to the Philippines as general storekeeper for the railroad constructing company. He was appointed assistant superintendent of the Panama Railroad, remaining until December 1909, when he decided he wanted to study medicine.

Having had no high school or college credits, he needed four years of the former and one year of college. Between March and September, 1910, he took exams in twenty-one subjects, receiving seventy-two credits before the Pennsylvania and New York boards. He entered Jefferson Medical College in Philadelphia on the last possible day, October 17, 1910. When he had finished, the Pennsylvania Superintendent of Public Instruction said, "This is the greatest scholastic achievement, four years of high school and one of college in eight and one-half months. If I did not know every detail of it, I would say it is impossible." He was president of the 1914 class when he graduated from Jefferson.

During his residency at Pennsylvania Hospital in Philadelphia he spent one year on mental cases and two years on medicine and surgery. He passed his Idaho medical licensing exam on April 6, 1917, and never forgot the date because the United States declared war on Germany that day. April to June he practiced medicine in Pocatello before going into the Army as a captain, and then major, and took Base Hospital 94 in France. In September 1918, within a three-hour period, 2400 casualties arrived from the Vosges battle. A flu epidemic struck on the day the Armistice was signed, November 11, 1918.

Major Sprague was discharged from the Medical Corps and appointed to the U.S. Public Health Service in charge of the Veterans Bureau for Idaho. October 6, 1921, he married Marietta Higson. Thanksgiving night, 1922, he gave the first dose of insulin (Isletin) ever given to a patient in the west. It was to a patient of Dr. George Spencer, Idaho Falls' Sacred Heart Hospital. Dr. Sprague had license direct from the inventor, Professor McLeod, and the shipment from Eli Lilly company. He remembered that it took him five hours to travel between Pocatello and Idaho Falls due to muddy roads. From 1918 through 1953 he took post-graduate courses at Harvard, Columbia, University of California, Northwestern, and the University of Oregon.

Other firsts included giving the first Thorazine at State Hospital South, Blackfoot, January 24, 1954, making it possible to take ten patients out of maximum security and to discharge fifty before the end of that year. He did the first red blood sediment rate (citrate and hypo vials) in 1919. He was a tissue pathologist from 1920 to 1925 at Blackfoot.

He was in Pocatello until 1925, when appointed medical director and superintendent of Broadlawn Hospital, Des Moines, Iowa. He returned to internal medicine practice in Boise from 1937 until 1942, when he went to Chicago as representative of American College of Surgeons until September 1948. He practiced for the next two years in Pocatello and was then chief psychiatrist at State Hospital South, Blackfoot, for nine years. From then until his death, at eighty, in 1962, he practiced in Pocatello.

DR. EMORY SOULE

Emory L. Soule was born September 2, 1904, in Salt Lake City, but his grade and high school classes were at St. Anthony, graduating in 1923. He worked during the summers on farms owned by his father and an uncle. After high school, he worked in the commissary at Yellowstone Park in the summer. He received a B.A. degree in science from the University of Utah in 1928. After three years of teaching in Idaho schools, he returned to Utah for two years and then entered Washington University Medical School in St. Louis, Missouri, to earn his M.D. degree. His internship was at St. Lukes in Denver, 1935–36.

Dr. Soule then practiced medicine in a C.C.C. camp, as a first lieutenant with the U.S. Army in Colorado Springs. He had twenty years with Selective Service and received Presidential Citations from four presidents. He started practice in St. Anthony in 1937. He believed he was the first doctor to use penicillin in Idaho. This was in the spring of 1939, when an eight-year old boy had osteomyelitis of the clavicle. The boy's parents were friends of U.S. Senator Henry C. Dworshak and appealed to him for the new "miracle medicine." The senator was able to have a supply released from Boston and it was immediately flown to Idaho.

Dr. Soule was the first to use cortisone, an experimental supply released to him from Chicago, where the son of a patient was studying medicine. He belonged to the Idaho Medical Society and was local president four terms and treasurer for twenty years. He was a national general practice delegate for three years and served on the Idaho Public Health Committee.

As a country G.P., he had many unusual experiences. He was calling on a patient who had delivered a baby the previous night in her home. He slipped off a dark porch into space through an open trap door into the cellar, and found he had broken an ankle. His calls for help were heard by a passerby on the street, who took him to Dr. Ellison. His ankle was put in a cast, he was given crutches and a sedative and sent home. Before morning he was called out on two deliveries, five miles apart. The deliveries and surgical repair were done by the light of a kerosene lamp. "Crutches were flying in every direction as speed was essential," he said. A blizzard was raging and he got out just before the roads were closed for an entire week.

Dr. and Mrs. Soule had two daughters and each had three children.

DR. FRED A. PITTENGER

Except for a five year period when he was associated with well-known Chicago surgeon, Dr. Charles Adams, Fred Pittenger practiced medicine in Boise since being licensed by Idaho April 4, 1905, until becoming ill several months before his death on February 13, 1964.

Dr. Pittenger and equally well-known Dr. J.L. Stewart, in the early 1900s, performed what apparently was the first coffee-type operation on a sufferer of extrophy of the bladder. They did this in Mountain Home under primitive conditions. There was no hospital there. The patient was alive and well thirty-two years later.

He was born in Cardington, Ohio, October 15, 1875, to Willis and Margaret Kern Pittenger. The father died at age thirty-four, and the widow and son, Fred, came to Boise in

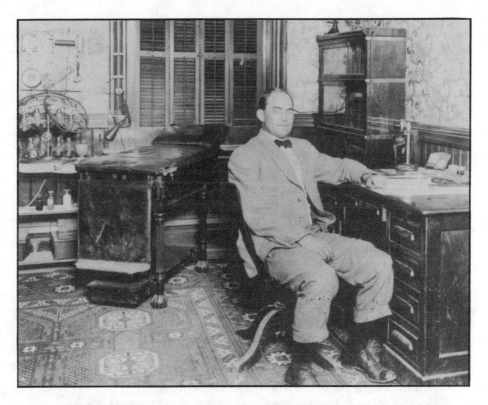

Dr. Fred Pittenger came to Idaho in 1909 from medical education in Chicago, married Dr. Alice Pittenger, gave years of medical care to residents in the Boise area, the Idaho National Guard, and the Soldiers Home. He died in 1964.
(Idaho Historical Society photo)

1890. The widow later became the wife of Dr. Harlan Page Ustick of Boise.

Fred received his grade and high schooling in Ohio and took four years of study, including two of medicine, at the University of Iowa. He was graduated from the Chicago Homeopathic Hospital in 1899, also interning there. He graduated from Northwestern Medical College, Chicago, in 1904, and joined Dr. Adams. In 1902, he married Alice Butterworth, also a medical graduate, in Chicago. Dr. and Mrs. Pittenger had an adopted daughter, Mrs. Oscar Yates of Boise.

He built a fine practice in Boise and was founder of the

Pittenger Medical Center and was senior physician at the time of his death. He was surgeon to the Idaho Soldiers' Home for thirty-two years and Boise physician for twelve years. He was a member of the Ada County, Idaho and American Medical societies, American College of Physicians and Surgeons and on the State Medical Examining Board for five years. Dr. Pittenger belonged to the Masons, with degrees in the Commandery, York, and Scottish Rites; Elks, Boise Commercial, Country, and University clubs.

As captain in the Idaho National Guard Medical Corps, he was at the Mexican Border from June 19, 1916 to January 23, 1917. From September 12, 1917, until January 2, 1919, he was a major with the Medical Officers Corps at Fort Riley, Kansas. After the Armistice was signed, he was commander of Army Sanitary Train 2.

DR. ROSCOE C. WARD

Dr. Roscoe C. Ward, born February 26, 1891 at Belleville, Kansas, the son of a farmer, also learned to farm. His secondary education was at Kansas University, 1909 to 1917, with a B.A. degree in 1913, and an M.D. in 1917. He joined Sigma Chi and Nu Sigma Nu. Internship was at Research Hospital, Kansas City, Missouri, 1916.

Dr. Ward was in the Medical Corps, U.S. Air Force, World War I. He became a member of "Ancient Order of Permanent Lieutenants." In 1919 he moved to Boise, and practiced until moving to Burns, Oregon in 1923. In 1925 he moved back to Idaho and practiced in Cascade until 1941, at which time he moved back to Boise. He was the first anesthesiologist in Idaho. He remembered having to travel by dog team, snowshoes, skis, saddle horses, sleighs, airplanes, and riding behind a motorcycle policeman in pursuit of patient care. He recalled driving forty miles in fifty-seven degrees below zero to deliver a baby.

He was a member of the executive committee of the Northwest Rheumatism Society. Dr. and Mrs. Ward had three boys (an M.D., a chemical engineer, and a sanitary engineer).

CHAPTER
10

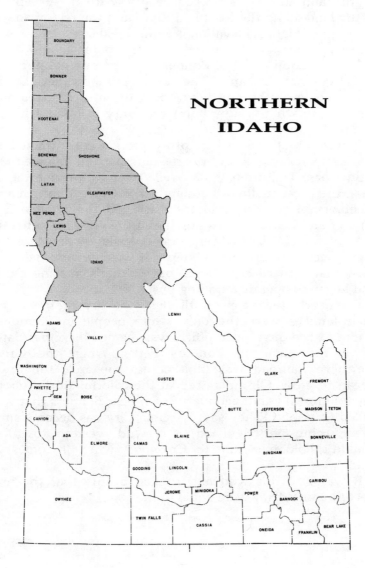

NORTHERN
IDAHO

BOUNDARY COUNTY

Idaho's northernmost county joins with British Columbia to form the Idaho section of the "blessed boundary," between the two great and friendly countries of Canada and the United States. Three different mountain groups, the Selkirks, the Purcells, and the Cabinets, divide the county and add to its rugged beauty. With the exception of the land along the Kootenai River and the region south, Boundary's highest elevation is about 7,000 feet.

First, Bonner was created out of Kootenai, and then Boundary County out of Bonner. It is the original home of the Kootenai Indians. The explorer-mapmaker David Thompson was the first white man to enter the area and went on to what is now Bonner County to build a house and trading post.

It was about 1860 when prospectors were attracted to the discovery of gold in British Columbia and followed the Wild Horse Trail from Walla Walla to cross the river at, or near, the present site of Bonners Ferry. Chief Abraham and members of his Kootenai tribe assisted the miners. E.L. Bonner and his associates purchased the crossing rights on the river and Idaho's Territorial Legislature later issued him a license to operate the ferry. It was ten years later, in 1874, that Richard Fry bought out Bonner's crossing rights and began to operate a trading post.

For nearly ten years, until 1884, the Fry brothers and their families were the only white people in Boundary County. The first post office was named Fry, but later given the name of Bonners Ferry. When the Great Northern Railroad was built across the area, the town began to grow. Oldtimers repeat the colorful stories about the tough, wild and legendary town near Bonners that was called Crossport. They say "Virginia City has become such a big thing on television as a wild western town. It couldn't hold a candle to Crossport when it comes to wild."

It was into this wild and rugged beauty that the first doctors came. They were equal to the task.

DR. EZRA ESHER FRY

There is an old saying that helps to put one's life into perspective: "Remember, the size of your funeral will depend entirely upon the weather." This was simply not true in the case of beloved and greatly admired doctor-physician E.E. Fry of Bonners Ferry. It was a cold and blustery February day in 1937 when his funeral was held and there were so many friends in attendance that it was necessary to hold it in the high school gymnasium to accommodate the crowd.

A tribute not likely to have been paid another white doctor in Idaho was the appearance at the funeral of the entire membership of the Kootenai tribe. The snow was extremely deep, but the Indians, most of them plodding on foot, came the several miles from the Mission. Dr. Fry had been interested in the Indians and their families, in their way of life, and in their health, doing what he could to be of help to them in every way. They recognized in him a stalwart friend. From the time of his arrival in Boundary County he would visit the Mission and came to know the Kootenais as friends. In the early days, they would row the river in their canoes to see him.

A many-faceted and fascinating man, Dr. Fry was born in New Berlin, Pennsylvania in 1875 to D.C. and Lydia Heist Fry, who had moved to the United States from Canada. He was graduated from the medical school of the University of Toronto in Canada. After taking additional training, he took a look at the money he had, bought a train ticket as far west as he could go and still have five dollars left in his pocket. When the train stopped in Bonners Ferry, he took his bag and stepped down to the wooden platform. He was home. And he had five dollars. Those dollars quickly diminished to three before he had completed his first walk down the main street. He met a couple of panhandlers and fell for their story of being down on their luck and needing money. He gave them each a dollar. He became known as an easy mark and gave away many hundreds of dollars in his life, but keep in mind that his funeral had to be moved to the biggest space in Bonners Ferry.

The year was 1902 and it was several months before the State Medical Boards would be held, so he worked with an

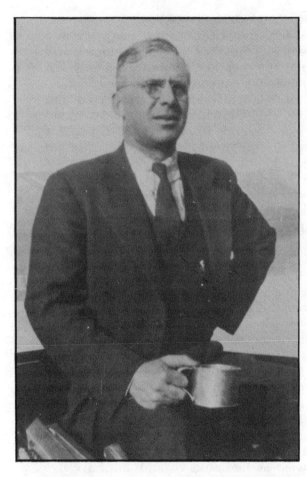

Dr. Esher E. Fry was an immaculate dresser who was unafraid of soiling his hands or clothing when it came to any necessary work for his community. Here he is having coffee from a tin cup as he travels by boat to a patient.

older doctor who had been licensed to practice. In October that year he passed the boards and was the 257th doctor to be licensed to practice in Idaho. In 1903, he opened his own office. Looking even younger than his twenty-eight years, he grew a mustache, hoping to give his older patients a sense of security when they came to him. He did not need the mustache for long. Once people came to know him, there was no one they trusted more.

Not only trust, but respect was given to the young doctor. He possessed an innate dignity that was quickly recognized and the greeting was, "Hello Doctor," and never, "Hiya Doc."

Early on the doctor walked to the homes of many of his

patients. When he could afford to buy a horse, he rode to his calls. Later came a team and a buggy and, finally, a little Maxwell runabout car.

Three years after the birth of Dr. Fry, the baby girl who was to become Mrs. Fry, Myrta M. Rickerd was born in 1878 in Eau Claire, Wisconsin, to C.W. and Emma (Roberts) Rickerd. Twenty-six years later she came west to Bonners Ferry to visit an uncle Rickerd, then manager of the Weyerhauser mill, and his wife. She knew virtually nothing about the Kootenai Indians and had what was, for her, a terrifying experience when she first met one of them. Soon after she arrived, she was carefully eying a group of Kootenais as she walked down Main Street in Bonners Ferry. One young man of the Kootenais noted her apprehension and decided to take advantage of it and give her a scare. When she walked by him, he reached out and grabbed for her handbag, not actually taking it. Then he laughed at her fright.

Had she not soon after that experience met the young and handsome Dr. Fry, dressed in his navy blue suit and wearing a snappy derby hat, she may have felt like hurrying back to Wisconsin. Dr. Fry was so kindly and charming that she wanted to stay. The courtship began and when he went to call upon Myrta, he carried a lantern as the streets were not yet lighted. She kept delaying her return to the midwest, and in 1906 they were married.

Meticulous in dress as he was, Dr. Fry was among those out with his shovel helping to control the waters during the 1916 flood of the town. No dikes had yet been built. Someone was heard to say, after glancing at the doctor aggressively wielding his shovel, "This is the first time I ever seen Dr. Fry with his coat and tie off and his white shirt sleeves rolled up."

That he cared deeply for people and would do anything he could to help out a patient, was shown by his making it a point to get acquainted with the families and learn of their lives and difficulties. He felt that he could not adequately treat a patient without knowing of his background. A lack of money to pay him never interfered with his treatment of the patients. One night he was called to see a patient in the "red light" district of the town. He fell through a damaged sidewalk plank while on his way and broke his leg. Like most doctors, he was not a patient-patient, and was driving his little car just as soon as he could walk with crutches. Wearing his bathrobe, crutches beside him, he would park his car by the entrance to his second floor office on Main Street, and see his patients right there.

While building the Spokane-International Railway through Bonners Ferry, the company constructed a small hospital to care for its employees. When the railway was completed, Dr. Fry secured the building for his own patients. Later it became a residence on the northside of the river. As the community and his list of patients grew, Dr. Fry purchased the Dawson property near his first hospital. He rebuilt and installed a hydraulic elevator to alleviate the problems of carrying patients up and down the stairs. In an attempt to make the larger hospital self-sustaining, he hired Al Cooper as caretaker of a large garden, Holstein cows, a small pig farm, and a smokehouse in which to cure meats, buildings for the animals, an isolation cottage, and cottages for the nurses and the caretaker.

Financial difficulties occurred when the Weyerhauser Company closed its large mill (about 300 employees) just a few months after Dr. Fry had done his extensive building. The major portion of the construction was financed through his contract with the mill workers for medical care at the cost of one dollar a month. While difficult, it was not impossible for Dr. Fry and he continued to care for the ailing. His buildings were sold a few years after his death to Boundary County. When a new hospital was opened, the Fry hospital became the Restorium, a home for the elderly.

Dr. Fry had high hopes of seeing Bonners Ferry a modern and growing town and he served in a number of capacities to reach that goal. For many years he served as a member of the school board and retained a keen interest in education all through his life. He was also called upon to serve as mayor for a few terms and was chairman of the board for the First National Bank. "Now, we'll have money enough to build up the town," was his enthusiastic comment when the Moyie Electrical plant was established.

On January 5, 1939, the new high school auditorium and

gymnasium at Bonners Ferry was dedicated to Dr. Fry, citing his many years on the school board and that he was chairman at the time plans for the new building were first drawn.

People still recount the legends that grew about Dr. Fry.

DR. ROY M. BOWELL

A lady by the name of Ida Holland wrote a poem in thanks to "Our Doctor Bowell," outlining how Bonners Ferry felt about a man who came there to associate himself in practice with Dr. E.E. Fry in the early twenties. Part of that poem is:

> We think of the lonely nights by a
> patient's bedside,
> When it seemed there was naught to
> do but hope and pray;
> But you faithfully claimed the help
> of the Great Physician
> And brought them through to the
> light of another day.
>
> This grateful mountain town will
> long remember
> The pleasant years of which
> you were a part;
> The flowers you gave, your acts of
> deep compassion
> And kindly deeds are written on
> each heart.
>
> You who have given your all to this
> mountain village
> Forsaking honor and glory in
> other lands,
> Your people rise up to pay you homage;
> Thankful that God has sent us
> such a man.

From his medical practice as a surgeon caring for Calumet-Hecla miners in Greencastle, Indiana, Dr. Roy Melson Bowell and his wife, Marie Callender Bowell, and their baby daughter, Mary Louise, answered the call of the west. They moved to Kuna, Idaho, but practice there proved a financial disaster. So the doctor answered with alacrity when an advertisement in the *Idaho Medical*

Journal announced that Dr. E.E. Fry of Bonners Ferry was seeking an associate.

Doctors Bowell and Fry enjoyed a long and agreeable relationship during which they ministered to hundreds of Idahoans, Canadians, and the Kootenai people. Both rode horseback, drove horse and buggy, railroad cars, or walked when called upon in order to answer all calls for medical help. They found it necessary to perform surgeries as the result of accidents in the woods and on the farms. Long before the state of Idaho required that they do so, they kept birth and death records. There was no limit to their service and a seven-day week was the norm. They also worked nights. When they could find the time, both doctors took part in community affairs. After a few years in practice, both bought agricultural land and were diligent overseers in the cultivation of the land.

Roy Melson Bowell was born on July 28, 1893 in Rolling Prairie, Indiana. His medical schooling was at the University of Illinois and he interned at Cook County Hospital. He was at the top of his class when he graduated. On June 15, 1918, he married Marie Callender in Greencastle, Indiana. They and their baby arrived in Idaho in 1920. On February 22, 1925 a second daughter, Dorothy Elizabeth, was born. It was often said that Dr. Bowell "was crazy about babies," and brought hundreds of them into the world.

During those years of long and hard practice, Mrs. Bowell not only kept the home fires burning, but she answered the telephone and never said that, "The doctor is not in." She found him if he was not nearby and he answered every call.

Dr. Bowell not only enjoyed seeing his farm productive and well kept, but he was an avid gardener at home. People drove by the Bowell home just to enjoy the beauty of the lawn and flowers, often comparing it to a park. Both the Bowells enjoyed travel and would take trips when they could get away. In later years, they drove thousands of miles in America and also traveled in Europe. Dr. Bowell kept a fine library, read avidly and kept up with the medical journals of the day. He was just as avid about sports and a splendid supporter of the University of Idaho athletics. He often drove to and from Moscow for basketball games.

The fish-filled rivers and creeks of Boundary County came to know Roy Bowell well. He would be out with his fishing gear by five o'clock in the morning and then put in a full day at the office and hospital. When he reached his fifties, he bought an Air Coupe and learned to fly. In 1961, when he retired from active practice he was honored by the American Medical Association for fifty years of devotion to medicine.

On September 15, 1969, Mrs. Bowell died and two years and two months later the doctor joined her. They are both buried in Bonners Ferry, the community they served so well and enjoyed so much for so many years. They enjoyed their family, which consisted of daughters and sons-in-law and six grandchildren.

DR. FRED W. DUROSE

Fred W. Durose was the youngest of seven children born to Charles H. and Mary Jane Wesson Durose, both of whom were born and reared in England. The father came to the United States in the 1880s and later returned to England to marry and bring his bride to Minneapolis, Minnesota. The family moved to Boundary County in 1920 and moved into the town of Bonners Ferry later. Charles Durose was a building contractor.

Fred graduated from high school with the class of 1922 and attended the University of Minnesota for one year. He took his pre-medical courses at the University of Washington in Seattle. He was graduated in 1926 with a bachelor of science degree and a five-year teaching certificate. After two years of teaching science at the Blaine, Washington high school, he entered the medical school at the University of Oregon. He received his M.D. degree in 1933. In 1930, he married Nelda Bender.

His internship was at the Deaconess Hospital in Spokane and his residency followed at Eastern State Hospital, Medical Lake, Washington. He then became associated with Dr. Max Smith and Dr. Paul Ellis in Wallace, Idaho. After Dr. E.E. Fry of Bonners Ferry died in 1937, he moved there. He later took a postgraduate course in surgery at Columbia University in New York City.

On September 1, 1980, Dr. and Mrs. Durose observed their fiftieth wedding anniversary. Their two daughters, Dolores Jean Tugby and Marilyn Jane Durose, both of Edmonds, Washington, joined them.

Dr. Durose belonged to several medical groups including the American Medical Association and the American Academy of Family Physicians (the latter required additional postgraduate study). He retired on May 1, 1969, but within a few months was back in activity. President Dwight D. Eisenhower had instituted a Physicians People-to-People Program which Dr. Durose joined. The group visited three countries behind the Iron Curtain and two free countries, seeing other physicians in a total of seven cities.

Dr. and Mrs. Durose made their retirement home at Talache on Lake Pend Oreille during the summers and autumns. The colder months of the year they spent in Mesa, Arizona.

DR. FRANK JOHN CORAM

Dr. Coram was born March 10, 1929, Yankton, South Dakota. His father was a salesman. He was raised in South Dakota, and the family moved to San Diego, California about 1936. He attended schools in San Diego, and summer jobs included seaman on a ferry boat, agricultural inspector for state of California, and spraying grape vines.

In 1950 he received his A.B. from San Diego State College; in 1955 an M.A. in botany from Claremont University College; M.D. in 1955 from George Washington University School of Medicine. He interned at the U.S. Public Health Service Hospital, Seattle, 1955–56. For two years, 1956–58 he worked at the Yankton Indian Hospital, Wagner, South Dakota.

He moved to Bonners Ferry in 1958. He was on the staff at the Bonners Ferry Community Hospital, and belonged to the Boundary County Medical Society.

The Corams have a son and two daughters.

BONNER COUNTY

Described as the most water-surfaced county in the state, Bonner is home to most of Lake Pend Oreille, which is, next to the Great Lakes, the largest freshwater lake in the country. It is also home to the pristinely beautiful Priest Lake, other lakes of various sizes, and to many creeks and rivers. The mountain ranges of the Bitterroots, Selkirks, and Cabinets add to the beauty.

It is now close to 200 years since the map-maker, explorer, fur-trader David Thompson arrived in 1809 at Lake Pend Oreille near what is now Hope and built the first two houses in Idaho. That was his trading post called "Kullyspell," for the Kalispel Indians, with whom he traded. He left the first good maps made of the area, although he spent a little over two months in Idaho, but what he did in that length of time was amazing. He was a trader for the Canadian North West Company which competed for furs with Hudson's Bay Company. He left big tracks wherever he walked.

The Jesuit Father Pierre Jean DeSmet came to Bonner County in the early 1840s to survey the possibilities of working with the Kalispels, the Kootenais, the Flatheads, the Coeur d'Alenes, and other tribes. His talent for working with the Indians brought international recognition.

Hudson's Bay Company built and operated a trading post near what is now Lacede. A mail and freight route across northern Idaho and Lake Pend Oreille came with the discovery of gold at Helena, Montana, later a part of the Idaho Territory. Boat builders moved in as the water route became important as the shortest way to Montana gold mines. The Northern Pacific, Great Northern, and Spokane International Railroads were followed by homes, hospitals, businesses, highways, and increasing numbers of people.

DR. WILBUR HENDRYX

Along with the developments of the late 1800s came the doctors. Bonner County history lists the arrival in the summer of 1884 of a young physician, Dr. Wilbur Hendryx, from Grand Rapids, Michigan. As it turned out, he spent as much time promoting and land developing as he did doctoring.

He heard about and visited the Bluebell Mine and its outcropping of galena ore on Kootenay Lake. Within a few months, Dr. Hendryx and associates had secured a half-interest in the property, formed a company called Kootenay Mining and Smelting with an office in New Haven, Connecticut. He and his company took over land for a townsite and named it Kootenai. He brought about a sawmill and bought timberlands. A tollroad was built from Kootenai to a short distance beyond Bonners Ferry and was called Galena Landing. A thirty-one-foot propeller steamer was shipped by his company from Chicago by rail and hauled by an oxen-pulled sled wagon from Kootenai to the river for launching. Many additions in buildings were made and the doctor built himself a fine home at Kootenai. By 1888, the tollroad was sold back to the county, the sawmill disposed of, and shortly thereafter Dr. Hendryx sold his home to Alfred Boyer, the postmaster, and it is assumed that he returned east.

PIONEER DOCTORS

Records show that a Dr. Will H. Potter, who was born on December 18, 1869, at North Collins, New York, and graduated from the University of Buffalo Medical School in 1897, practiced in Kootenai. He received his Idaho medical license October 6, 1911 and held it until 1922.

Four doctors are mentioned as having practiced at Laclede. **Robert A. Allen**, born May 30, 1877 and a graduate of Northwestern University in 1906, received his Idaho license on October 7, 1913. **M.R. King**, a graduate of Stanford University in 1917, was in Hope from April 1919 until 1922. **William N. Norris** graduated in 1894 from Louisville Medical College and licensed to practice in Idaho October 2, 1918; and **Earl S. Prindle**, a graduate of Hahnemann Medical College in 1893, was licensed on April 3, 1902 and held it until 1924.

Former physicians in the town of Hope include **Talleyrand Martin**, who settled in Hope in 1888, opened a drugstore and other businesses; **Heber W. Coulter**, born November 13, 1878 in Ontario, Canada, and a graduate of Trinity Medical College in 1903, licensed October 4, 1912. **Edward Desmond**, a graduate of Tulane in New Orleans in 1906, was licensed in October. **Earl Eames**, was born at

Menan, Idaho in November 1890; graduated from Rush Medical College, Chicago, 1917; licensed February 1920. He cancelled his license in 1922, but was reinstated in 1948. It is believed that he died in 1953. **W.M. Knapp**, an 1872 graduate of St. Louis Medical College, was licensed in 1902. **Mark Loop**, an 1893 graduate of Baltimore Medical College, was licensed on October 3, 1899.

AT PRIEST RIVER

Among the former physicians at Priest River are listed: **Carl P. Getzlaff**, born October 24, 1888, Good Thunder, Minnesota, graduated from California Eclectic Medical College in 1914, licensed in October; and an **Edward E. Getzlaff**, born March 17, 1892 at Warmington, Washington, graduated from Walla College in 1916, and practiced from October 1923 until October 1928; **W.J. Ingram**, graduate of Hashville, 1902, licensed April 1916; **P.A. Lillie**, Rush Medical College graduate in 1891, licensed April 1918, and held until 1924; **Elba McCarthy**, born in Michigan, March 2, 1875, graduated from the University of Michigan in 1903, licensed April 6, 1910, until 1922; **Harold C. Soucey**, born August 2, 1894 at Battle Creek, Michigan, graduated, College of Medical Evangelists in 1927, practiced from April 3, 1930 until his death in 1946. There is also listed a Dr. Bond at Priest River.

DRS. PAGE AND WESTWOOD

The people of northern Idaho remember Doctors Ones F. Page and his sister, Dr. Ethel Page Westwood. Their activities were colorful and their accomplishments great. Ones and Ethel, along with Joseph Barrett, who was a dentist and fisherman (and expert at both), were the children of John Hardy Page and Frances Barrett Page.

It would be difficult to forget a doctor who had been an acrobat with the Ringling Brothers Circus before he went into medicine. Both Ones and Joseph did that. Joseph passed on his entertainment gene to his son, John, who is remembered for riding his gear-driven Pierce Arrow bicycle, with no chain or sprocket in the Sandpoint parades.

Ones had a number of firsts to his credit as he built the Page Hospital on the bank of Sand Creek shortly after arriving in Sandpoint from Pullman, Washington in 1900.

He operated the hospital until 1939, when it was sold and renamed the Community Hospital. He organized Sandpoint's first band, was the town's first elected mayor. When Bonner was split from Kootenai County, he became the first state senator from that county, serving as a Republican for the 1910 and 1911 sessions.

Dr. Page got his M.D. from the Marion Sims College of Medicine in St. Louis, Missouri in 1897, and served as a surgeon with the U.S. Army during World War I. He bought a ranch at Wrencoe, where he raised purebred Black Angus cattle. He died at seventy-four, just three and one-half months before the United States went to war following the bombing of Pearl Harbor, December 7, 1941. The Pages had four children: Olive, who married Harry Nesbitt and lived in Sandpoint until her death in 1977; Hardy, Benjamin, and Frances.

When Dr. Page retired to his ranch, he sold the Page Hospital to **Dr. W.R. Werelius**, who operated it.

DR. ETHEL PAGE WESTWOOD

Ethel Page Westwood was born at Fort Dodge, Kansas, April 18, 1875. She received her medical training at Northwestern University Women's Medical College, from which she was graduated in 1899. She married a native of Kirkcaldy, Scotland, the Reverend William Westwood, June 1, 1898, one year after he received his Doctor of Divinity degree from Chicago's McCormick Theological Seminary.

When he was invited to serve as pastor of the First Presbyterian Church in Sandpoint, the Westwoods and their daughters, Martha and Page, moved from Bend, Oregon, and Dr. Westwood set up her practice as a specialist in eye, ear, nose, and throat. The Reverend Westwood died on April 27, 1937. Dr. Westwood continued her practice until 1946. She then divided her time between the family home on Dover Highway and the summer cottage on Lake Pend Oreille, which she had given the Scots name of "Dubbie Braes."

Her grandson, Jim Parsons Jr., relates that she was actively interested in wildlife, trees, and flowers. She had an extensive knowledge of geology. Among the land purchased by the Westwoods, was the site of the summer cabin in Bottle Bay and the shoreline east of the mouth of

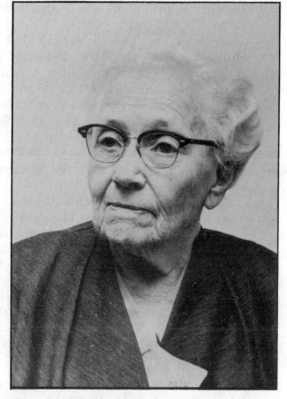

Dr. Ethel Page Westwood was an eye, ear, nose, and throat specialist in Sandpoint for many years. Her brother, Dr. Ones F. Page, who had been an acrobat with Ringling Brothers Circus before going into medicine, was also in Sandpoint. They often practiced together.
(Photo courtesy Jim Parsons, Jr.)

the bay. It is believed that the cabin was the first summer home built on the lake in either 1903 or 1905. Lumber and other supplies were barged in by one of the lake steamers and the daily mail boats, the Western or Northern, would stop when a flag signal was given.

Dr. Westwood died August 2, 1964.

DR. J. P. MUNSON

J.P. Munson graduated from the University of Oregon Medical School in 1949. After internship in 1950, he left to serve during the Korean War, returning in 1952. He went to Sandpoint to open a general practice in association with Dr. F.G. Wendle and his son, Dr. C.C. Wendle, and Dr. Wilbur C. Hayden at the North Idaho Clinic.

He married a native of Bonner County, Ellen Shear, born at Westmond to Mr. and Mrs. Joe Shear. Before his death, Joe Shear was known as the longest continuous resident of

Bonner County. Ellen was graduated from the university of Idaho in 1945, with a bachelor's degree in education. It was while attending the University that she and Jasper Paul Munson met in 1943. He later attended the University of Oregon Medical School and it was in Portland they were married on August 18, 1945. She and Dr. Munson had eight children and now have nine grandchildren.

Dr. Mike Hamilton joined the clinic for a three year stint. When the Doctors Wendle retired, Drs. Hayden and Munson operated the clinic at 502 North Second Avenue. They were joined by **Dr. Fred Marienau**, who later opened his own office on Dover Highway.

Dr. Munson moved into a new building across the street from the Bonner General Hospital in 1968. He was joined for about two years by **Dr. James Arthurs**. Later he and **Dr. Steven Puffer** bought the building and Dr. Munson practiced there until retiring in 1984. During his practice he had as his private nurses two well-known Sandpoint residents, **Pearl O'Donnell** and **Nancy Hagadone**. Drs. Neher and Puffer retained offices in the San Creek Medical Building.

DR. E. B. PATTERSON

Edward B. Patterson had much medical experience before arriving in Sandpoint in 1908. He was born at Elyria, Ohio, December 22, 1858. He was first graduated in the literary and chemistry courses at Oberlin in Ohio, and became assistant professor of chemistry there. He accepted a position with Parke, Davis and Company, one of the largest drug firms, and moved to Detroit. For several years he was manager of the compounding laboratory. While there he determined to study medicine, and entered the University of Michigan and graduated with an M.D. in 1886. He took postgraduate work in New York City at the Manhattan Eye and Ear Hospital.

He was a member of the staff of physicians for the Calumet and Hecla mines at Lake Linden, Michigan, and it was there that he married Sara K. Kaufman in September 1893. They soon moved to Michigamme, Michigan, where their son, Howard, was born in 1895. In 1901 and 1902 the three of them traveled over most of Europe, spending the winter in Vienna, where the doctor studied at the University Medical College. Later, he and Howard spent a winter in the Orient, traveling in China, Japan, and the Philippines.

In 1902 they moved to Phillipsburg, Montana and he practiced for six years until moving to Sandpoint. Their second son, Edward K., who was born shortly after their arrival, died by drowning in a tragic accident the following year.

Dr. Patterson was active in the Elks, El Katif Shrine, Modern Woodmen of America, and Woodmen of the World. At age sixty-one, he died in Sandpoint, November 1919. Mrs. Patterson was an activist in her own right and after his death divided her time between Sandpoint and Seattle. She taught music in the Sandpoint schools, was dean of women at the University of Washington and held the same position at the Southern Branch of the University of Idaho in Pocatello. She died in November 1942, in Seattle. Her request to be cremated and have her ashes sprinkled on the grave of her husband was met.

DR. FLOYD G. WENDLE

Frances Wendle Miller, remembers the two-month camping trip that first brought their family from Chicago to Sandpoint. Her father was suffering from what today is called "burnout" after years of daylight-to-dark practice.

Dr. F.G. Wendle decided that the family would get away and booked train tickets throughout the country. When they got to Sandpoint, they liked it so well that they camped on the lakeshore near Hope. While camping, the doctor realized that there was much lacking in apartment living and the feverish schedule of practicing in Chicago.

After returning to Chicago, he accepted an offer of physician for the Hope Lumber Company, and they returned west to stay. Dr. Wendle was born at Moline, Illinois, February 16, 1882. He received his M.D. degree in 1904 from the University of Chicago. He was married to Susie B. Jones while a student, and their son, Cornelius C., also a doctor, was born January 10, 1904. The Wendles became the parents of two other sons, Chud and Rex, both of Spokane; and one daughter, Frances Miller, Sandpoint.

In June 1934, with a father's pride showing, Dr. Wendle ran an ad in the *Pend Oreille News* titled "An Open Letter to My Patients." A portion of it is: "My son will be associated with me in the practice of medicine and surgery after July 1. The young physician is a home grown product . . . . earned his living and education by hashing, bridge painting, fire fighting, . . . then rode a sheep train to Chicago . . . common courtesy requires that a physician Dad should extend to his son an invitation of affiliation. I did, never dreaming that he would accept. He writes me that he is coming to teach me some things that I should know about the business. So it is to be a battle between this thirty-year-old, blood-transfusing, bone-grafting, spinal puncturing, serum-squirting, up-to-the-minute son and the dad who for all these years had depended upon the old reliable, tried-and-true onion poultices, nannie berry tea and castor oil, with you as the referee. Why anyone would put in ten years hard work . . . to practice medicine when there are such wonderful opportunities (and new automobiles) in bootlegging and politics, is more than I can figure.

"So when you phone No. 8 (day or night) . . . and are asked, 'Which doctor do you want?' Please keep in mind old folks are very sensitive and my feelings are easily hurt."

DR. FRANK BUTLER EVANS

Dr. Frank Evans came to know Idaho well, practicing at American Falls, Sugar City, Genesee, Dover, and Sandpoint. He was a general practitioner, but obstetrics was his chosen field. One morning in the Sandpoint area, he delivered three babies in three different homes before breakfast.

During the flu epidemic of 1918-19, he was one of two doctors in the entire area surrounding Sugar City and went for days without going to bed. He would sleep as he could in the backseat of an old Ford, while a driver would take him from patient to patient.

Some of Frank Evans' memories of his boyhood were of going with his doctor-father on his medical rounds, a small boy in the horse-drawn buggy, next to his father's old-fashioned, black medical bag. As they jogged along the dirt roads from farm to farm, he discussed with the boy the illnesses and care of the patients. Frank knew before he

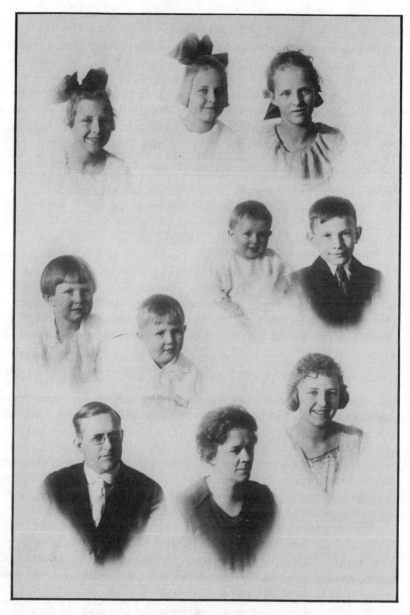

Dr. and Mrs. Frank Evans of Sandpoint had a combined family of eight children and had cared for many others over the years. Top three in the photo are Ida, Dot and Harriet, with Adah and Chuck just below. Mary and Frank Jr. are situated above the parents and Sylva is on the right. The photo was taken in the 1930s.

(Courtesy Jane Pier Evans)

graduated from high school at sixteen that he wanted to become a doctor.

Frank Evans was born to Dr. and Mrs. B.W. Evans, Dow City, Iowa, May 12, 1881, and as a boy he worked for neighbor-farmers and saved earnings to help pay for a medical education. After two years at Iowa State College, he taught a few terms to save money for Northwestern Medical School in Chicago, graduating in 1904, the second youngest in his class. He had a long bicycle paper-route during college and washed dishes at a restaurant for breakfast and lunch. His one luxury was a fifteen-cent gallery seat to a concert or the opera. After graduation, he assisted his father for a few months before opening a practice in Dow City. He married Harriet Davis of Grinell in 1905 and they became the parents of four girls.

The family lived in Dixon, Nebraska for several years and the doctor developed business interests and served as senator in the 1912 Legislature. The family moved to Idaho at the urging of his brother, Burton, and located near American Falls. Mrs. Evans died Christmas Day, 1916. Dr. Evans returned to Nebraska where he met and married a young widow, Clara Chubb Sargent. She had a son, Charles, who became part of the Evans family.

They decided to return to Idaho and take over the practice, home and twelve-bed hospital of a Sugar City doctor. A son, Frank Jr., and two daughters were born to them. Following World War II, Dr. Evans returned to Northwestern for a course in diagnostic medicine. After a short stay in Genesee in 1922, he went to Dover to take over the practice of Dr. R.N. Jackson, who had been drowned when his car went off the Laclede ferry. He was the doctor for the A.C. White Lumber Company.

In addition to taking care of the family, Clara helped with the patients and often assisted him with night calls in the country. In 1926, they moved to Sandpoint where he practiced until just ten days before his death in 1936. He served in the Idaho Legislature in 1934.

DR. WILBUR CURTIS HAYDEN

Dr. Hayden was a member of the Medical Evacuation unit with the first U.S. military group to Australia, New Guinea and the Philippines after the bombing of Pearl

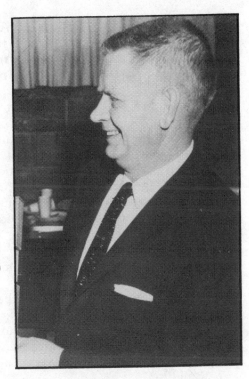

Wilbur C. Hayden, M.D. in 1962 takes time from his Sandpoint practice for a social event. Younger doctors could always look to Dr. Hayden for support and advice.
(Courtesy Penny Armstrong)

Harbor, December 7, 1941. He had been called to duty with the Army Reserve that year and was at Fort Lewis, Washington. His unit practiced triage, which has become so well known to viewers of the "M.A.S.H" television series. He also delivered so many babies on Mindanao and later, in Sandpoint, he became known as the "baby doctor." While in the Pacific, he met Dr. C.C. Neal Wendle and Dr. Dave Cornell. Dr. Wendle sang the praises of Sandpoint and convinced the other two doctors to join him there at the end of the war.

Dr. Hayden was born November 26, 1905, at Donna, Oregon, and was graduated in 1932 from the University of Oregon Medical College. He interned at Harborview in Seattle. At one time he served as doctor for a Civilian Conservation Corps camp.

After the death of his first wife, Dr. Hayden married again. When he died in 1969, he was survived by three daughters, Karen, Patty and Claire, and sons, Roger and Michael.

DR. WILLIAM TYLER

Dr. Tyler was never sure that he had not deliberately missed the Northern Pacific train to the west coast as he explored the magnificent docks on Lake Pend Oreille during a stopover. He had graduated from Syracuse University Medical School in New York and practiced in the east before coming west in 1928. He was heading for California, but during the train stop in Sandpoint, took a walk that changed the course of his life and provided the county with a general practitioner who became one of the best diagnosticians in the northwest. In 1937 he married Edith Lowry, sister of Jessie (Mrs. Harry) Lyons. He had a daughter, Louella, by a previous marriage and he named his handcrafted cabin cruiser "The Edie Lou" for his wife and daughter. It was one of two boats built for him by builder Harry Eiteman, whom the doctor befriended and supported in his old age.

Dr. Tyler was born November 13, 1883 and died May 14, 1966 at his Sandpoint home. He never turned down a request for a house call and was a physician at Page Hospital. He was honored by the naming of the Idaho Public Health building in Sandpoint the 'Tyler Medical Building.'

DR. CORNELIUS C. WENDLE

Better known as "Neal," C.C. Wendle spent his boyhood in Sandpoint, graduating from high school in 1923. In 1927, he received his bachelor of science degree from the University of Idaho and spent the next year as an assayer at Bunker Hill and Sullivan zinc mines in Kellogg. He enrolled at Northwestern University and took his M.D. degree in 1934. He completed his internship at the Chicago Shriner Hospital and Harbor View in Seattle, and still was able to join his father in 1934.

On May 12, 1933, he married Gladys Brower, a professional nurse, in Seattle. They became parents of three sons, Bruce C., Mark William, and Jan Neal, all of whom were active in Boy Scouts and all achieving the Eagle award, and attending World Jamborees. Dr. Wendle was active in scouting while the boys were growing and held several positions with the organization in the Inland Empire.

Several years after the death of Mrs. Wendle, the doctor married Susie Huss Williams of Coeur d'Alene. They owned the land upon which the chimney of David Thompson's old Kullyspell House still stood and took a great interest in its history and preservation. The doctor was past president of the Bonner and Boundary counties medical boards; director of the American Academy of General Practice; and Idaho and American Medical associations. He died several years ago.

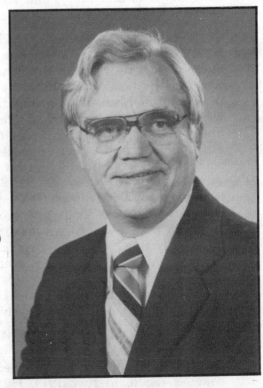

Dr. Fred E. Marienau was one of the many medical practitioners who were attracted to the mountain, stream, and lake country in northern Idaho. He practiced for many years in Sandpoint.
(Courtesy Penny Armstrong)

DR. FRED ELWOOD MARIENAU

Dr. Marienau was born December 11, 1929, in Sioux City, Iowa, to Fred and Christine Seitz Marienau. He was the second of three children. In 1948, he was graduated from Akron, Iowa, high school, and continued his education at the University of Iowa School of Medicine, graduating in 1955. He served in the U.S. Navy until 1958.

In January 1959, Dr. Marienau moved to Sandpoint and joined Drs. C.C. Wendle, Wilbur C. Hayden, and J.P. Munson in the North Idaho Clinic. He built his own office on the Dover Highway in 1967, remaining there until 1991. He is now emergency room physician at Bonner General Hospital. He has belonged to the American and Idaho Academies of Family Practice and was president of the latter.

He married Delsie Harmon of Sac City, Iowa, August 30, 1953, and they have six children, Fritz, Eric, Mathew, Rebecca, Sara, and Mary, and have eleven grandchildren. Over the years, they have had many foster children.

DR. R. N. JACKSON

Dr. R.N. Jackson of Dover, one of the oldest physicians in Idaho, was drowned in the Pend Oreille River December 6, 1924. It is not known how the accident happened, but the doctor and his nurse, responding to an emergency call, were crossing the river on the ferry. He must have been under pressure to get to his patient, as when the ferry was about one hundred feet from the shore, he started the engine and drove into sixty feet of water.

He was born in New York in 1855, graduated from Long Island Hospital Medical College in 1880; practiced in Leander, New York for two years; to Fairbault, Minnesota, for more than twenty-five years; coming to Sandpoint in 1908. He was elected as a Democrat to the 1917–18 Idaho Senate, and was appointed later that year as superintendent of the mental hospital at Blackfoot, where he opened an office after two years. He returned to Sandpoint in 1922, as surgeon for the A.C. White Lumber Company.

DR. MALCOLM McKINNON

Dr. Malcolm McKinnon, who had practiced medicine at Laclede and Sandpoint, was killed in a car accident near Baker, Oregon, in July 1919. He was fifty-two. Born on Prince Edward Island, Canada, he attended McGill and Trinity universities and received his M.D. from the latter in 1895. After ten years at Fosston, Minnesota, he came to Sandpoint in 1906 and located later at Laclede. He was a captain in the Marine Reserve was and at Camp Funston when the Armistice was signed. He served as president of the Bonner Medical Society.

KOOTENAI COUNTY

Until 1881 there had not been the necessary fifty citizens to organize a county in this lake, river, and tree-clad area that was to become Kootenai. In that year, at the Pony Express station Westwood, near present Rathdrum, fifty qualified men got together and signed the petition, forwarding it to Boise. The second Territorial Legislature passed the Country Creation Act and had already named the area for the Kootenai Indian tribe.

Father Pierre DeSmet had visited the shores of Lake Coeur d'Alene in 1842 to meet with Coeur d'Alene Indians relative to establishing a mission. Captain John Mullan surveyed the lakeshore in 1859, prior to building the famed Mullan Trail. Gold seekers stopped enroute to British Columbia in 1860, and later to Montana. The Northern Pacific Railroad put down tracks through Kootenai County and new settlement, that has not stopped, began. Lakes, rivers, creeks, fertile farm and recreation lands abound.

DRS. SABIN, ELDERKIN, AND DWYER

The first licensed civilian doctor in Kootenai County was Dr. John Sabin, who graduated from Buffalo, New York, University in 1867. He was one of the nearly 200 doctors who had applied for licenses when the law went into effect on June 20, 1899. Dr. Sabin received license number 147.

The second to appear was Dr. Heber R. Elderkin, the first physician to be licensed in 1901 and the 200th to apply. He received his medical degree from the Medical School of the University of Louisville in 1858. He practiced in Coeur d'Alene until his death.

Dr. John Condit Dwyer graduated from the University of Illinois as a physician and surgeon in 1901. He received Idaho license 241 on April 3, 1902 and practiced in Coeur d'Alene until his death, sometime in December 1932.

DR. JOHN TRAVERS WOOD

The ten-year-old boy, John Wood, would have had to be clairvoyant to have known that something extremely important to his future was happening at the very hour and place the train upon which he and his family were traveling through Kewatin, Lake of the Woods, Ontario,

Canada, on June 9, 1889. At that hour, a baby daughter, Margaret, was born to Mr. and Mrs. George C. Thomson.

Sixteen years later, Margaret Thomson and John T. Wood were married in Coeur d'Alene and spent most of their lives there. John T.'s parents, William and Sarah Heaton Wood, three sons and two daughters, had left their home in Wakefield, England, and sailed on a ship to Quebec. They took the train to what they believed was their homestead in Saskatchewan, only to later find they were one mile across the United States border near Sarles, North Dakota.

By anyone's standards, John T. was an unusual person. He stood six feet, four and one-half inches tall and weighed 260 pounds. A classmate at Detroit College of Medicine, a Dr. Watts, graduated one year ahead of John T., moved to Coeur d'Alene and wrote asking John T. to join him in his practice. After graduating in 1904, he did so. Watts moved to Pendleton to specialize in eye, ear, nose and throat.

In 1905, John T. went to Orofino, where he was coach for the husky and good players, but the doctor's coaching career was a short one. He took the team to Pendleton, Oregon to play. There was also a circus in town and five of the farm boys became so enamored of the circus that they left when it did. As a result, John T. left and came back to Coeur d'Alene.

He became the physician for Stack-Gibbs Lumber Company and its successor, the Blackwell Lumber Company, and the Milwaukee Railway, in a capitation plan, under which the companies pay a certain amount each month per employee. Dr. Wood received five dollars per employee. Dr. Wood built the Coeur d'Alene Hospital, on West Garden Avenue, and later added a wing. His first office was in the hospital. He later sold his interest to Dr. Alexander Barclay.

Dr. and Mrs. Wood had three children, a daughter who died in her youth, and two sons, Dr. William T., physician and surgeon, and Dr. George, a Spokane dentist. They bought the beautiful three-story Blackwell home at 817 Sherman Avenue in 1924 and raised the boys there. Doctor Wood converted a portion of it into an office and, with the exception of two years while he served as Idaho's First

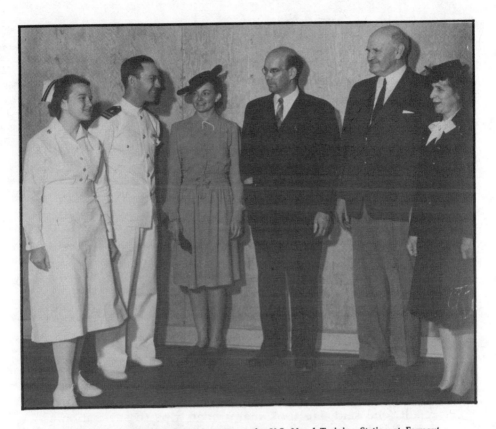

This picture was taken in the early 1940s at the U.S. Naval Training Station at Farragut, Idaho, on Lake Pend Oreille during an informal open house. Staff members escorted visitors around the hospital at Farragut. *Left to right:* Ensign Genevieve Bryant, Nurse Corps; Lieutenant Atlee Hendricks, Medical Corps, USN; Mrs. William T. Wood, Dr. William T. Wood, Dr. John T. and Mrs. Wood. The Wood men are father and son and both practiced in Coeur d'Alene for many years. Dr. Wood Sr. is deceased and Dr. William Wood is semi-retired.

(Photo courtesy Dr. Wm. Wood)

District congressman in Washington, D.C., practiced there until his death in 1954. His son, Bill, said that his father saw twenty-one patients in his office the day he died. "That's the way he wanted it," Bill said.

When Dr. Wood ran for the congressional office his campaign manager was his daughter-in-law, Dolores.

DR. WILLIAM T. WOOD

Bill Wood attended Coeur d'Alene schools and graduated from the University of Idaho with a bachelor of science degree in pre-med. In both high school and at the university, he was interested and active in track and music. He was an excellent swimmer and was swimming against Jack Medica in 1934 when Medica set a new world record. He turned out for track and played trumpet in Coeur d'Alene High School band, with the Idaho pep band and university orchestra.

He took pre-med at the University of Idaho and went on to Western Reserve University in Cleveland to earn his doctor of medicine degree in 1938. He joined Phi Rho Sigma fraternity. Dr. Bill had a two year rotating internship and six month assistant residency in pediatrics at the university hospitals, and a six months residency in contagious diseases at Cleveland City Hospital. After that he took many special courses at the University of Oregon and University of Washington to study the most unusual cases in pediatrics and family practice review courses at Zion Hospital in San Francisco.

Dr. Bill well remembers spending forty-eight snowbound hours with a patient in prolonged labor with no forceps available. "However, everything came out fine. A happy result," he said. He took many boat trips to see patients who lived on the lake and once brought a man on a stretcher on a tugboat to Coeur d'Alene through a howling blizzard.

His medical activities include being secretary-treasurer and president of the Kootenai Medical Association; chairman of the program committee of the Idaho Medical Association, and trustee to Northwest Medicine. He was an auxiliary officer for the U.S. Coast Guard; president, Coeur d'Alene Rotary Club and of the Kootenai district of Boy Scouts of America; six years on the Coeur d'Alene school board, two as chairman.

While studying in Cleveland, Bill met and married a vivacious brunette nurse, Dolores VanDyke, who was across the campus park at Mount Sinai Hospital. Dolores first noticed Bill because he wore a typical Idaho "lumberjack" jacket. They were married in the Presbyterian Chapel in Cleveland on June 11, 1938. His parents and brother George, then in dental school in Minnesota, were among those attending.

Bill and Dolores decided to make Coeur d'Alene their home and they became the parents of twins, Jacqueline Lee and John VanDyke, and Jennifer Lynn. All three are married and each has two children.

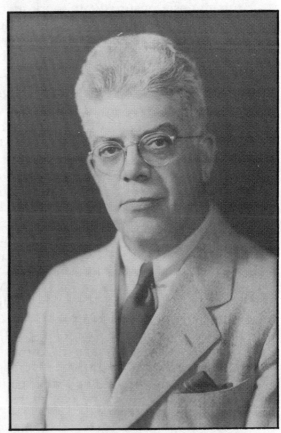

Dr. Alexander Barclay Sr., often known as "Lec," was one of the best-known physicians and surgeons in Coeur d'Alene. He was active in organizing the Kootenai County Medical Association and was a member and worked in the state association. Both his son, Alexander Jr. and C. Gedney, became doctors and returned to Coeur d'Alene to practice.
(Photo courtesy Dr. Gedney Barclay)

THE DOCTORS BARCLAY

Dr. Alexander Barclay spent the early years of medical practice in Cloquet, Minnesota, coming to Coeur d'Alene in 1917, when he purchased the Coeur d'Alene Hospital. He was born August 12, 1882 in St. Paul, Minnesota and had his preliminary schooling there. He received his M.D. degree from the University of Minnesota in 1907. The following year he married Agnes Gedney and the couple had three children, Alexander Jr., in 1910; Barbara in 1911; and Charles Gedney in 1921.

Dr. Barclay Sr. earned a degree in eye, ear, nose, and throat from the University of Vienna in 1926. He served as president of the Idaho Medical Association in 1928 and was on the Board of Councilors for many years. He took tuberculosis postgraduate work at the Phipps Institute in 1936 and was tuberculosis consultant for north Idaho after that time. He retired from active practice in 1939 because of ill health. He died at the family ranch in Arlington, California on February 27, 1942.

DR. ALEXANDER BARCLAY, JR.

Born to a physician father, Dr. Barclay Sr. and Mrs. Barclay, at Cloquet, Minnesota the day after Christmas in 1911, "Bud," as he was known by family and friends for the rest of his life, was later joined by a doctor brother.

He attended grade and three years of high school in Coeur d'Alene and was graduated from Moran School on Bainbridge Island, Washington in 1928. He received his bachelor of science degree in 1932 from the University of Washington, where he affiliated with Delta Upsilon. The great depression was in full swing in 1933, and he took a year and ran a service station in Coeur d'Alene before renewing his medical studies. His M.D. degree was from Vanderbilt University School of Medicine in 1937. There he joined Alpha Kappa Kappa. His internship was from 1937 until 1938 at Virginia Mason Hospital in Seattle.

Dr. Barclay Jr. married Alma Dews of Nashville, Tennessee in 1937 and they moved to Coeur d'Alene. They had three sons, Alexander, Richard and Stuart.

He practiced medicine in Coeur d'Alene from 1938 until he retired in 1964. He was president of the Idaho Medical Association in 1954-55 and a delegate to the American Medical Association.

DR. C. GEDNEY BARCLAY

The youngest of the Doctors Barclay, Charles Gedney, better known as "Ged," was born in the Coeur d'Alene Hospital in the room which became his office in later years. He attended Coeur d'Alene schools and was graduated from Webb School, California, and entered the

University of Washington for pre-med. Injuries from an automobile accident took one school year, so he actually had three years of pre-med. He was graduated from the University of Washington with a bachelor of science degree in 1940. He associated with Delta Upsilon fraternity. His M.D. degree was from the University of Oregon Medical School in 1943 and he joined Alpha Kappa Kappa.

Dr. Barclay's internship and residency were at the Good Samaritan Hospital. He found it interesting that Good Samaritan had to be persuaded to get the twenty vials of penicillin they were allowed, as it cost twenty-one dollars per 100,000 units (or each vial) and they were not sure it was worth it. They thought it was a lot of money for a drug they might not have much use for. Penicillin, as everyone now knows, became known as a miracle drug.

He began practice in Coeur d'Alene in 1946, joining his brother, Alexander Jr. Ged became chief of staff at the Lake City Hospital 1959-61 and was president of the Kootenai County Medical Society, member of the Idaho Medical Association and the Medical Disciplinary Board, for which he served as chairman.

During World War II, Dr. Gedney was lieutenant j.g. for the year 1944-45 in the U.S. Navy and was lieutenant commander until August 1954.

Dr. Barclay and his wife, Helen, became the parents of two sons, Scott and Steve, and one daughter, Barbara. The Barclays now live at Hayden Lake, where they indulge their great liking for golf.

DR. JOHN BUSBY

Dr. Busby practiced medicine at the scenic town of Harrison on the southeastern shore of Lake Coeur d'Alene and was known as "the doctor who practiced medicine on the lake," as he made a floating houseboat into a hospital to attend people living along the lake. Born June 14, 1868 in Montreal, Canada, he grew up in timber country and practiced medicine in the same type country.

John attended McGill Medical School and received his M.D. at age twenty-two. Because he was so young, he took two years of surgery and graduated with a masters degree in 1890. After practicing in Michigan, he came west and traveled to Harrison aboard a paddle wheel steamer. He liked it and wired his wife, Grace, and daughters to join him. He had all the patients he could handle and rode horseback when patients couldn't be reached by lake or river travel. He loved horses and always kept two of the finest.

He had many injury cases by loggers and other timber workers. Like many other early doctors devoted to their profession, he was a poor bill collector and would say, "pay when you can and what you can." He was paid in produce, home-cured meats, chickens and eggs. In 1904, he built the largest home in Harrison, before or since, and it is now on the National Historic Register.

After another home burned, the Busbys moved to Coeur d'Alene and later to Spokane. Many of his Harrison patients continued to travel to Coeur d'Alene to see him. Many Coeur d'Alene patients later traveled to Spokane to see him.

DR. FREDERICK FORREST HORNING

It could have been the genes that sent Fred Horning into the study of medicine. His maternal grandfather William Martin Owsley, who may have been the first doctor into Idaho Territory, was born August 21, 1819 in Lincoln County, Missouri. Dr. Owsley is said to have gone to California in the gold rush, but returned to Missouri, where he married on October 27, 1853. He and his bride went west by covered wagon, where one child was born in 1862 in Carson City.

From Nevada, the Owsleys moved to Boise, where Fred Horning's mother, Elizabeth Price Owsley, was born February 15, 1864. From Boise, the Owsleys moved to Oregon, where he died in Lakeview on May 12, 1893. Dr. Horning's paternal grandfather, Frederick Augustus von Horning, came from Germany to Missouri and joined a wagon group heading to Corvallis, Oregon. He married Mary Johnson, whose brother, John, was the first Oregonian to attend Yale. He became the first president of the University of Oregon. F.A. Horning was one of the signers creating the land grant college of Oregon State and his homestead was on the O.S.U. campus. Their son, James Robert, who was to become the father to Dr. Horning, was born in Corvallis in 1854.

Fred Horning was born January 25, 1898, in Silver Lake, Oregon, and was about to finish high school when the board declared that all boys who enlisted to fight the Germans would be graduated. Carol Horning Stacey said, "My father, who figured he would never pass algebra, joined the Army May 1, 1917 and served in the First Division, Artillery, in France." He and two brothers, Robert and Keith, returned in September 1919, unscathed.

Fred and Keith went to Moscow to attend the university, where their sister, Odalite Vincent, was married to a professor of agriculture. Both boys joined Phi Gamma Delta and Fred was on the wrestling team. He had hoped one day to be a vet and graduated in animal husbandry in 1923. He taught at Valleyford High School near Spokane. April 1, 1925, he married Carolyn Olsen Booth and they moved to Seattle, where he took pre-med at the University of Washington. He graduated from the Washington University School of Medicine in St. Louis, June 8, 1931. In his last year, Fred found he was eligible for a LaVerne Noyes Fund scholarship for World War I veterans, and it paid his final year tuition and reimbursed him for all that he had already paid.

The Hornings moved to Rathdrum in 1932, where he was doctor for the railroad and in private practice. In 1936 they moved to Coeur d'Alene and bought a home at 1017 Sherman Avenue. His office was in a building between Third and Fourth streets that burned in 1943. He then bought a stucco house at Fifth and Coeur d'Alene and converted it into an office, complete with minor surgery and X-ray rooms.

The Hornings' daughter, Shirley, was born at the lying-in hospital at First and Indiana in 1937. Carol was born at Sacred Heart in Spokane in 1934. The 1930s were not easy. Dr. Horning often took pay in cordwood, venison, cream, quilts and even doilies. House calls into the country were frequent, and Mrs. Horning went along to administer anesthesia, which the doctor had taught her to do. He stitched up wounded farmers on their kitchen tables and performed other necessary operations. With World War II, things changed, the population more than doubled, many doctors were drafted and others put in extra time, some of it at Farragut Naval Training Station examining recruits.

With the new Lake City General Hospital opening after the war, Dr. Horning did lots of surgery and thought of it as his specialty. His daughter, Carol, says, "He loved surgery, describing it as like working on a car with the motor running." He built the home at 806 South 11th Street, now occupied by Dr. Jack Riggs. Dr. Horning died of a coronary March 20, 1950.

DR. JOHN HUNT SHEPHARD

Dr. Shephard was born in Iowa in February 1879, and attended Grinnell College there. He received his medical education and degree at Rush Medical College in Chicago. After his internship, he came west by train in 1906 to visit a sister in Cheney, Washington. He left the train at St. Maries and came on to Coeur d'Alene by steamship. It was coincidental that one of the first people he met was Dr. John T. Wood, who told him of the need for more doctors because of many injuries to those working in mills, mines and logging. That, added to the usual births and deaths, put a strain on the doctors on hand.

His first night in town, he went to the hotel and signed for a room. He noticed a card game going on, and asked, "What are you playing?" Someone said, "Solo." Dr. Shephard said, "There's a pistol on the table. What is that for?" "That," said the player with a nod toward the gun, "is to keep the peace and silence onlookers!"

After visiting his sister, Dr. Shephard returned to Coeur d'Alene and set up his medical and surgical practice. He, as many young professionals, became interested in politics and on April 5, 1907 was elected to the city council. Councilmen served for two years and earned fifty dollars annually. Dr. Shephard served on the lights and streets committee. On May 14, 1909, the streets were ordered cleaned and repaired and "all males 18 to 50 ordered to pay a tax or work on the streets." He later served as mayor of the city.

Dr. Shephard married Vera Nevers and they built a beautiful home on West Lakeshore Drive, now occupied by another doctor, Ernest Gumprecht and family. They became the parents of a son, John, now a retired attorney who with his wife, Mary, divide their time between California and Hayden Lake. They also had a daughter, with both children being born in Coeur d'Alene.

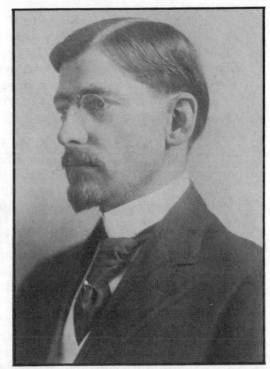

Dr. John Hunt Shephard arrived by steamboat in Coeur d'Alene early in the century and helped build a hospital. He was elected mayor or the town. He and Mrs. Shephard built a lovely home fronting the lake at 613 West Lakeshore Drive, which is now occupied by another doctor, Dr. Ernest Gumprecht, and his family.

(Photo courtesy John Shephard)

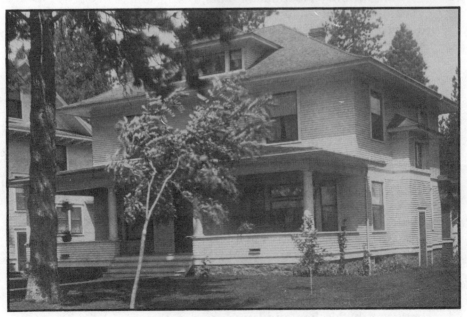

Doctors Shephard and John T. Wood built the Coeur d'Alene Hospital from an old Fort Sherman barracks building, and had the first X-ray machine in the county. Dr. Shephard left in 1916 and went to the Mayo Clinic where he had a fellowship in the study of neck and breast surgery. Later the Shephards moved to San Jose, California to spend the rest of their lives.

DR. E. R. W. FOX
Dr. E.R.W. Fox with his wife, Ellen Susan, and baby son, John Gatewood, came to Coeur d'Alene and opened his medical practice in 1939. He is still in practice and shows no sign of stopping. A few years after their arrival in Coeur d'Alene, they added son, David, to the family and both sons have since added grandchildren for Dr. Fox. When Ellen died they had been married forty-seven years.

As with many other young doctors of the time, Dr. Fox worked his own way through medical school, with summer duties consisting of counseling at boys camps in northern Wisconsin. He earned a bachelor of science degree from Rush Medical College at the University of Chicago in 1934 and his internship and medical residency were at Ancker City and County Hospital, St. Paul, Minnesota.

The Fox family had scarcely become settled when Coeur d'Alene changed almost overnight into a boom town, due to the close proximity and the building of Farragut Naval Training Station on the shores of Lake Pend Oreille. There were 50,000 "boot" sailors at Farragut, which had its own hospital, but only seven physicians in Coeur d'Alene. This brought with it the usual quota of interesting illnesses, ranging from rheumatic fever to "cat fever."

The boom atmosphere was not the only thing in which the doctor had to accustom himself. He entered practice with Dr. Otto Husted in his fourteen bed hospital, fresh from his residency in a 500-bed hospital. Brother Doctors Harold J. and W.H. Sturges, graduates of the College of Medical Evangelists, came to Coeur d'Alene in 1924, and owned the Lake City General Hospital. There was rivalry between the two hospitals and Husted eventually bought out the Sturges brothers, and built an extension on the hospital. The new facility had twenty-four beds and eleven bassinets, one X-ray machine, and a basement laboratory between the kitchen and laundry.

Dr. Fox practiced with Dr. Husted for twenty-one years.

He is a fellow of the American College of Surgeons and the American College of Obstetricians and Gynecologists. Dr. Fox served as president of the Idaho Medical Association, the Coeur d'Alene Rotary Club, and chief of staff of Kootenai Memorial Hospital. He is a charter member of the Idaho Cancer Coordinating Committee, the Coeur d'Alene unit of the American Cancer Society, and Hospice of North Idaho.

A talented writer, he is editor for Idaho on the editorial board for the *Western Journal of Medicine* and a contributing editor to the *Coeur d'Alene Press* with a weekly column on health subjects. Dr. Fox is equally talented at landscape gardening and his home grounds are viewed with appreciation.

THE DOCTORS GUMPRECHT

Dr. Donald Max Gumprecht, and his wife, Dr. Jane Doering Gumprecht, arrived in Coeur d'Alene in 1951 to open a joint practice. They have three sons, all of whom are doctors; and one daughter, Ruth Ellen Carlson, a graduate of Montana State University with a double major in music. Doctors Don and Jane were born in Montana, he at Helena on February 12, 1921 and she at Lewistown, February 6, 1922. Dr. Donald was raised on the family farm west of Helena, and he won several blue ribbons as a 4-H member for the vegetables he raised.

At Montana State College, where he received his B.S. degree in 1942, he was a cadet colonel in ROTC, member of Scabbard and Blade and Senior Septum Viri. He received his B.M. and M.D. from the University of Minnesota Medical School, which he attended 1944-47. His rotating internship was served in 1948 at Minneapolis General Hospital. At Officer's Candidate School, Fort Benning, Georgia, he was given the rank of second lieutenant, infantry, and was a captain with the U.S. Air Force from 1949-51.

The doctors were married September 3, 1944, while attending medical school. Both have been president of the Kootenai Medical Association and held committee appointments with the state association. He was chief of staff at Lake City General Hospital. They both practiced at

Three Forks, Montana, Fairchild Air Force base in Washington and in Coeur d'Alene.

From the time she was four until age eleven, Dr. Jane's family moved nine times as her father managed stores in California, Utah, and Montana. She graduated valedictorian of her high school class and with honors from Montana State College, where she received her B.S. degree in 1942. Her B.M. and M.D. degrees are from the University of Minnesota Medical School, 1942–46. A fifteen months rotating internship was at Minneapolis General Hospital.

Both the Gumprechts remember amusing incidents in their practice. Don tells of a couple of years after being in Coeur d'Alene, the family was seated at the Christmas dinner table. The phone rang and a woman asked him if he would make a house call. He said, "Your name isn't familiar to me and I don't think you are a patient of mine." She said, "No, but I wouldn't think of bothering Dr. Fox on Christmas!"

Jane remembers a day when Dr. Don was fishing and a patient of his phoned with an emergency. The caller was in 4-H and some of her piglets from a prize sow were dying. She pleaded, "Dr. Jane, would you please come and see them? The vet isn't able to come." So, Jane went out and slogged through the barnyard mud to the pigs. The piglets still alive were dragging their hind quarters. Questions brought out the fact that the vet prescribed a combination of penicillin and streptomycin for "milk fever," but the dosage was for an adult pig. Dr. Jane said, "With streptomycin a neurotoxin, I had the diagnosis. The piglets were having trouble breathing, so I gave shots of adrenalin. They survived. Of course, I was given credit for saving their lives but it also may have been luck!"

DR. DONALD GEORGE GUMPRECHT

Donald G. Gumprecht was graduated from the University of Washington Medical School and took his residency in internal medicine at Southern Illinois Medical School, where he was chief resident. He was granted a fellowship in pulmonary medicine at the University of Washington Medical School, and is board-certified in internal and pulmonary medicine. He practiced as pulmonologist in Coeur d'Alene for ten years before going to Springfield,

Illinois, where hs is practicing and clinical instructor in pulmonology at Southern Illinois Medical School and an affiliated hospital.

DR. THOMAS FRANK GUMPRECHT

Thomas graduated from the University of Washington Medical School and took his residency in internal medicine in San Diego and at the school from which he had received his M.D. His general surgery residency was for one year in Pueblo, Colorado, and in eye, ear, nose, and throat at the University of Colorado in Denver. He is board-certified in internal medicine and E.E.N.T. He first practiced in Lewiston and is now located in Bellevue, Washington.

DR. ERNEST CHARLES GUMPRECHT

Ernest graduated from the University of Washington Medical School and took his residency in internal medicine at Rutgers Medical School and was resident in cardiology at the Heart Institute in Kansas City, Missouri. He is board-certified in cardiology and internal medicine. He is practicing in Coeur d'Alene.

DR. EDWARD LEO GALLIVAN

Dr. Gallivan was born in Helena, Montana, February 4, 1908, and attended grade and high school, and Carroll College there.

He received his M.D. from St. Louis School of Medicine in 1932. Dr. Gallivan had a general practice in Helena, until returning to St. Louis for a degree in radiology.

The Gallivans moved to Coeur d'Alene in 1956, and he was the only radiologist in the Panhandle. Besides Coeur d'Alene, he traveled to Bonners Ferry, Sandpoint, Wallace, Kellogg, and St. Maries. His family kidded about his living in his car. Often films from these towns arrived at the Gallivan home, having traveled by bus and taxi. Dr. Gallivan would read the films at home, and call in the results to the waiting doctor. At that time Shoshone County was on mountain time, and that meant he had to get up at 2:00 A.M. to get to Shoshone County in time. Traveling during the winter was not one of his favorite pasttimes.

At that time the hospital in Coeur d'Alene was the small

Lake City General. The hospital was so small, that on one occasion he had to share his hospital office with a corpse.

As a child Dr. Gallivan had polio and was unable to go into the military service. In 1935 he married Ellen Sullivan in St. Louis. They had two sons and four daughters.

DR. REX T. HENSON

Dr. Henson was born August 23, 1900 at Athol, Idaho. His father was a school teacher. He went to grade school in Athol and Lewis and Clark High School, Spokane. In 1926 he received an A.B. degree and in 1931 his M.D. from George Washington University Medical School. Dr. Henson interned at Deaconess Hospital, Spokane. He practiced in Phoenix, Arizona, and Coeur d'Alene. He was on the staff at Lake City General Hospital and Coeur d'Alene General Hospital. In Phoenix he was on the staff of the U.S. Public Health Hospital. From 1942–46 he was in the U.S. Air Force.

The doctor belonged to the American, Idaho State and Kootenai Medical associations. He and his wife, Edna, had a daughter.

DR. HARREL DON MOSELEY

Dr. Moseley was born March 6, 1917 at Oklahoma City and received his grade and high school educations there. He attended Central State College in Edmond; University of Oklahoma in Norman, and earned his M.D. degree in 1943 from the University of Tennessee Medical School in Memphis. His internship and residency were from 1943–45 at St. Anthony Hospital in Oklahoma City.

As an Army captain, he was stationed as chief of surgery services at the 183d General Hospital at Fort Richardson, Alaska, twelve miles from Anchorage during a part of World War II. It was there he met Kathleen McGarvie, Army nurse from Oakland, California, and they were later married. They are the parents of a daughter, Donna Kay Crumb, and two sons, Charles William and David Jefferson.

Dr. Moseley practiced in Oklahoma City in 1947 and in St. Maries, Idaho, where he was manager and chief surgeon at the hospital for Western Hospital Association, 1947–50. He also served as district surgeon for the Milwaukee Railroad at the same time. The Moseleys moved to Coeur d'Alene in 1950 and he opened a general

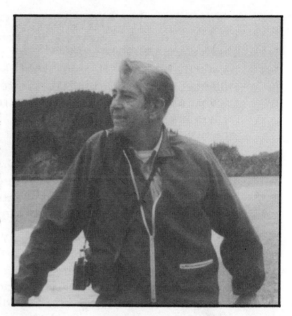

Next to practicing medicine, the late Dr. H. Don Moseley of Coeur d'Alene enjoyed fishing. He is on a fishing boat near Seward, Alaska, in 1975. It was while fishing along the Little Salmon River that he was killed in a rockslide, loosened by the previous night's rain.

(Courtesy Kathy Moseley)

surgery and family practice until 1978, when he became field representative for the Joint Committee on Hospital Accreditation.

Dr. Moseley was a member of the Idaho Board of Medicine, 1973–79; and chairman of the Idaho Medical Disciplinary Board, 1977–79. He was a member of the American, Idaho and Kootenai-Benewah Medical associations; American Cancer Society and Idaho division president and delegate; American Association of Family Practitioners; and a Fellow of the American Society of Abdominal Surgery.

He had the experience of performing two successful amputations for gas gangrene within one year, 1947–48, in St. Maries. Dr. Moseley had traveled by boat, jeep, airplane and railroad section car to reach his patients. On one occasion in 1950, he performed an emergency appendectomy on a scarlet fever patient at his apartment in St. Maries. The man's wife assisted the doctor.

Dr. Moseley raised wild turkeys and gave them to the fish and game department for release or to his friend, Lloyd Jones, dude ranch operator at Harrison. It was while he was fishing on the Little Salmon River on August 8, 1981, that he was killed by a rockslide.

DR. HOWARD A. HUGHES

Dr. Hughes was born in Steubenville, Ohio, March 22, 1914. He lived in Canton, Ohio, until 1932. In 1936 he received his B.S. degree from Mount Union College, Alliance, Ohio; M.D. in 1941, Western Reserve University, Cleveland. He interned at E.W. Sparrow Hospital, 1942, and University hospitals, Cleveland, 1945. From 1945-64 he practiced in Coeur d'Alene. He was on the staff at both the Lake City and Coeur d'Alene General hospitals. From 1942-45 he was in the U. S. Navy; Southwest Pacific theater; Solomon Islands; New Guinea; Marshalls; Marianas. He and Laverne Ruth Withers were married May 7, 1938 in Cleveland, Ohio. They have a son and two daughters.

DR. WILBUR H. LYON, JR.

Dr. Lyon was born November 8, 1924 in Miraj, India, where his father was a Presbyterian missionary. His sister, Dr. Lois Neumann, was assistant professor in pediatrics at New York University Medical School.

He went to Woodstock High School in India, and came to the United States in 1941. In 1942 he went to Princeton. From March 1943 to December 1945 with the Air Force he was a navigator, radar operator, and bombardier with the B-29 509th bomb group; and squadron navigator in 325th troop carrior squadron 20th Air Force, Tinian. He was a captain and received the Air Medal.

In 1947 he received his B.A. from Wooster College, Ohio. He went to Hartford Medical School from 1947-51 and got his M.D. in 1951. For three years he had a surgery internship and residency at Roosevelt Hospital, New York City. He had a surgery residency at Boston V.A. Hospital, and teaching fellowship in surgery at Boston University Medical School.

He practiced in San Raphael, California from January 1958-June 1959. From August 1959-July 1961 he was chief of surgery, Hospital of American Samoa, Pago Pago. He started his private practice in Coeur d'Alene August 1961.

He was doctor aboard the yacht "Gerda" for a month in 1952, and treated many fishermen and Eskimos in Newfoundland, Labrador, and Greenland. In Samoa the villages were reached only by mountain trails or outrigger canoes. Dr. Lyon made an unusual house call to Swain's

Island, 200 miles from Samoa, via Coast Guard buoy tender, to see a seriously ill patient and bring her to the hospital. He helped evacuate the hospital for American Samoa during a tidal wave resulting from an earthquake in Chile. He was honored by a special resolution of the senate in American Samoa expressing appreciation for his work there as chief of surgery.

Dr. Lyon was on the staff at Marin General Hospital, San Rafael General, and Ross General; staff at Lake City and Coeur d'Alene General hospitals. He is a member of the American, Kootenai and Benewah Medical societies.

He and his wife, Joan, have three sons, and a daughter.

DR. DUANE A. DAUGHARTY

Dr. Daugharty was born on June 17, 1925 in Minneapolis, Minnesota, where his father was a forester. After high school graduation, he spent three years in the U.S. Navy. He was graduated with an A.B. from Carroll College, Helena, Montana in 1950; an M.D. from St. Louis University Medical School in 1955; and joined the medical fraternity Alpha Kappa Kappa, as well as Sigma Alpha Epsilon.

Dr. Daugharty's internship and residency were at the St. Louis City Hospital from 1955-59. His residency was in internal medicine. His last year in residency he was chief at the VA Hospital and chief of medical service at St. Louis City Hospital. He started practice in Coeur d'Alene on October 15, 1959 and continues to practice.

In medical and community activities, Dr. Daugharty served two years as president of the Idaho Heart Association, on American Cancer Society of Idaho board of directors; on the Kootenai Medical Center board of trustees since 1978; instrumental in starting first coronary unit at the medical center; district one trustee for the Idaho Medical Association; medical director for Kootenai Cancer Society; and member, Spokane Society of Internal Medicine.

DRS. BARBARA AND SUSAN DAUGHARTY

Dr. Duane and Mrs. Daugharty are the parents of seven children, two of whom are doctors. Barbara has an M.S. in nursing and an M.D. from the University of North Dakota School of Medicine. She served her residency in internal medicine at the University of Utah Medical School.

Susan received a B.S. in zoology at Idaho State University and an M.D. at the University of Washington. Her residency in internal medicine was at the Utah School of Medicine. The other five children are Jan, Stacey, Amy, Duane, and Paul.

DR. JOHN M. LANHAM

Dr. Lanham was born in Nebraska, and raised in central Idaho on an eighty-acre farm in Long Valley, near Cascade. He graduated from the College of Idaho in 1952, and taught public school four years before entering the Army for two years. A personal tragedy stimulated in him a desire to study medicine, when their baby son had water on the brain and they learned it was inoperable. He entered George Washington School of Medicine in Washington, D.C., and graduated in 1962. He later wrote, "Medical school was one of the most exciting times of my life. Each day was a day of new discovery. I was . . . amazed at the amount of material to read, digest, reorganize, apply and reapply."

After graduation he accepted an internship at Thomas Dee Memorial Hospital in Ogden. He practiced in Coeur d'Alene and was chief of staff at Kootenai Memorial Hospital. In 1975, he withdrew from the practice of medicine in protest over the malpractice crisis and governmental encroachment into the field, saying that a physician must compromise his principles to function within the demanding bureaucratic system.

Later the Lanhams and their four children moved to Michigan where he practiced industrial medicine.

DR. JAMES WESLEY HAWKINS

Dr. Hawkins was born March 10, 1909, to Mr. and Mrs. James V. Hawkins who had moved to Coeur d'Alene from St. Joe during the devastating fire of 1910. He attended grade and high schools in Coeur d'Alene and received his bachelor and master degrees from the University of Idaho. He graduated *summa cum laude* from Harvard Medical School in 1935 and interned at Cincinnati General Hospital.

In 1937, he was named by Governor Barzilla Clark to direct the Idaho Public Health Department, during which he established well-child clinics and health units throughout the state. He returned to Harvard for further studies as

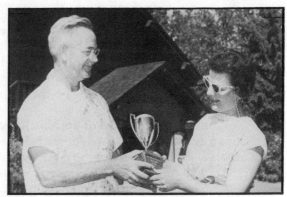

surgical house officer at Peter Bent Brigham Hospital in Boston, and received master and doctorate degrees in cancer research at Harvard.

Commissioned an officer in the U.S. Public Health Service, he was in charge of epidemiologic studies of cancer at the National Cancer Institute, the cancer control program, and was one of the first physicians to promote self-examination for detection of breast cancer, which was then controversial. Dr. Hawkins did the original fluoride studies on tooth decay.

As senior medical officer during World War II, Dr. Hawkins served three years of sea duty in the South Pacific, where his ship was involved in major naval battles, including Leyte and the Coral Sea. Following the war and returning to cancer research at the institute and serving as resident surgeon at Pondville Cancer Hospital in Walpole, Massachusetts, he established and directed the Boston unit of the National Cancer Institute, was associate professor of pathology at Harvard, associate pathologist at Children's Hospital, and junior associate at Peter Bent Brigham.

Prior to returning to Coeur d'Alene in 1947, Dr. Hawkins spoke to the United Nations on the cause and management of epidemics in Third World countries. From 1948 until 1957, he was in partnership with Drs. Otto Husted and E.R.W. Fox. He then purchased the Coeur d'Alene Medical Clinic. He was affiliated with Kootenai Memorial Hospital and Sacred Heart in Spokane until his death April 3, 1972. He left his widow, Ida Daugharty Hawkins; three daughters, Carol, Betsy and Mary; four sons, William, John, Ronald and Richard and stepson, Robert.

DR. LYNN C. FREDRIKSON

Dr. Fredrikson was born in Davenport, North Dakota January 15, 1914. His father died in the 1919 flu epidemic. His mother taught school to raise her five boys, four of whom received college, two professional degrees. The doctor had worked his way through college and medical school.

From 1932–36 he went to North Dakota State University and received his B.S. degree. In 1940 he received a B.M. degree from Northwestern University, and his M.D. in 1941. He interned at St. Joseph's Hospital, Chicago from 1947–50, and Carle Hospital Clinic, Champaign, Illinois, in surgery, 1945–47. From 1947–59 he practiced in Spirit Lake, and moved to Coeur d'Alene in 1959.

One winter, the doctor and a helper donned snowshoes to move a woman with a fractured pelvis on a toboggan from an island in the middle of frozen Spirit Lake to a point where the road had been plowed.

He was on the staff at the Spirit Lake Community, Lake City General, and Coeur d'Alene hospitals. He belonged to the Kootenai County Medical Society. From 1941–46 he was a major in the U. S. Army Medical Corps in the European theater. He received four battle ribbons, three overseas stripes, and the Purple Heart for valor under fire.

The Fredriksons have three sons. They now make their home in Arizona.

DR. FRANK WENZ

Dr. Frank Wenz was born in Wurttemburger, Germany, where he received his grade and high school education, before immigrating to Galena, Illinois, with his parents, Mr. and Mrs. Christian W. Wurttemburger. He attended the Detroit College of Medicine and became a medical doctor in 1889. With his diploma in his pocket, he came west in 1890, with Spokane, Washington as his destination. When the train stopped at Rathdrum, Dr. Wenz stepped out on the platform, liked what he saw, and stayed there.

He bought a medical practice and drugstore (perhaps from Dr. D.D. Drennan, according to Dr. Frances S. Heard's chapter on health care which is part of a social history she is writing: *North Idaho Scrapbook*). He mixed his own prescriptions in the drugstore. Dr. Wenz became active in the town of Rathdrum, serving as trustee and clerk of the school board; city health officer; member of the council; physician for Modern Woodmen of America; member of the Masonic Lodge.

Dr. Wenz became county health officer when Kootenai encompassed what are now Boundary, Bonner, and Benewah counties. Multi-talented, the doctor contributed definitions for the 1915 unabridged *Funk and Wagnalls Dictionary;* achieved much success in treating victims during the flu epidemic of 1918–19; developed a special bicycle with flanged wheels to ride the rails from Rathdrum to patients in the area. He also traveled by horse and buggy as well as sleigh. Dr. Wenz opened a creamery in 1895 with twelve horsepower boilers, cream separators, butter maker, and cold storage. He also had interests in farming and in the Continental Mine near the Canadian border.

Dr. and Mrs. Wenz had five daughters.

DR. EDWARD N. HAMACHER, JR.

Eddie Hamacher, Jr. was not yet born when his father became one of the thousands that died during the flu epidemic of 1918. Eddie was born in Spirit Lake on February 7, 1919, where his father managed the laundry for the corporation operating Panhandle Lumber Company and the Spirit Lake Land Company. There was also a box factory. Together the lumber companies hired nearly 450 workers in the town that began in 1907. There were also large railroad machine shops where the powerful double-piston Mallet engines could be installed.

There were many different types of injuries in such work, and the corporation had built a hospital and con-tracted with doctors to serve in it. Among those were Doctors Pringle and Lewis. A Dr. Spooner was also a druggist and operated the store and medical office on Main Street. Phil Dolan, close friend of young Eddie Hamacher, remembered Dr. Pringle using the school gym as an operating room and removing tonsils of about sixty people in one day.

Eddie remembers lying on the green grass of the Spirit Lake Park, across the street from the hospital, on warm summer days and liking the smell of ether that came wafting his way. "I thought it must be a wonderful thing to be a doctor, to heal sick people, and to repair broken bones," Dr. Hamacher reminisced many years later. He had reason to know of the setting of bones, for he suffered a broken arm in jumping off the barn roof. He played football in high school and was given a scholarship to Gonzaga University in Spokane. The second year he injured his shoulder and turned to serious study as a pre-med student. He was elected student body president and was awarded a scholarship to study medicine at Georgetown University, Washington, D.C., beginning in 1936.

He met a skilled plastic surgeon, Dr. Moran, and did his residency in the east. Dr. Bob Rotchford of Spokane, also a plastic surgeon, had helped and encouraged the young doctor all the way through his studies. He joined Dr. Rotchford after medical service with the U.S. Army at Fort Campbell, Kentucky, in World War II. It was not long before people were talking of the skill of Dr. Hamacher who was performing delicate surgery on many crippled children. He developed new types of bone surgery, and was always available for emergency surgeries.

In Washington, D.C., Dr. Hamacher met and married a nurse. They became the parents of six children: Bob, Eddie, Tom, Paul, Christine, and Regina.

DR. ALEXANDER CAIRNS

John Harrison of Hayden Lake, whose parents came to Coeur d'Alene in 1904, two years before John's birth, remembers Dr. Alexander Cairns as a "big Scotsman, six feet, four or five inches tall. He played the bagpipes and marched back and forth on his front porch at 615 Wallace Avenue. He wore the kilts, and all the trappings, and annoyed the neighbors with his piping."

Dr. Cairns practiced medicine in Coeur d'Alene from 1910 until 1920, when he died.

DR. ALEXANDER HUNTER

Dr. Hunter was graduated from McGill University Medical School in Montreal, Canada. His first practice in Idaho was at Juliaetta, where two children, Clifford and Eleanor, were born to him and Mrs. Hunter. They moved to Coeur d'Alene in 1906 and he established an office on the second floor of the Clark Building, Sherman and Fifth.

The family home was at 501 Foster Avenue. Dr. Hunter developed multiplesclerosis and retired from practice in 1912. He died in 1914. Mrs. Hunter moved to Chicago to live with her daughter and died in 1956. They were members of the Presbyterian Church.

DR. OTTO MAXWELL HUSTED

Otto Husted was born August 7, 1897 in Rooks County, Kansas, where his parents operated a farm. Elementary school was at Codell, Kansas, junior high and high school at Madera, California. He attended the University of Redlands Prep School, where he also took his pre-medical training. Dr. Husted was at the University of Southern California Student Army Medical Corps from 1918 to 1920. He graduated from the University of Nebraska in Omaha with his M.D. He was a member of Phi Chi. He interned at University Hospital and did his residency at Seattle General and Orthopedic hospitals in Seattle in 1924–25. Postgraduate work was done in 1933 at Peter Bent Brigham in Boston and one semester each in 1934 and 1936 at Toulaine, France.

Dr. Husted practiced in Marmouth, North Dakota in 1923; Clearwater County, Idaho from 1925 to 1931, and in

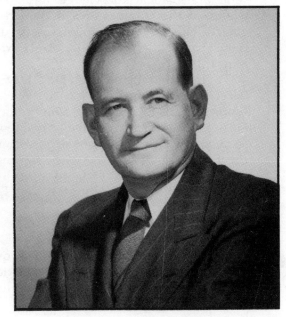

Dr. Otto Maxwell Husted, practitioner in northern Idaho for many years, was born August 7, 1897, and died January 17, 1962. He was the primary builder of the Lake City General Hospital in Coeur d'Alene.
(Photo courtesy Enid Nissen)

Coeur d'Alene from 1931 until retirement in 1961. He died on January 17, 1962. He built and operated Lake City General Hospital and brought Dr. E.R.W. Fox from Chicago to be associated with him for a number of years. Other doctors also practiced with Dr. Husted.

In North Dakota he performed tonsillectomies and appendectomies in his office and in Idaho delivered many babies in homes. He remembered the devastation of the influenza epidemic of 1918. Dr. Husted used a variety of methods of travel: horseback, horse and buggy, and a Model T; and was stuck many times in the "gumbo mud" of North Dakota. He was president of the Kootenai County Medical Society in 1934; member, Northwest Arthritis Society; and a Fellow in the International College of Medicine.

His children are Dr. Dean Husted, dentist; Dr. Robert M., internist; Michael and James Paul, and two daughters, Mrs. W.S. Barnett and Connie Johnson.

KOOTENAI-BENEWAH MEDICAL ASSOCIATION

"To promote the harmony and unity of action of the medical profession, to join with other such associations, to stimulate the advancement of medical science, to disseminate medical knowledge, and to guard and foster the health of the communities in which we serve," were the objects cited by a group of Coeur d'Alene doctors when they formed the Kootenai County Medical Association on May 1, 1920.

Original members were Drs. D.D. Drennan, Alexander Barclay Sr., John T. Wood, W.H. Holden and C.E. Worthington. Dr. Drennan was named president; Dr. J.M. Finney of Harrison, vice president and Dr. Barclay, secretary-treasurer, an office he resigned from at the next meeting, May 31. He was back signing the minutes as that officer in November. They adopted a constitution and by-laws. Drs. Wood, Worthington and F.L. McCauley of Post Falls were elected censors.

Invitation was extended to the Idaho Medical Association to hold its summer meeting in Coeur d'Alene on June 10 and 11. The state meeting was quite an event with a banquet at Hayden Lake, a launch ride on the lake, and a rental of films from Stoddard Dray line. The total bill was

$99.70. Minutes reveal the dues of five dollars per year covered most expenses, with some members adding funds when needed. Stenographers were paid from seventy-five cents to $1.25 for taking notes at meetings.

The state association returned to Coeur d'Alene for the annual session June 27 and 28 in 1930. Kootenai members voted to charge a registration fee of five dollars and that the secretary send an invitation to every member in Idaho. All invitees were urged to "bring your bathing suits." All were taken to the Boy Scout camp by launch and a noon meal was served there. The Friday evening banquet was at Bozanta Tavern. By that time an active medical auxiliary had been formed, and the Kootenai members planned the entertainment for wives of the visiting doctors. Business meetings were held at the Masonic Temple on Sherman Avenue.

Just as the program and festivities had expanded, so had the costs. Boat hire and the Scout camp lunch totaled thirty-five dollars; refreshments at Bozanta $85.55; and banquet, $112.50.

The society added one or two members each meeting. Members added include Drs. P.J. Scallen, F.W. Thurston, Harold T. Anderson; F. Wentz of Rathdrum, J.C. Dwyer; T.J. Stauffer and H.F. Schrader of Rose Lake, S.W. Didier of Plummer; E.S. Prindle, C.W. Martin and Robert Gerlough of Spirit Lake. J.H. Sturges (who was continued as an honorary member when he moved his practice to Bukama in the Belgian Congo in 1929), C.A. Spooner, Nelson T. Hersey, Jones, Eugene Spohn, who later moved to Priest River; Karl May and H.R. Baukerd of Harrison. In 1932, members added: Dr. Otto M. Husted transferred from the Tri-County Medical Association, Dr. John Schori, Spirit Lake, transferred from Spokane County, and Dr. Rex T. Henson.

In latter years the Kootenai and Benewah associations joined in one unit.

SHOSHONE COUNTY

The original Shoshone County was created by the Territorial Legislature of Washington, of which Idaho was then part. When Idaho became a territory, including Montana, Wyoming and parts of the Dakotas, the boundaries were changed to those of present Shoshone and Clearwater counties, the latter being changed to a single county in 1904. The Coeur d'Alene mining district in Shoshone became one of the most important in the world for its silver, lead and zinc. The first settlement at Wallace, in 1864, was called Placer Center. Wardner, Kellogg and Mullan soon followed. Much of Idaho's history occurred in, or is associated with, events in Shoshone County.

DR. WARREN F. DAVIS

Dr. Warren F. Davis, who was born September 25, 1849 in Quakerstown, Pennsylvania, was one of the very first of the Shoshone County doctors. He was graduated from Penn State Medical school in 1872, moved to Portland, Oregon in 1885 and practiced until 1895. He moved to Wardner in 1886 and practiced until 1892, when he moved back to Portland.

Dr. Davis was urged to move to Shoshone County by a close friend, Simeon Reed, at one time the largest stockholder in Bunker Hill and Sullivan Mining Company.

DR. CHARLES E. SEARS

An early-day surgeon in Wallace was Dr. Charles E. Sears. He married Irma Mentz Sears in Chicago in 1905, then left by train for Wallace.

Dr. Sears was born in 1880 at a town named for his family, Searstown, Illinois, now Rock Island. His father had the first flour mill west of the Mississippi. He had one sister, Heginoria. From the age of twelve, when his father died of cancer, he determined to become a doctor and see if he could help prevent such deaths. He was graduated from Rush Medical and Northwestern universities. He interned at Cook County Hospital, Chicago, where he was contacted to come to Wallace and operate the hospital there.

Dr. and Mrs. Sears arrived in Idaho about the same time as other newlyweds, Mr. and Mrs. John P. Gray, and

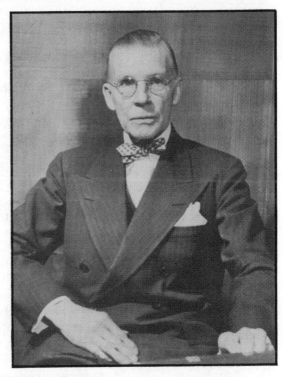

Dr. Charles E. Sears of Wallace was described to the author as "perhaps the first clean doctor in Shoshone County." He was a meticulous man, as can be noted by his dress, and he has the "born physician hands." A perfectionist who demanded the best from himself and others, he became a noted physician.
(Courtesy his daughter, Norma Sears Lee)

formed such a solid friendship that it is being carried on by their children. John P. Gray was to become an international mining attorney, and Sears an equally well-known physician and surgeon.

The Sears' daughter, Norma, and the Grays' daughter, Mary Lee, later attended Miss Bennett's School in Milbrook, New York together. Dr. Sears brought Katherine, the Grays' oldest daughter, and his own two daughters, Marcella and Norma, into the world of Wallace. Mrs. Sears used to tell Norma that she "was born between night and day" as the Days lived on one side of their house and the Knights on the other. Mrs. Sears not only had a sense of humor, but was an accomplished vocalist and often performed for friends and groups.

Dr. Sears was fascinated with automobiles from the day the first was invented and had the first car in Idaho, and one of the first in Oregon, where he later established his own hospital and clinic. Dr. Sears taught at the University of Oregon Medical School at Eugene, where he was head of the internal and diagnostic medicine studies for forty-eight years. On two separate occasions, he was also president of the Oregon Medical Society.

Norma Sears Lee, now of Monterey, California, said, "I am sure daddy's beginning in Wallace, with the variety of illnesses, surgery, and patients, prepared him for his future. He loved the adventure of driving all over that country in those very early, primitive days and he had some harrowing experiences."

A common thread that seemed to link so many of the early day physicians and surgeons was one of high intelligence, curiosity in diverse fields, and a desire to continue their education. Thus they were omnivorous readers. Most were perfectionists with themselves and others, with the exception of keeping good financial records. Mrs. Sears told her daughters of the doctor's total disregard or interest in sending bills to his patients. If she had not been observant, "we would have starved," she said, "except for those patients who paid their bills with produce." Dr. Sears joked with John Gray saying, "They pay me with potatoes and you get mining stock!"

Dr. Sears was a friend and contemporary of the brothers Mayo and Dr. Menninger. He knew and admired Sir William Osler and preached his philosophy of "living in day-tight compartments." Sears had a brilliant mind (some said "a genius in medicine"), and patients came to him from all over the country. His many interests included fishing, hunting (at a rifle range in his basement he loaded his own shells), cars and carpentry, with a complete shop in his garage. He wrote many articles on medicine for magazines and books. Because of his perfectionism in so many fields few could match his expectations.

The Sears had packed and stored their belongings, including twenty-four packing cases of his books, in Wallace before leaving for Vienna to live, when thousands of acres of tinder-dry trees exploded into more than three-thousands blazes in August, 1910. The town of Wallace was left an ashen gray specter. The Sears belongings, including his collection of books and papers, formed a part of the ash. Later, Dr. Sears became an avid collector of books, and became a true Shakespearean scholar through his study of all Shakespeare's writings.

DR. HUGH FRANCE

During the labor troubles in 1893 and 1897 when violence threatened the mining industry of Shoshone County, Dr. Hugh France of Wardner was physician and coroner. Charged with incompetence, the sheriff was deposed and the duties of that office, by law, settled upon Dr. France. He did not shrink from the job and gathered strength from his responsibilities. He was twice elected mayor and in 1906 was nominated by the Republican party for the office of governor.

He was born at Kattaning, Pennsylvania, July 9, 1867, later moving with his family to Nebraska, where he finished school and taught for three years. He went to work for Dr. Smart in Seattle where he studied medicine in the summer. In the winter and spring he studied and was graduated from Bellevue Hospital Medical College in 1892. He immediately came west to Wardner. He was associated with Dr. R.P. Sims at Wardner and Wallace.

In 1894, Dr. France assumed medical and surgical charge of the Bunker Hill and Sullivan employees and for a short time housed patients in a frame building a short distance below the mine tunnel. In the same year, he built the Wardner Hospital which was used until 1908. He was supervisor of the building and chief surgeon for Providence Hospital in Wallace and the Wardner Hospital. He was an active member of the Idaho Medical Society and was of great assistance to the legislative committee on medical education, for which he was chairman.

In 1897, he married Hattie Johnson. They had no children. He was of robust health until 1909 when he thought he had a "slight problem". Exploratory surgery revealed cancer of the liver. He died in Seattle October 26.

DR. CALEB S. STONE

Dr. Caleb Stone arrived in Shoshone County from Colorado in September 1889. He located at Burke, where he became surgeon for the mines of Canyon Creek, receiving as a salary one dollar a month paid by each miner. When Providence Hospital in Wallace was completed, the Sisters took over the contract with the mines in the district and Dr. Stone was hired to work there. He received a percentage of the monthly dues from the miners until 1905, and also carried on a private practice for residents.

For a number of years he was city health officer and at one time county health officer. During the labor troubles in 1899, he provided medical care to the prisoners in the "Bull Pen," where several hundred miners were confined.

During the years 1905–07, he took an absence from Wallace, and on his return rejoined the hospital staff. He remained until August 1934, when he retired from practice. He was a member of the Idaho Medical Society and active in its affairs.

Dr. and Mrs. Stone had two children, both born in Wallace: Dr. C.S. Stone, Jr., Santa Barbara surgeon, and Mrs. J.C. McKisseck, San Francisco. Dr. Stone moved to Santa Barbara after his retirement.

DR. PAUL MARVIN ELLIS

From the time he was a boy on the farm at Odell, Nebraska, Paul Ellis wanted to become a doctor. He was born July 17, 1897 in the farmhouse, the son of Thomas H. and Frances Singleton Ellis. He remembered his mother driving a horse and wagon to Beatrice to shop. In 1904, Paul and three sisters, Ruth, Zella and Frances and their parents took the train to Eugene, Oregon to live.

After high school, he had one year at the University of Oregon, Eugene, where he volunteered for the Students' Army Training Corps. He worked in shipyards, sawmills and harvest fields in Washington, Oregon and Alberta in 1917–18, and when the Armistice was declared in November, he went to Twin Falls, Idaho, where his parents had moved during the war. His father farmed near Filer and worked on the first irrigation system built in that area.

Paul's sister, Zella, was attending the University of Idaho and he decided he would register there. He was graduated with a B.S. degree and a commission as first lieutenant in the Infantry Reserve in 1922.

He taught science and math and coached football at Twin Falls High in 1922–23, and this was where he met an intelligent, attractive and witty teacher, Elizabeth Davies, whom he married in Spokane on May 27, 1927. He went back to the University of Oregon to receive his M.D. in 1929, and was a resident physician at St. Luke's Hospital in

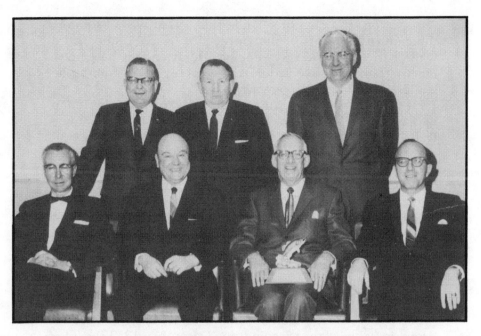

Dr. Paul Ellis was honored by fellow members of the Idaho State Board of Health when he received the Clean Water Award from the Idaho Sportsmen's Association in 1966. *Front row, left to right,* Hugh Wagnon, Dr. Ellis and Dr. Terrell Carver, director, Idaho Health Department. In the back row are Fran Blomquist, Westerman Whillock and George Watkins.
(Courtesy Paula Stephenson)

Spokane until 1930. He joined the staff of the Wallace Hospital that year and remained until the hospital was closed in 1963. The Ellises were members of the Episcopal Church where he served as vestryman and lay reader.

Dr. Ellis was a Fellow of the American College of Surgeons; associate fellow, Spokane Surgical Society, 1938; studied under the senior member of the Wallace Hospital, Dr. Max T. Smith, an associate of the American College of Surgeons, to become an associate; member of the Wallace School Board; was named by Governor C.A. Robins to the Idaho Board of Medicine when it was set up in 1947; in June 1958, was appointed by Governor Robert E. Smylie as chairman of the new Idaho State Board of Health, from which he received a citation in 1968; 1942 president, Idaho Medical Association, which gave him the Robins Community Service award; and president of the U of I Alumni

Association. His daughter Paula said, "Dad was absolutely rabid in his support of the University of Idaho and had a wall of pictures and memorabilia. He attended the games, meetings of the association and kept up with friends he had made during his university days."

He also received the Clean Water Award from the Idaho Sportsmen's Association. He was a member of Phi Gamma Delta, Nu Sigma Nu, Wallace Gyro Club, Elks Lodge and the Masonic Order. The doctor was an amateur thespian and enjoyed acting with the Valley Community Theatre.

Dr. and Mrs. Ellis had three daughters and one son: Paula Jane Pettengill, wife of Thomas Stephenson of Osburn; Marcia Gertrude, wife of Gwin J. Hicks of Walnut Creek, California; David Thomas Ellis, Spokane; and Shirley, wife of David Garness, Anchorage, Alaska. Dr. Ellis died in the Silverton hospital on January 31, 1984 at age eighty-six.

DR. ORLAND BREBNER SCOTT

Born to pioneer parents, Orland and Margaret Brebner Scott, in Chewelah, Washington, December 13, 1916, O.B. Scott was known to his grade and high school friends as "Bud" and later to associates as "Scotty." His father was a minister who served in a number of small communities in the Inland Empire until settling in Coeur d'Alene, where the future doctor received most of his preliminary education.

He attended the University of Idaho, 1935–40, where he was a member of Alpha Epsilon Delta, and the University of Chicago, 1940–44, a member of Alpha Omega Alpha. His medical education included a one-year internship and one-year residency in the University of Chicago clinics, 1944–46; and another residency at the King County Hospital (University of Washington) from 1949–52.

Dr. Scott practiced in Kellogg from 1948–49, before entering the U.S. Army Medical Corps for two years. From 1952–87, he returned to his Kellogg practice. He has been semi-retired since 1987, and still spends two days a week on emergency duty at the Shoshone Medical Center. To do this, he commutes from his home at the foot of Red Hog Mountain overlooking Lake Coeur d'Alene, which he and his second wife, Karin Rottenwallner of Germany, built a few years ago.

Dr. Scott was on the active and consulting staffs, and chief of surgery in 1959 and 1961 at Kellogg. While serving as captain in the medical corps he was stationed in Chicago; Fort Riley, Kansas; Fort Sam Houston, Texas; Camp Beale, California; and Fort Worden, Port Townsend, Washington. He was president of the Shoshone County Medical Society in 1961 and served on numerous committees.

Dr. and Virginia Scott were parents of a son, Dale, Redmond, Washington, daughters, Janet, Columbus, Ohio, and Ann Marie Hunter, also of Red Hog Mountain.

DR. H. E. BONEBRAKE

Dr. Bonebrake was born in Philomath, Oregon, October 23, 1910. His father was a preacher. He lived in Portland, and went to Jefferson High School.

He graduated from the University of Oregon Medical School in 1936. He had a rotating internship at Multnomah County Hospital 1936–37. He practiced in Wallace from 1937–59, moving to Osburn in 1959. He was on the staff at Wallace Hospital, Providence Hospital, and West Shoshone Hospital. Dr. Bonebrake belonged to the Shoshone County medical Society and Idaho State Hospital Advisory Board. he and his wife Mildred had two daughters and one son.

DR. CHARLES V. GENOWAY

Charles V. Genoway, physician and surgeon in Wallace and Boise, Idaho and Spokane, Washington, was reared by his paternal grandmother, after his mother died when he was two. He was born October 27, 1863, to Daniel C. and Ruth MacGuire Genoway in Cincinnati, Ohio. He stayed with his grandmother until he was eighteen years of age.

Charles became a teacher, earning the necessary funds to become a doctor. He then entered the medical department of Cincinnati University, graduating in 1888. After a year of postgraduate work in Cincinnati Hospital, he went into general practice there. After one year, he moved to Nashville, Tennessee, remaining until 1892.

Lured by the northwest, he moved to the mining town of Wallace, staying until 1900. The next two years he furthered his study in Vienna and Paris. This time, he came west to Spokane, practicing for eight years. He served as health officer, and was instrumental in getting into law new dairying regulations for Washington.

Dr. Genoway liked to travel and in 1908, he began an extended tour to China, Japan, other Asiatic countries, and while in Europe he again took short courses in medicine. Going on to London, he pursued four months of post-graduate work. Upon returning to the United States, he stayed in New York for further study at Bellevue Hospital.

Upon his return to Spokane, he was married to a Montana native, Helen Curran, on August 25, 1909. They were members of the Roman Catholic Church. In May 1912, Dr. and Mrs. Genoway moved to Boise. He established his offices in the Mode Building, specializing in X-ray and electro-therapeutic work.

He maintained his membership in the Elks Lodge at Wallace, where he had been exalted ruler for three years; belonged to the Idaho and American Medical associations and the Boise Physicians and Surgeons Club.

DR. T. R. MASON

Friendly, outgoing and "mildly profane," was the way one friend described Dr. T.R. Mason, who doctored many in the Kellogg area in the early 1900s. He was typical of his genre in mining towns with grubstaking prospectors, buying interest in some mines, bringing hundreds into the world, generation after generation, and serving the community in any spare time.

He was on the Sunnyside school board, mayor of Kellogg from 1917 to 1929, and director of the First National Bank there. He seldom sent a bill and many patients made sacrifices to "pay him first, because he is so decent." He liked the special relationship he had with his patients.

DR. ERNEST E. GNAEDINGER

Dr. Gnaedinger was born in Wallace, August 1, 1919. His father was a mining engineer.

The doctor attended Wallace High School, and graduated from the University of Idaho with a degree in chemical engineering. He worked for Alcoa in Vancouver, Washington until entering the service in 1944, as an electronics technician. He went back to Alcoa after the war, but decided to change professions. From 1946–47 he went

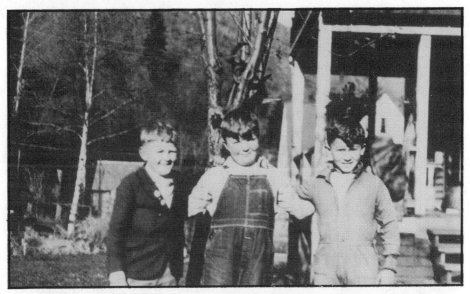

THEN AND NOW: They are changed a bit in circumference and perpendicularly, but Dr. E.E. "Ned" Gnaedinger, Max T. Smith Jr. (son of the late Dr. Max Smith), and Dr. Mike Weyer are a happy trio of boys about 1927 in Wallace. In the second picture, taken in 1990, they pose in the same lineup in a happy reunion. Max Smith Jr. lives in Florida and Dr. Weyer is in Spokane. Dr. Gnaedinger and his wife still live in Wallace.

(Photos courtesy Dr. Gnaedinger)

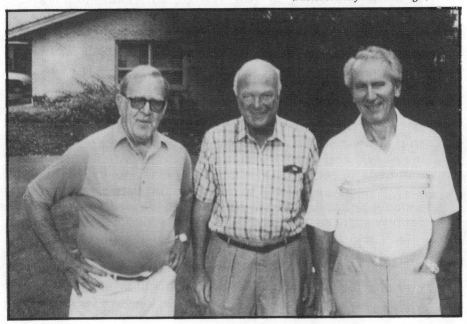

to Washington State College, Pullman, for pre-med. He attended the University of Oregon Medical School 1947-51. From 1951-52 he interned in San Bernadino County Hospital. He was a member of the American Academy of General Practice.

He started practicing medicine in Wallace in 1952.

The Gnaedingers have two sons and two daughters. Mrs. Gnaedinger said, "We are pleased to think, in this day and age of change, we are bringing up our children in the house that Dr. Gnaedinger's father built, and that the boys can play on the same mountain and fish in the same streams."

DR. CLARENCE IRWIN GIBBON

For three and one-half years before entering the University of Colorado Medical School, Clarence I. Gibbon used the knowledge he had gained in securing his B.S. and masters degrees in chemical engineering at Oregon State College as director of the Solutions Division of Cutter Laboratories in Berkeley.

He earned his M.D. degree at Colorado in 1946. He spent 1947 at the U.S. Marine Hospital in San Francisco, and was with the U.S. Army at Fort Warren, Cheyenne, in 1949, with the rank of captain. He then went to Kellogg to begin general practice. He served as both secretary and president of the Shoshone Medical Society and a member of the Idaho Board of Medical Examiners from 1961-67.

Immediately following the war years, Shoshone County became a hotbed of Communist activity, with *Life* magazine publishing a national map showing that county as one of the highest, per capita, in Communist membership in the country. Dr. Gibbon joined a number of others in a vigilant anti-Communism movement that had hundreds of recruits. Dr. Gibbon gave so much thought, energy, work and worry to the program, that his widow, Jean, feels that it hastened his death. "He cared about this country so much," she said. He died in 1970.

Jean told of her husband's caring for the people who needed a doctor. She said that he liked, best of all, sitting around a kitchen table, having a cup of hot coffee and a visit after he had taken care of someone ill at their home. "Sometimes, he would get into such a long conversation that it would be after midnight before he returned from calls out in the country."

The Gibbons had three sons and one daughter. It was for them and, even more so, for the doctor that Jean agreed to purchase a summer getaway in the mountains above Bonners Ferry. Their three sons became associated with healing arts: Larry, an M.D. at Post Falls, where he and his dentist brother, Rick, share offices; and Tom, an osteopath in Wisconsin. Their only daughter, Sally, is married to John Montandon of Coeur d'Alene.

DR. W. S. SIMS

Dr. Sims had a colorful arrival and a colorful leaving from the town of Wallace. He was from the deep south, and he had the accent to prove it. The Episcopal Church had founded the Holland Memorial Hospital, named in memory of the late husband of Mrs. Frances Holland, who Holland, who had contributed most of the funding in 1890.

Within a few months the church found the operation less than a money-making proposition and disposed of its interest to Dr. Sims. Immediately, Dr. Sims started a complete renovation of the hospital and had it completed by June 1891. He announced to the press that "The hospital is open to all respectable physicians and is controlled by no religion sect nor creed." To prove he meant it, on August 1, 1891 a Mrs. Callahan arrived from Chicago to be supervisor, and her assistant, David Strouder, was the first black man to reside in Wallace. His duties included cooking, nursing and assisting Dr. Sims with operations, and making beds.

Dr. Sims continued to operate the hospital for twenty-five years and served as coroner by appointment of Governor Frank Steuenberg, who was assassinated as an outgrowth of the labor wars in the mining district. In 1915, a policeman charged a patron of the Old Opera House with smoking in the gallery. The man pulled a gun and started shooting. Dr. Sims was struck by a stray bullet and died.

A Dr. St. Jean took over the hospital and was associated with Dr. Charles T. Mowery for a short time before Dr. Max T. Smith and Dr. Leonard Hanson took it over. Dr. Mowery moved to Spokane; Dr. Hanson died in 1925; and Dr. Smith retired in 1945.

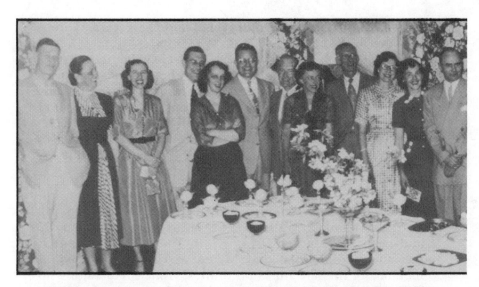

Shoshone County doctors and their wives often gathered for dinner parties and this is one of them. Left to right: Dr. Robert Staley, Willowdeen Hunter, Dr. Bob Revelli, Marie Whitesell, Dr. Glen Whitesell, Dr. E.J. and Marian Fitzgerald, Dr. Paul Ellis, Mildred Bonebrake,

DR. ROBERT W. STALEY

Dr. Bob Staley, Kellogg physician for many years, was born August 13, 1904. His father was a farmer in a rural Iowa area, where the future doctor spent his youth. He received his B.A. degree after two years, 1924-25 at the University of Nebraska and his M.D. at the Nebraska Medical School in 1930. He interned for one year at Swedish Covenant in Seattle, and had a three months residency at Seattle Orthopedic Hospital.

Dr. Staley practiced at Enumclaw, Washington from 1931 until 1939, when he and his wife, Dorothy, and their daughters moved to Kellogg. He became the owner of the Wardner Hospital in Kellogg. Dr. Staley held membership in the Shoshone County and Idaho State Medical associations. He served as president of the state group.

One of his colleagues said he was a man of direct action. To illustrate the description he told of the time Dr. Staley was in the hall of the hospital at noon, on his way to lunch, when a drunk staggered in with a face that looked like he had been run over by a truck. The drunk was very belligerent and insisted that the doctor do something right then to "fix my nose." The doctor said, "I'll fix your nose!"

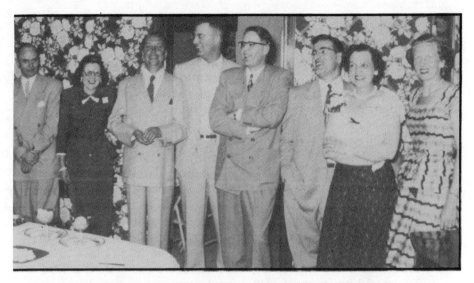

Shirley Landreth, Dr. Lewis B. Hunter, Margaret and Dr. Pete Peterson, Dr. Robert Cordwell, Dr. Hubert Bonebrake, Dr. Landreth, Dorothy Staley, and Jean Gibbon.
(Photo courtesy Marie Whitesell)

He hit the drunk and knocked his nose back into shape, and without another word, went to lunch.

One son-in-law, Dr. William Maston of Denver, is a physician. Another daughter became a physiotherapist, and a third daughter, Virginia, is married to Burgess "Bud" McDonald of Coeur d'Alene. The Staleys also had two sons.

DR. EDGAR JAMES FITZGERALD

A founder of ski facilities on Lookout Pass between the Idaho-Montana border, providing free ski school for hundreds of children; used one of the first water skis on Lake Coeur d'Alene, made out of cedar slab; "nuts about raising begonias," he said; flew his own plane, fished, hunted, loyal supporter and former president of the Board of Regents of his Alma Mater, Gonzaga University. All of these help describe Dr. Eddie Fitzgerald of Wallace. He once said, "I like everything."

As a physician he was equally versatile. While playing golf a few miles down valley from Sunshine Mine, he was called on emergency when a large ore slab fell and crushed a miner. He rushed to the mine and descended one mile underground, to be taken by mine train to the miner whose body was free except for one arm, crushed and held against another rock by a slab the size of a small room. It was necessary for the doctor to amputate on the scene.

In 1943, he delivered a pair of twins every month for eight consecutive months, and delivered only one set from then until he retired.

Dr. Fitzgerald was born in St. Paul, Minnesota, October 3, 1904. His father was an attorney and later a judge. He attended grade schools in Spokane, Culdesac, Kooskia, Orofino, and Gonzaga High School and University, Spokane, with B.A. and B.S. degrees. His M.D. was granted at St. Louis University, 1930, and he interned at City Hospital there. His residency was at Children's Hospital in Los Angeles. He said that he practiced in Wallace from 1932 "until November 20, 1961 at 4:50 p.m." Dr. and Mrs. Fitzgerald have one daughter and a son.

DR. GLEN MARTIN WHITESELL

University of Idaho pep band leader, Army Medical Corps captain, husband, father and grandfather, and a medical doctor who had delivered more than 3,000 babies: this was Dr. Glen Whitesell of Kellogg. At the time of his death, September 15, 1978, a longtime friend, Barbara Craig, was moved to compose a ditty called,

"See You Later, Doc"
For twenty-eight years a friend you've been,
Delivering my babies, and others, again and again.
You've listened to complaints, sighs and regrets.
Standing with tears in your eyes at some upsets.

This is a small portion of a lengthy poem, but well describes a part of the life of an Idaho doctor.

Born September 22, 1916 in Spokane, Dr. Whitesell went from the Spokane schools to the University of Idaho for a B.S. degree in zoology. He was a member of Sigma Nu, Silver Lance and Blue Key. His M.D. degree was from the University of Chicago and he interned at Billings Hospital, Chicago, and Denver General in Colorado.

When discharged in Missoula, Montana at the end of World War II as captain in the Army Medical Corps serving overseas with the 167th General Hospital, Dr. Whitesell settled in Kellogg. When he joined the clinic, which had a contract with Bunker Hill and other mining companies including Sunshine, he found he was working with a group of outstanding, well-educated physicians. They included Drs. Glenn McCaffery (Loma Linda College, Los Angeles), Robert E. Staley (University of Nebraska), Robert Cordwell (University of Rochester, New York), Clarence I. Gibbon (University of Colorado), and O.B. Scott (University of Chicago and University of Washington). Later they were joined by Dr. Hubert Bonebrake (University of Oregon). Most of the doctors took yearly refresher courses.

Glen Whitesell and Marie Haasch of Twin Falls were University of Idaho classmates and it was there they became engaged. They were married after graduation, September 4, 1939, at Twin Falls, where they boarded the train for Chicago and his medical education.

Dr. and Mrs. Whitesell had one son, William, and two daughters, Mary and Julie, and fourteen grandchildren. Mrs. Whitesell lives in the lake home, "Loch Hurst," overlooking Bennett's Bay on Lake Coeur d'Alene which they bought from the late Ramsay and Abbie Walker in 1953. They used it as a family summer place until 1962 when they made it their permanent home. Until his death, Dr. Whitesell commuted to Kellogg to maintain his practice.

DR. ROBERT J. REVELLI

Robert Revelli was born in Wallace, Idaho, November 13, 1919. His father was a mine safety engineer. Dr. Revelli went to grade and high schools in Wallace. In high school he won an award for "All State Basketball Guard." He worked as an orderly at Deaconess Hospital in Spokane.

He attended the University of Idaho from 1937–40, and received his B.S. degree. He received his medical degree from Jefferson Medical College in 1944, and was rated second in his class. He was president of Phi Delta Theta; member, Alpha Kappa Kappa; president, Alpha Omega Alpha. He interned at Jefferson Medical College Hospital, Philadelphia, Pennsylvania. From October, 1946 to March 1947, he was in residency at Altoona Hospital, Altoona, Pennsylvania.

For two years, 1944–46, he was a captain in the U. S.

Army, stationed in general hospitals, Spokane, Washington, Fort Lewis, Washington, and Tuscaloosa, Alabama.

In 1947 he started private practice in Wallace. He has held various staff offices, including president of staff of Providence Hospital in Wallace; president of Shoshone County Medical Society. From 1976–79 he was a member of the State of Idaho Board of Health and Welfare.

Dr. Revelli retired in 1982. He now lives in Hayden Lake, where he once owned an 1,800 acre cattle ranch. The Revellis have one daughter, an attorney.

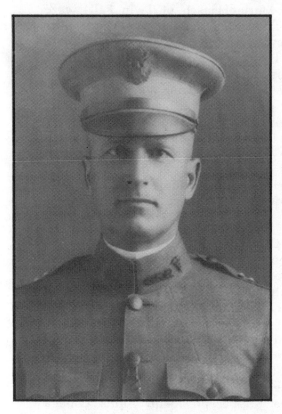

The Mowery name was prominent in northwest medicine. Dr. Herbert, who practiced with brother Charles in Wallace, enlisted in the U.S. Army medical service in World War I and served at many posts and hospitals. He became a captain and later major in the medical corps, and in 1920 became an investigator for the Intelligence corps. He was sent to investigate conditions in Mexico. He returned to Wallace in 1921 to continue practice.
(Courtesy Sylvia Mowery)

THE DOCTORS MOWERY

Dr. Charles R. Mowery was born in Ottumwa, Iowa, March 1, 1875, to John W. and Mary Wilson Mowery. Other Mowery children were Herbert, who also became a doctor; Kenneth, William, and Harry. After grammar and high

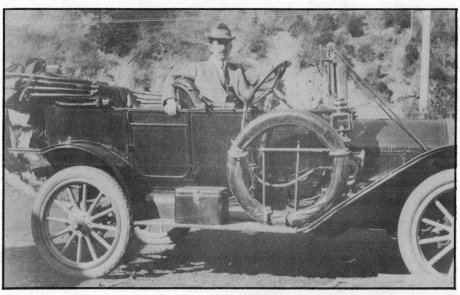

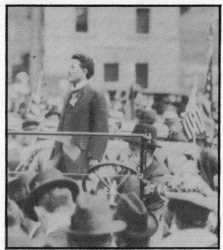

Dr. Charles Mowery, bareheaded and surrounded by hundreds, is giving a talk
following his election as mayor of Wallace
about 1920. Note the American flags raised by
some of his supporters. He has put on his hat
for the photo with his new 1911 two-seated
touring car. His daughter-in-law, Sylvia
Mowery, remembered he had often to turn
the car around and back up the mountain
roads in order to reach his destination.
(Courtesy Sylvia Mowery)

school in Ottumwa, Charles took pre-med at the Uni-
versity of Iowa and graduated from Creighton Medical in
Omaha. His postgraduate work was at the Rotunda
Hospital in Dublin, Ireland, and the University of Vienna,
Austria.

In 1909, Dr. Charles was hired by the Spokane International Railway as surgeon in Wallace, and later in

Spokane. In 1912, he married Doris Mathewson, whose father was the railway engineer. They became the parents of Betty, who married Dr. Donald Harvey, a dentist; John A., an attorney in Spokane and married to Sylvia Svornish, a Spokane dietitian; Charles Jr., who became a doctor.

In 1922, Dr. and Mrs. Charles Mowery moved to Spokane and purchased the historic Hutton home on Seventeenth Street. The doctor continued to commute to Wallace to take care of patients as he established a Spokane practice. He belonged to many medical and civic groups and lodges. In 1933, the Boy Scouts of America awarded him their highest honor, the Silver Beaver.

Charles enjoyed the Wallace practice and urged his brother, Herbert, with whom he had studied in Vienna and London, to join him. Herbert also became a railroad surgeon in northern Idaho. He was the Shoshone County health officer and coroner and practiced at Providence Hospital. On June 30, 1917, he married Mary Clark in Coeur d'Alene. She died during a diptheria epidemic during World War I and he never remarried.

Dr. Herbert became captain and major in the Army Medical Corps, during World War I and served at many post hospitals, traveling by the early-day planes. He served in the Cavalry on the Mexican border and was sent to Mexico in 1920 by the Intelligence Department to investigate conditions in that country. He returned to his Wallace practice in 1921 and lived there until his death in the 1960s.

DR. MAX TRUMAN SMITH

Dr. Smith practiced medicine at Wallace and at one time owned the Wallace Hospital. He and his wife, Mary Beryle Batchelor Burch, built the large log building in Casco Bay on Lake Coeur d'Alene as a summer home. Of peeled cedar, with cathedral ceilings and hardwood floors, it is a handsome structure, now owned by Duane and Lola Hagadone.

The Smiths became parents of one daughter, Cybil, and a son, Max Jr.

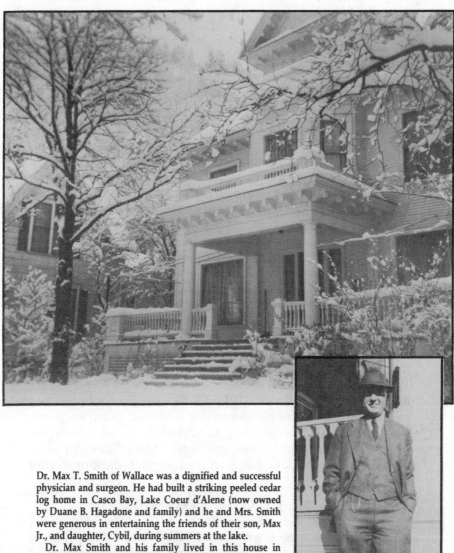

Dr. Max T. Smith of Wallace was a dignified and successful physician and surgeon. He had built a striking peeled cedar log home in Casco Bay, Lake Coeur d'Alene (now owned by Duane B. Hagadone and family) and he and Mrs. Smith were generous in entertaining the friends of their son, Max Jr., and daughter, Cybil, during summers at the lake.

Dr. Max Smith and his family lived in this house in Wallace from 1926 until 1946. The house was built by Wallace attorney C.W. Beale in 1904, and lived in by Dr. Paul Ellis and his family after the Smiths sold to them. It is now owned by Wallace school teachers Jim and Linda See.

(Courtesy Paula Stephenson)

BENEWAH COUNTY

Four-season scenic lovers will find Benewah County a paradise. It is a rolling, hilly area with three higher mountain ranges separated by three picturesque rivers flowing into Lake Coeur d'Alene, the southern tip of which lies in Benewah County. Smaller, but pretty as a speckled trout, lakes include Chatcolet, Benewah, Bells and Swan Lake.

Benewah's early history is tied with that of Kootenai, from which it was carved. With the completion of the Mullan Road in 1860, the settlers came into the area. The discovery of placer mines near St. Maries in the 1880s saw a big advance in people moving in. Lumbering, mining, and farming were well underway when the county was created by legislative act. The shadowy St. Joe River, the highest navigable river in the world, is nationally known. To this land of beauty came medical men and women who had a passion to heal and care for the people of their community.

Zella Goodwin, director of the Benewah Historical Society in St. Maries says that a Dr. Darnell was likely the first doctor to arrive in the area. Dr. Kinsolving arrived in 1900 and St. Maries Hospital was started in August 1911 and finished in February 1912. Until then doctors operated in their office or the homes of the patients. "Rain or shine, sleet or hail, Dr. Kinsolving would ride horseback to the remotest area to give medical help," Mrs. Goodwin said, "often having to make his own trail in pitch dark or during snowstorms."

DR. DELOS E. CORNWALL

Dr. Cornwall was born in Richland County, Wisconsin, on February 17, 1883, and when six years of age moved with his parents to Moscow, Idaho, where he attended public schools. As a boy, he earned his first money by working in the harvest fields. He continued this type of work, saving his money until he entered the University of Idaho, from which he graduated in 1903. At the age of twenty he entered Rush Medical College of Chicago, from which he graduated in 1907.

He interned for eighteen months at Cook County

Hospital, for practical experience and clinical study. For one year he practiced in the timber town of St. Joe on the river of the same name. After a year, he moved downriver to St. Maries to become district surgeon for the Milwaukee Railway and to take charge of the hospital.

The doctor's father, Frank E. Cornwall, was born in Ohio and moved to Moscow in 1889, where he engaged in real estate and took an active part in politics and public affairs. He was secretary of the Board of Regents for the university, mayor of the city, county treasurer, and leading member of the Odd Fellows Lodge. Of the four children of the Cornwalls, the doctor was the eldest.

At Rush, the doctor joined Phi Delta Theta and the medical fraternity Nu Sigma Nu. He joined the Masons and Elks.

DR. OWEN DALE PLATT

Fifty-four years ago, in November 1939, Dr. Owen D. Platt, St. Maries' country doctor, delivered premature triplets born to Mr. and Mrs. Sam Sampson at Fernwood, which brought him nationwide fame. He had driven twenty-two miles through thick fog over a curving mountain road at two o'clock in the morning. Without electric lights, without antiseptic facilities, he toiled five nonstop hours to successfully deliver those tiny babies.

It was necessary for him to use artificial respiration to bring life into the last-born. With only a hot water bottle and heat from a wood burning kitchen range he kept the temperature in the frame shack above ninety degrees, while outside it was far below freezing. He didn't take time to bathe the triplets, but smeared their tiny bodies with melted cocoa butter and wrapped them in soft blankets.

He borrowed hot water bottles from neighbors in the village a mile away to improvise an incubator from an old baby bed, lined it with blankets and packed it with the hot bottles. When he had safely tucked the wee ones into the incubator, he gave a few drops of diluted brandy and rum, with a medicine dropper, to each one. Dr. Platt had also delivered the two previous children of the Sampsons.

He had been answering day and night calls to deliver babies on the farms, in logging camps, and in towns of Benewah and Kootenai counties. He knew nearly every miles of the rugged timberland on both sides of the St. Joe

River and used horseback, teams and automobile. He had an affectionate feeling for the log cabins, shake shacks and humble farm homes where he would deliver some future citizen.

When asked about all the late night and early morning calls, he said, "I answer every call and admit every case which comes to the hospital. In these days there are many who can never pay. It isn't like it was after the war (World War I) when everybody was working and there was plenty of money. Nearly all of them paid doctor bills then. Now the town is full of dust-bowlers who are on relief or the WPA." He wasn't complaining, just stating the facts.

Dr. Platt graduated from the University of Nebraska Medical School in 1903 and started practice. Six years later, he moved to St. Maries and remained, with the exception of thirteen months as a medical officer with the 68th Engineers in France during the war. He helped organize the American Legion post in St. Maries and served a term as commander.

Dr. Platt was a hospital builder and was owner and builder of three of them during his time in St. Maries. St. Maries Hospital was located where the Presbyterian Church now stands. Another hospital, one block off the Main Street had three stories and a standup attic. Dr. Platt occupied the second and third floors and the Alcorn Drug Store occupied the first.

DR. EDWARD M. SULLIVAN

Dr. Edward Sullivan, of St. Maries, Idaho, used all his medical skills in the delivery of a one pound-eleven ounce baby boy. The baby was so premature it didn't seem possible he could survive. But he did. Still, Dr. Sullivan, in filling out the questionnaire on early hospital experiences wrote "routine."

Dr. Sullivan was born May 7, 1911 in Chicopee Falls, Massachusetts. His father was assistant manager of the U.S. Rubber Company, Fisk Rubber Company division. As a youth he was active in the Boy Scouts and other youth organizations.

He went to the University of Pennsylvania for three years, then to Yale University School of Medicine. He interned one year at Mercy Hospital, Springfield,

Massachusetts. From 1936 to 1952 he practiced in Massachusetts, then moved to St. Maries, Idaho. He was assistant surgeon at Mercy Hospital, Springfield from 1936-50. He was on the general staff of the Benewah Community Hospital, St. Maries. He spent three years as an Army captain in the European theater.

He had five sons and three daughters.

DR. WALTER DYCE THURSTON

His given first name is Walter, but everyone calls him Dyce, his middle name. He was born at Wheatland, Wyoming February 7, 1919. His high schooling was at Rapid City, South Dakota, graduating in 1937. He graduated from the South Dakota School of Mines in 1939, with a degree in chemical engineering. He took his pre-med course at Denver University, graduating in 1941, with a bachelor of arts degree. His M.D. was earned at the University of Colorado Medical School in 1944. He was president of both the junior and senior classes at the medical school.

Dr. Thurston interned at the Oakland Naval Hospital in 1944-45. He was a surgical resident at the University of Colorado in Denver, 1946-47; Childrens Hospital, Denver, 1947-48; Corwin Hospital in Pueblo, Colorado, 1948-49; and chief surgical resident at the State Hospital in Pueblo, 1949-50. His fraternities are Pi Kappa Alpha and Nu Sigma Nu.

In September 1944, Dr. Thurston was married to Barbara Kroeger of Durango, Colorado. They had three sons and two daughters, Kay, Bob, Kathy, Bill and Rick. The entire family enjoyed living in the lake and stream country of Benewah County and the Thurstons' large home over-looked the river. They all liked hunting, fishing, camping and boating. Dyce has been chairman of the St. Maries school board, and Elder in the Presbyterian Church and a member of the Kiwanis Club.

He has used a row boat and a helicopter to get to patients who were in need of a doctor and has learned to cope with the deep snow and high water that comes with the annual runoff.

Dr. Thurston was with the 133rd Sea Bee Battalion, 1945-46; and at the Naval Training Center in San Diego and aboard the U.S.S. Boxer, 1952-54.

The entire community of St. Maries and friends from far and wide grieved at the tragedy which struck the Thurston family when their wife, mother and grandmother, Barbara, called "Bobbie" by most, lost her life in a fire. The blaze, which apparently sparked from a short in basement wiring, destroyed the large and old home which they had purchased from the St. Maries pioneers Jim and Anna Brebner, when they first came there. They had done a great deal of renovation and Bobbie had made a genuine old country home of it.

Dr. Thurston practiced surgery in Pueblo, 1950–52 and from 1954–57. He and his family arrived in St. Maries in 1957, and have resided there since then. He has a general practice and in 1991, his youngest son, Dr. Rick Thurston, and his family moved to St. Maries from California. The two Doctors Thurston practice together.

DR. BERGEN RAPP

Dr. Bergen A. "Barney" Rapp moved from Alaska to St. Maries on May 1, 1947, to fill the medical vacancy left when Dr. C.A. Robins became governor and moved to Boise. He had been an Army medical officer at the 183rd General Hospital at Fort Richardson, Anchorage, Alaska, and with a fellow doctor, Captain Don Moseley, decided to practice in St. Maries. They worked for the Western Hospital Association, a branch of the Milwaukee Railway, and under the system established years before when logging dominated the area, they received one dollar and fifty cents per month from the woodsworkers and one dollar and fifty cents from the logging contractor for taking care of all medical needs. For a short while, Dr. Harvey Smith of Boise also practiced in St. Maries, returning to Boise in May 1947.

Dr. Rapp was born June 24, 1917, at Manhasset, Long Island, and received his M.D. as a general practitioner from New York University. After a rotating internship at Brooklyn's Swedish Hospital, he joined the Army and went to Alaska. He married Army nurse, Margaret Darcy, and they became the parents of son, Greg, and daughters, Darcy, who works with a family medical practice in Spokane, and Tracey, who works with a Portland, Oregon hospital. Dr. Rapp later married Joann Angelo of St. Maries. He retired in December 1982, but practices part time.

LATAH COUNTY

Latah is the only county in the United States created by an act of Congress. In 1864 the Territorial Legislature passed an act to create Lah Toh (later Latah), which, like Kootenai County, was attached to Nez Perce for legal reasons. Even after Lah Toh was annexed to Nez Perce and vanished, the founding of the town of Moscow began a lengthy battle for a county organization separate from Nez Perce. Three attempts to form their own government went down before rigid resistance of Lewiston. In 1887, Fred T. Dubois, Idaho's delegate to Congress introduced a bill to create Latah County, got it passed, and the President signed the bill in 1888.

Latah is divided by the Thatuna range of hills and is great wheat, pea and lentil country. The rolling hills are as fertile as the valley and prairie lands.

A few dozen families had settled in and near Moscow when **Dr. James H. McCallie**, a dentist, arrived in 1877. The next year, **Dr. Henry Blake**, a physician, joined him. By 1886, the six hundred residents included four physicians and two dentists.

Moscow doctors practiced out of their homes or offices until 1893, when Dr. Charles Gritman, who arrived in 1892, and Dr. R.C. Coffey purchased the former McGregor House on South Main Street and converted it into a hospital.

DR. EDWARD NORTH DUNN

Dr. Dunn was born in Corvallis, Oregon September 16, 1902. There were several doctors in his family; son, Ronald Edward Dunn, El Paso, Texas; brother, M. J. Dunn, Florence, Oregon; nephew, Wallace W. Dunn, Northwestern University Medical Center, Chicago; niece, Mrs. W.W. Dunn, Chicago, pediatrician.

He was graduated from Oregon State College in music and pharmacy, and taught music at Oregon State School of Education at Monmouth, Oregon. He was a driver for National Park Service and played in National Park Service Hotel orchestras. For three years he was pharmacist at the University of Oregon Medical School Hospital.

He had a pharmacy degree from the Oregon State College and his M.D. from the University of Oregon. He interned at the University of Oregon Medical School

Hospital for one year in 1931. Three and a half years later he was staff physician at the University of Oregon Medical School Hospital. He started his practice in Moscow in 1934.

He belonged to the American Academy of General Practice; Idaho and American Medical associations. He was president, American Association of General Practitioners for Idaho in 1955. Music, travel, and photography were his hobbies. The Dunns had one daughter and one son.

DR. ROBERT C. COFFEY

When Robert Coffey of Cottonwood decided to study medicine, he talked to Dr. J.W. Turner, who became his preceptor. Dr. Turner loaned him a human skeleton and a *Gray's Anatomy* book. He studied both and recited to Dr. Turner on Sundays for three months and then went to medical school in Louisville, Kentucky, graduating in 1892. That year he opened a practice in Moscow and was a charter member of the Idaho Medical Society. August 9, 1893, he married a second cousin, Clarissa Ellen Coffey, and they went to the Louisville City Hospital for a year of graduate study.

They returned to Moscow in October 1896, and he was elected vice-president of the Idaho Medical Society in 1897. October that year they moved to Colfax, Washington, and in 1900 to Portland, Oregon, where he practiced until November 9, 1933, when he was killed in a plane crash while on an errand of mercy.

DR. CHARLES LEE GRITMAN

Charles Gritman was born in Illinois in 1862 and worked as a sheep herder and farmer until moving with his family to Dayton, Washington in 1881. Late in the decade, he decided to study medicine and moved to Ohio to enter the Cincinnati College of Medicine and Surgery. He practiced two years in Ohio before moving to Moscow as one of the first doctors in the Palouse. He had the town's first hospital, performed the first appendectomy and first tonsillectomy. He may have been the first owner of an automobile in Latah County and rival doctors joked with him about building a bigger business in broken bones by owning a machine that caused horses to bolt.

In 1885, he married Bertie Cox, Waitsburg native and a registered nurse who helped the doctor in the hospital.

They had a large apartment in the building and she planned all the hospital meals. The Gritmans kept cows in an adjoining field and milk was a basic food at the hospital. Growing up in a working home, Dr. Gritman understood that patients often did not have money to pay, so he accepted farm-grown food or other items in lieu of cash.

After Dr. Coffey left in 1900, **Dr. C.O. Armstrong** became Gritman's partner and they made house calls to the far corners of the county. During the 1918 flu epidemic, Gritman maintained two teams of horses and two drivers, and would sleep while a driver took him from one house call to another. He often worked twenty-four hours a day.

Both Charles and Bertie Gritman were active in civic and social affairs and belonged to many organizations. In 1933, the doctor announced his retirement, and within a week died in his sleep of a heart attack. They had just moved out of the hospital into their first home on East B Street. Mrs. Gritman operated the hospital for several years, selling out in 1938 to the Moscow Hotel Association, which was raising money for a larger, modern community hospital. Mrs. Gritman sold the building and land at a greatly reduced price, with the agreement that the new structure would be called the Gritman Memorial Hospital.

DR. JOSEPH W. THOMPSON

Another early-day Latah County doctor was Joseph W. Thompson who was born half-way around the world on February 7, 1875, in Appleby, England. He received his early education in England, not coming to America until the age of nineteen and with the intention of studying medicine.

In 1894, he entered the Washington University Medical School in St. Louis, Missouri, graduating in 1898. He interned for one year at the St. Louis City Hospital, then returned to England for postgraduate study in London. On returning to the United States, he first practiced in Nilwood, Illinois. In 1905, he entered the Eye, Ear, Nose, and Throat College in Chicago, thereafter practicing in Wasau, Wisconsin.

Dr. Thompson moved to Idaho, locating in Moscow, in 1908. The next year he moved to Potlatch, where he practiced until 1938, when he moved back to Moscow. He specialized in E.E.N.T. until retirement in 1952. In 1905, Dr. Thompson married Kathryn Hoecker of Carlinville, Illinois, and they had four children, Josephine, Edward, Donald and Willard, all born in Potlatch.

DR. DOYLE M. LOEHR

Born September 4, 1902 on a farm near Wintersed, Iowa, Doyle M. Loehr, did not arrive in Moscow to practice medicine until thirty years later. He attended the Wintersed grade and high schools and was graduated from Simpson College, Indianola, Iowa; the Iowa State University School of Medicine in 1931, and became a Phi Chi there.

His internship was at St. Luke's Hospital in Spokane and residency at the Shriner's Hospital there. Moscow was nearby and he arrived there to open a practice in 1932. He was a member of the Idaho and American Medical associations. During World War II he served as a commander in the U.S. Navy.

He married Phyllis Wright and they had a daughter, Roxanne, graduate of the University of Arizona with a master's degree; and one son, David, who studied ocean-ography at the University of Washington and was in the regular Navy R.O.T.C.

DR. JOSEPH G. WILSON

Joseph Wilson, who arrived in Moscow at the same time as Doyle Loehr, was also born, reared and worked on a farm, this one in Kent, Oregon. He was born December 6, 1905 and worked on the family farm until entering the University of Oregon. With the exception of a summer he spent working at Pacific Christian Hospital in Eugene, he returned to the farm.

He graduated from Kent High School in 1923; University of Oregon, 1927; and Oregon Medical School in 1931. His internship, as was Dr. Loehr's, was at St. Luke's in Spokane. He practiced in Moscow from 1932 until 1962. He ran two small hospitals in Moscow before associating with Gritman Memorial, where he held all staff positions.

Dr. Wilson used all modes of transportation, walking, by sleigh, and flying to take care of patients. With one case, he used a sled as far as it would go in the deep snow, and then walked to the home. He helped organize the Moscow Hospital Association which operated the hospital there; was president, North Idaho Medical Association and Idaho Chapter, American Academy of General Practice.

He served with the Medical R.O.T.C. at the University of Idaho from 1931-41. Dr. and Mrs. Wilson had two girls and three boys.

DR. WILLIAM YOUNG

Dr. William Young cast his fortunes with Idaho in 1911, establishing residence and practice in the logging town of Bovill. He was born at Elkhorn, Wisconsin, November 15, 1883, taking grade and high school there. He entered the University of Wisconsin at Madison, where he studied liberal arts and then took a four year medical course at Northwestern University, Chicago, graduating in 1910. He interned at Monroe Street Hospital, Chicago.

When he arrived in Bovill, he was the only doctor. He became a Mason and joined the Episcopal Church. During college, he joined Alpha Kappa Kappa medical fraternity and enjoyed sports, and played on the university ball team at Madison and Chicago.

June 29, 1910, at Elkhorn, Wisconsin, Dr. Young married Linn Sprague, daughter of Mr. and Mrs. Geo. B. Sprague. Dr. and Mrs. Young had one daughter, Helen G.

DR. PETER S. BECK

Dr. Peter Beck, former mayor of Genesee, was a homeopathic physician, which he felt brought prejudice and opposition, but overcame it to become successful in Latah County. He was a native of Pennsylvania, born March 28, 1852, of German ancestors. Jacob Beck, his father, was born in the same county in 1820, and his mother, Sophia, in 1821. Jacob Beck was a Dunkard, and his mother a Methodist. They had six sons and a daughter.

The doctor was raised on his father's farm, and attended public schools. At the age of nineteen he was certified to teach. Thus he earned enough to complete his education, and study medicine at Iowa State University. After receiving his M.D. degree he practiced in Kansas.

In 1893 Dr. Beck came to Genesee, and joined his brother, Dr. John Beck, in practice. August 13, 1892 Dr. Beck married Ida A. Thomas of Michigan. They had two sons, Orrin Roy and Joseph Edward. Mrs. Beck was a Seventh Day Adventist. Dr. Beck was a Mason; Knight of Pythias; Odd Fellow; and a Woodman of the World. He was a school trustee and councilman in Genesee, and in 1897 was mayor of the city. He built a residence on ten acres and grew fruit and vegetables and raised poultry.

DR. A. F. WOHLENBERG

Dr. Wohlenberg, physician and surgeon of Kendrick, was a native of Lyons, Iowa, born April 27, 1862. His parents, Ludwig A. and Maria (Vollbehr) Wohlenberg, were both born in Germany and came to America as children. Dr. Wohlenberg was educated in the public schools, worked on a farm, clerked in a store, and was determined to become a doctor. He graduated in 1894 from the College of Physicians and Surgeons, Chicago.

He began practice in Seattle, and soon went to Kendrick, where he enjoyed an increasing practice. He studied leading medical journals and belonged to the Idaho Medical Association. He was a member of Woodmen of the World and Knights of Pythias. In 1886, Dr. Wohlenberg was married to Julia Canfield, of Marshalltown, Iowa, a daughter of Dr. and Mrs. Mosley Canfield.

DR. CORNEY J. KLAAREN

Corney Klaaren had been doctoring in Latah County four years when it was customary to do home deliveries. He was called to a small motel-residence to deliver a baby. After the birth, he asked the nurse to get the name of the child from the father in order to save a return trip to complete the certificate.

When she asked him, he replied, "I don't know what to name him. I didn't even know my wife was expecting a baby!"

On another occasion, while he was cauterizing a small growth on the hand of a patient, he remarked, "Smells like roast beef," The patient said, "It should, my name is Bull." And so it was.

Dr. Klaaren was born on a farm at Oskaloosa, Iowa, and farmed with his father until age twenty. He then decided he should get on with becoming a doctor and attended Penn Academy until 1924, and received his B.S. degree from Penn College in Oscaloosa in 1927. His M.D. degree was granted in 1931 from the University of Iowa, where he joined the Phi Chi fraternity.

His internship and residency were at Tacoma General and Pierce County hospitals from 1931–33. He was in Army service from 1933–35 and came to Moscow in 1935. In 1952 he was named chief of staff at Gritman Memorial Hospital; president of the North Idaho Medical Society, 1945–46; on the national commission of the American Association of General Practitioners, 1957–59; and secretary-treasurer of the state A.A.G.P. in 1954.

Dr. and Mrs. Klaaren had two daughters and four grandchildren.

DR. R. D. BROOKS

Dr. Brooks was born February 14, 1926, Elgin, Kansas. His father was an oil field pumper. The doctor grew up in the country of oil fields, and worked weekends and summers paying for his education. He had the highest grade point average in high school, and he played on the state championship softball team.

In 1949 he received his B.A. degree from the University of Kansas, and his medical degree in 1953. For one and a half years he was histology instructor at the University Medical School. From 1953–54 he interned at Madigan Army Hospital, Tacoma, Washington. He was a first lieutenant in the Army Medical Corps.

The Brooks have three boys and two girls.

DR. JUSTUS MILLARD FLEMING

Dr. Fleming was at the University of Idaho Health Center and practiced medicine in Moscow from September 1955 to March 1962. He was born October 16, 1899, at Elkhart, Indiana, where his father and an uncle were physicians. Years later, his son, Dr. Peter Fleming, was to be surgical resident at Mary Hitchcock Hospital in Hanover, New Hampshire.

He attended Elkhart grade and high schools and received a B.S. degree in 1921 from Dartmouth, where he became a member of Chi Phi. His M.D. degree was granted in June 1929 from the University of Michigan Medical School, where he joined Nu Sigma Nu. His internship was at Blodgett Memorial in Grand Rapids, where he practiced from 1930 to 1955, before coming to Moscow.

Dr. Fleming had assisted his father in several "dining-room table appendectomies" and had several difficult forceps deliveries of babies in his own practice. Called out on emergencies during an Ohio River flood of 1937, he traveled by launch and rowboat to get to the patients. During World War II, he entered the Navy Medical Corps as a lieutenant commander and was discharged in 1945 as a captain.

DR. DOUGLAS ALFRED CHRISTENSEN

After moving from Salt Lake City, Utah where he was born November 15, 1903, Dr. Christensen lived in southern Idaho until the age of thirteen. His family relocated to Tremonton, Utah where he attended high school at Brigham City, Utah. He went on to the University of Utah and received his B.A. in 1927. He completed two years of medical school at the University of Utah and finished at the University of Pennsylvania graduating with his M.D. in 1930. After beginning his internship at City Hospital in Seattle he completed his work at the new Harbor View Hospital in 1931. He then moved to Kendrick, Idaho in October 1931 to begin practice.

He repaired a third degree perineal laceration in a shack with only a dim flashlight for illumination. Methods of transportation were on horseback, sled, wagon, tractor, jeep, car and foot. Unusual weather made unusual methods of transportation necessary. He never experienced a severe epidemic. He is the past president of the North Central Idaho Medical Society for one term. In addition, he has been a director of the American Pheasant Society for four years. Married to Irene Snowling on September 18, 1928 just before entering the University of Pennsylvania in Philadelphia, they had two sons and one daughter.

DR. OMER H. DRURY

Dr. Drury was born October 21, 1922 to an Emmett farming family. The doctor worked his way through high school and college as a baker.

He received his B.A. degree in 1944 from Walla Walla College, Walla Walla, and his M.D. degree in 1947 from Loma Linda University, California. For a year, 1947-48 he interned at Porter Sanitarium and Hospital, Denver, Colorado. He spent two years at El Reno, Oklahoma, in public health service, rank of senior surgeon. He started his practice in Troy in 1949. He has been a regular member of the Gritman Memorial Staff, and served in each of the elective offices.

The Drurys have two sons and three daughters.

DR. DONALD E. ADAMS

Dr. Adams was born March 6, 1922, Hingham, Massachusetts. He attended the University of Wyoming and St. Louis University. For one year he interned at Sacred Heart Hospital, Spokane. In 1956 he moved to Moscow to start his practice.

The Adams have two boys and two girls.

DR. JOHN M. AYERS

Dr. Ayers was born in May 1918 in Grangeville and received his pre-med education at the University of Idaho, 1935-38; studied at the University of Chicago, 1938-40; and received his M.D. from Rush Medical College in 1942. His internship and residency were at Highland-Alameda County hospitals in Oakland, with an interim of two years as captain in the U.S. Army Medical Corps in Europe.

Captain Ayers was awarded five campaign stars with the bronze arrowhead (invasion), the Bronze Star with Oak Leaf Cluster and the Combat Medical badge. Dr. and Mrs. Ayers had three sons.

DR. J. BURT BRITZMAN

Dr. Britzman was born August 8, 1930, Canton, South Dakota. He attended high school at Hawarden, Iowa. In 1953 he received his B.S. degree and in 1957 his medical degree from the University of Iowa Medical College. For one year he interned at St. Benedict's Hospital, Ogden, Utah.

He joined the staff at Gritman Memorial Hospital, Moscow.

He was a captain in the Marine Corps in Germany, and in charge of dispensary that served 5,000 troops and 5,000 dependents.

Skiing, hunting, and fishing are his hobbies. The Britzmans had four boys, and two girls.

NEZ PERCE COUNTY

Nez Perce, named for the tribe of the famed Chief Joseph, was formed in 1861, by the Territorial Legislature of Washington. It is "mother" to all the other Idaho counties, in that it was one of the seven in 1864, from which all present Idaho counties were created. Size of the county changed many times until present boundaries were set by Idaho Legislature in 1911. History abounds in Nez Perce, to which Lewis and Clark brought the first white men. The Reverend Henry Harmon Spalding and his wife, Eliza Hart Spalding, established the first mission in 1836 near the confluence of the Clearwater River and Lapwai Creek. Lewiston became a busy landing where steamers were unloaded of goods onto pack trains for delivery to the mining camps.

Lapwai was the site for the U.S. Military Post in 1861. The Nez Perce Indian Reservation was created in 1863 and within the next two years farms and villages sprang up, opening the rich farm land. The geography is startling, ranging from 741 feet at Lewiston to 5,000 in the Craig Mountain and high plateau areas. The Snake River forms the western boundary and joins the Clearwater at Lewiston, named for Captain Meriwether Lewis.

The medical men and women who have been attracted to the county were, in themselves, as strong and colorful as the history and terrain.

DR. JAMES M. LYLE

Dr. James M. Lyle whose father started medical practice in 1885 in Murphy, North Carolina, knew from the time he was a small boy that he wanted to become a doctor. His Idaho home and medical office were at Peck, but he covered hundreds of miles in the area, caring for the ill.

James Lyle was born September 16, 1876 in Franklin, North Carolina, where he attended grade and high schools. When he was sixteen his father died, and he worked for several years on farms and contributed to the support of his widowed mother. He determinedly kept his mind on becoming a doctor and began to save as much of his earnings as possible. Eventually he entered the medical department of the University of Nashville, Tennessee and received his Medical Doctor degree in 1901.

After graduation he headed for Peck, Idaho, to visit a cousin, Henry Crawford, and found the town surrounded by mountains. Many years later, his son, Jim Jr., remembered his father telling of that visit and saying, "I went on the train and didn't get into Peck until 3:15 in the afternoon. I looked up at nothing but walls on both sides and ends of Peck and thought 'If there were any way to get out of here, I would!'" He had planned to practice in North Carolina. But, instead of getting out, he remained and built up an extensive medical practice.

He started courting an attractive school teacher, Elizabeth Rogers, daughter of Mr. and Mrs. R.D. Rogers of Nez Perce County. Her father and brother had started homesteading on Central Ridge in 1896. Elizabeth taught at the village of Lookout, which Dr. Lyle described as being, "Fifteen miles and two grades over from Central Ridge." After making the drive every weekend, the doctor said to himself, "By gosh, she should have a better job than that. She should marry me."

She did, on April 29, 1903 in Butte, Montana. They became the parents of two sons and a daughter, James M. Jr., Donald R., and Elizabeth Louise, all born at Peck. Dr. Lyle became a hero to the townspeople in 1910 when, during a flood and at the risk of his life, he rescued a woman and her six children from a dwelling near the river. The house was soon washed away by the rising waters.

Jim Jr. remembers two of his cousins at Peck, and one, Harry Jones, dying within two days of contracting spinal meningitis in 1912. Paul Jones practiced in Peck from 1912 to 1914. While there he married a nurse from Rhode Island. "I still remember them getting on that horse-drawn stage to head for Rhode Island. What a trip that must have been."

The Lyles bought a farm at Reubens in the 1930s, and a wheat and pea farm in the 1940s. "We always kept driving teams and one or two good saddle horses," Jim Jr. said, "and my job from age seven on was to feed, curry and water the horses. Then I cleaned the stables and greased the buggy wheels. Dad bought an old Maxwell Tarrytown car with brass trim over everything and a righthand drive. Dad said he'd bought it from an auctioneer, so he knew it must've been a good deal."

Dr. Jim Lyle Sr. retired in 1951 and died in July 1958. Mrs. Lyle had died in November 1953.

He became a member of the North Idaho, Idaho and American Medical associations. He was a Democrat and active in political and community affairs. He joined the Peck Commercial Club and served on the city council. Interested in education, he became a member of the school board.

In October 1992, the University of Idaho Alumni Association established the Jim Lyle Service Award for dedication to the university, and Jim Jr. was the first recipient.

DR. JOHN N. ALLEY

Dr. John Alley was one of the leading forces in the building of the Lewiston Clinic, 11th and Main, in Lewiston in 1918. Associated with Dr. Alley were his brother-in-law, Dr. Elmer G. Braddock, Dr. Paul W. Johnson, and Dr. O.C. Carssow. Establishment of the clinic made specialization in several fields possible. Dr. Alley and Dr. Braddock had married sisters.

For a number of years, Dr. Alley and his family made their home in Lapwai. He had two sons, John Jr., and Ralph, who also became a doctor. His daughter, Margaret, lives in Seattle. Dr. Alley was an elder in the Episcopal Church in Lapwai, along with rancher John Kennedy, a close friend whose daughter, "Jack" Stellmon remembers the doctor with great affection.

She tells of John Kennedy buying a new Hupmobile sedan from a salesman whom he convinced that he could drive, although he had never driven a car in his life. The salesman must have doubted him, because he went along when John took his family for their first ride. "He turned too sharply at the top of Beaver Grade," Jack said, "and turned that new Hupmobile over, dumping everyone out. Maudie's (Mrs. Kennedy) leg was broken and we kids had abrasions and skinned ourselves. We called and Dr. Alley came and gathered us all up. All the way to Lewiston, he kept singing, 'Shall We Gather At the River.'"

Jack Stellmon says that she owes her life twice to Dr. Alley. He brought her into the world at the Kennedy home on north Tom Beall Road out of Lapwai. When she was about twelve years old, another doctor gave her a dose of castor oil to relieve what he thought was a stomach upset. It resulted in a ruptured appendix and although not a surgeon, Dr. Alley assisted Dr. Braddock with the surgery. The little hospital in Lewiston was operated by two Irish nurses, Sister Innocence and Sister Immaculata, and they permitted Jack's mother, Maudie, to sleep in the hospital. They thought Jack was going to die, and they had lighted candles around the bed.

Jack remembers that an old honey merchant and friends came to her room and knelt around the bed to pray. "No sooner had they finished the prayer than I sat up, threw up, and began to get well," she said.

OTHER DOCTORS ARRIVE

Dr. Charles Phillips, associated with **Dr. White** in Lewiston, said upon his retirement, "It is an exacting profession. The worst of it is, people expect so much of you and you have no time to yourself."

On December 10, 1886, the *Lewiston Teller* made reference to a **Dr. Stirling**. Many small towns were springing up in northern Idaho and some doctors were not mentioned in newspapers and others barely noted as practicing in the town. Mention was made of **Dr. Emanuel Vodney**, in the village of Morrow. He owned and operated the town's drugstore.

Doctor Joseph W. Stoneburner was a popular physician in the Nez Perce County office at Leland.

DR. M. A. KELLY

Soon after Fort Lapwai was established and the soldiers had arrived, a brief item made mention that a Doctor M.A. Kelly had arrived in Lewiston. Other than the facts that he had arrived in 1862 and had died in 1903, nothing is known. Whether he was graduated from a medical school or received medical knowledge as an apprentice is not known. A medical apprenticeship consisted of grinding powder, mixing pills, going with the doctor on his rounds to see patients, holding the basin when the doctor bled patients, aided in surgery, and adjustments of plasters. By watching the doctor, he learned to suture wounds. When not actively engaged with the doctor or patients, he studied from what medical books were available, swept out the office, cleaned empty bottles and jars, and answered the night bell. Or, he may have learned from books alone. Whatever, he was as busy as the doctor.

It can be assured that Dr. Kelly was kept busy from the time he arrived as many families had arrived or drifted into the Clearwater area and by the summer of 1862 the population was over 14,000. Illnesses came from many places where families ate from a common platter and drank from a common tin cup; flies and mosquitoes spread malarial fevers; hungry miners craved half-baked bread and washed it down with whiskey, resulting in severe indigestion and dysentery. Vegetables were scarce and scurvy raged.

DR. BURTON R. STEIN

Dr. Stein was born in Oakfield, New York, April 11, 1917. His father was a physician in Oakfield, and his brother a surgeon in Buffalo. He attended Oakfield High School, University of Rochester, where ill health forced him to drop out. He later went to the University of Arizona four years. He was graduated from the University of Buffalo with an M.D. degree, and then received a M.S. in medicine from the University of Minnesota. He earned Phi Beta Kappa membership. From 1943-44, Dr. Stein interned at Huntington Memorial Hospital, California, and from 1944-47 had a fellowship at Mayo Clinic. He started practice in Lewiston in 1947. He was on the staff at St. Joseph Hospital.

The Steins had two daughters and a son, adopting the boy and one girl.

DR. DAN E. STIPE

Dr. Stipe was born in Dodge City, Kansas July 29, 1927. His father was a pharmacist. In 1945 he was graduated from high school in Wichita. Dr. Stipe served in the U.S. Navy for two years in the Pacific theater. He was machinist mate 3rd class.

He attended Wichita University 1948-50 and Kansas University, Lawrence, 1950-51, graduating with an A.B. degree. In 1957 Dr. Stipe was graduated from Kansas University Medical School, Kansas City, with his M.D. degree. He interned at Pierce County Hospital, Tacoma, Washington, 1956-57.

Dr. Stipe moved to Lewiston, in 1957, to begin practice.

He was on the staff at Tri State Memorial, Clarkston, Washington, St. Joseph Hospital, Lewiston, and belongs to the American Academy of General Practice. He has been secretary-treasurer of St. Joseph staff and North Idaho District Medical Society, and delegate to the State Medical Society.

He and his wife have a daughter and two sons.

DR. OLIVER M. MACKEY

Dr. Mackey was born in Lewiston on December 8, 1920. He attended public schools in Lewiston; the Lewiston State Normal School, and completed his pre-medical education at the University of Idaho. He attended the Washington University School of Medicine, St. Louis, Missouri, and received his M.D. degree in 1945.

Dr. Mackey interned at the Deaconess Hospital, Spokane, and received license No. M-1759 to practice medicine and surgery in Idaho on June 24, 1946. Except for the two years he was on active duty with the military, Dr. Mackey maintained an active practice in Lewiston.

He was a delegate from the North Idaho District Medical Society, a member of the Insurance Advisory Committee, and president of the North Idaho District Medical Society.

He had three daughters and two sons.

DR. JOHN FREMONT HULBURT

John Fremont Hulburt was born in 1861 at Dalton, Wisconsin, attended public school at Portage, Wisconsin, and was graduated from Hahnemann Medical College in 1886. He married Jessie Webster in 1888.

He practiced in Duluth, Minnesota from 1887–92, and in Eureka, California from 1892–1901. He took further studies at Physician's and Surgeon's College, San Francisco, 1901–03, gaining an Allopathic degree.

He practiced in Lewiston from 1903 until death in 1914.

DR. ROBERT L. OLSON

Dr. Robert Olson was born October 1, 1930, in Lindsborg, Kansas where his father was a blacksmith. A brother, Dr. Erwin T. Olson, practiced in Newton, Kansas. Lindsborg was a small Scandinavian community, and he went to grade and high schools there.

In 1952 he received his B.S. degree from Bethany College,

Lindsborg. He was graduated from the Kansas University of Medicine in 1956 with an M.D. degree.

He spent two years in the U.S. Army. In 1956–57, when stationed at Fort Lewis, Washington, he interned at Madigan General Hospital. Then he was transferred to Larson A.F. Base, Moses Lake, Washington, where he was promoted to captain.

From 1959–61 he had a residency at Kansas University School of Medicine, Kansas City. In July, 1961 he moved to Lewiston. Dr. Olson was a member of the general staff at St. Joseph's Hospital.

The Olsons have two sons.

DR. MALCOLM JOHN McRAE

Dr. McRae was born October 3, 1904 in Nez Perce, Idaho. He went to grade school in Nez Perce; high school at Gonzaga in Spokane; pre-med at Georgetown University, Washington, D.C. and University of Washington, Seattle.

After getting his medical degree, he interned at Altoona General Hospital for one year before moving to Lewiston in 1931 to practice. He was on the staff at St. Joseph's Hospital. Dr. McRae belonged to the local and state medical societies, and the American Medical Association.

The McRaes had two girls and a boy.

DR. SAMUEL A. ROE

Dr. Samuel A. Roe, sixty-one, a former Lewiston physician, died July 14, 1937 of a heart attack in Corvallis, Oregon. He was born at Hannibal, Missouri in 1876 and received his medical education at Missouri Medical College, St. Louis, graduating in 1897. He went to Lewiston in 1902 and practiced there until 1933 when he moved to Corvallis.

DR. JAMES H. BAUMAN

The son of a furniture store owner, James Bauman was born March 30, 1914 in Lewiston and attended area schools until after his second year of college at the Lewiston Normal School in 1931. He studied at the University of Idaho from 1932–34, and on to Northwestern University to earn his B.S. degree in 1937. His M.D. degree came from St. Louis University School of Medicine in 1942. He worked to support himself as a waiter, switchboard operator and in the first aid department of a street car company. Internship and residency were at St. Vincent's and Providence Hospitals in Portland, Oregon, 1942–43.

He took postgraduate work in dermatology at the University of Illinois, Northwestern University and the University of Chicago, 1947–48. His residency was at the V.A. Hospital in Hines, Illinois, 1948–49. He served in the Army Medical Field Service School in 1943 and was battalion surgeon and commander in the 8th Armored Division; assistant surgeon in the Portable Surgical Hospital, 4th Army Headquarters Evacuation Hospital, European theater; chief of Medical Service Station, 279th Station Hospital in Berlin, Germany, attaining rank of major there; received battle stars in Ardennes, Rhineland and central Europe. He was a past president of staff at St. Joseph's Hospital and a member of the North Idaho District Medical Society. He had five single children and a set of twins. His wife was an R.N. and one daughter a nurse.

DR. GEORGE GAIGNARD

Dr. George Gaignard was born in New Orleans in 1868, moving to Chicago in his boyhood. He died at Lewiston, Idaho, September 27, 1937, after a prolonged illness.

He obtained his medical degree from Harvey Medical College, Chicago, in 1901. In 1902 he located at Lookout, and later moved to Reubens until 1919, when he located in Culdesac.

For ten years, 1927–37 he had been contract physician for the Indian Sanatorium at Lapwai.

DR. DONALD DAVID McROBERTS

Lewiston physician Dr. Donald D. McRoberts, was born at Stillwater, Oklahoma, January 29, 1909. At the age of three he moved with his family to Wichita, Kansas, where he attended public schools. He earned B.S.and M.S. degrees from the University of Wichita, where he was teaching Fellow and president of the senior class. He belonged to the Mens' Honor group.

Following one year of medicine at Northwestern University in Chicago, he became Associate Professor of Zoology at the University of Wichita in 1934. He continued at Northwestern University, receiving an M.B. in 1937 and an

M.D. degree in 1938. He was a member of the Phi Beta Pi medical fraternity.

He served an internship at St. Joseph Hospital, Chicago, 1937–38. Further training was at Peter Bent Brigham Hospital, Harvard, with postgraduate training in X-ray in 1940. Training in X-ray and radium therapy was received at Los Angeles Tumor Institute in 1946.

In 1938 he became staff member at St. Joseph's Hospital, Lewiston. Following a year as Nez Perce County physician in 1941, Dr. McRoberts entered the armed services, serving with the Army in Africa, Italy and France. In 1945 he returned to Lewiston as radiologist with the Lewiston Clinic. He served as radiologist at St. Joseph's Hospital 1946–55; Tri-State Memorial Hospital, Clarkston; General Hospital at Grangeville; and Clearwater Valley Memorial Hospital, Orofino. He was a member of Pacific Northwest Radiological Society and the Radiological Society of North America.

He served as president of the North Idaho District Medical Society in 1957, and of the Idaho Radiological Society in 1959. He was president of the St. Joseph's Hospital Staff in 1947. He served as Potentate of the Calam Shrine Temple in 1957. He was a thirty-second degree Mason. He and his wife had three daughters.

DR. C. STAMEY ENGLISH
Dr. English was born in Hutchinson, Kansas in December 1927. He spent two years in the Navy before entering the University of Colorado in Boulder in 1947. He transferred to a pre-med program at the University of Kansas where he joined the Phi Chi fraternity. He graduated from the University of Kansas Medical School. His internship was at St. Lukes in Kansas City, Missouri and surgical residency was at Providence Hospital in Portland. Dr. English opened his practice in Lewiston in 1957.

DR. ROY W. EASTWOOD
Born on September 9, 1910 and raised in Lewiston, Idaho where his father was the manager of a flour mill, Dr. Eastwood returned in 1947 to set up practice after completing his education and military service. He was at the University of Washington, 1930–43 and the University of

California, 1934–37. After earning an A.B. degree he went to Syracuse University, College of Medicine, 1937–41 and graduated with his M.D. degree. His internship was at the Duval County Hospital in Jacksonville, Florida, 1941–42; assistant medical resident at Grady Hospital, Atlanta, Georgia, 1942–43. He was in the U.S. Army, 1943–46, as captain on staff of the 80th General Hospital, returning to Lewiston in 1947. He is the father of two boys.

DR. JOHN J. E. CARSSOW

Dr. Carssow was born in Tacoma, Washington, April 24, 1905. His grandfather and an uncle were both doctors. A nephew, Charles Norland had his M.D. in internal medicine. Dr. Carssow attended the University of Idaho, Gonzaga, Spokane, and University of St. Louis. He interned at City Hospital, St. Louis and St. Luke's in Spokane.

He started practicing in Lewiston in 1936. He was base surgeon in the Army Air Force, 47th AAG, 33rd San Bernadino, and 47th in India. He was flight surgeon at Davis Field, Tucson, Arizona and physician for the Northern Pacific Railroad and Union Pacific.

He and his wife, Dorothy, had one son.

DR. JOHN W. ARMSTRONG

Dr. Armstrong was born in Houston on January 25, 1914. He took his pre-med at Rice Institute, and received his M.D. from University of Texas Medical School.

From 1941–46 he was a captain in the U.S. Army. He served in Africa, Italy, France, Germany, and won the Bronze Star.

He had a residency at Cleveland City Hospital from 1946–48; Southern Pacific Hospital, Houston, 1948–49. He moved to Lewiston in 1958. He was on the staff at St. Joseph's. Dr. Armstrong belonged to the American Board of Internal Medicine and the North Idaho Medical Society.

The Andersons had four sons and two daughters.

DR. PAUL WARDNER JOHNSON

Dr. Paul Wardner Johnson was claimed by Clarkston, Washington and Lewiston, Idaho, and had lived and practiced in both places before his death from an ailing heart on March 22, 1947. He had officiated at the birth of more than 4,500 babies in the Lewiston-Clarkston area. He was a charter member and past president of the Lewiston-Clarkston Kiwanis club, and a 32nd degree Scottish Rite Mason.

Born January 23, 1875, at Stonefort, Illinois, he received his bachelor of science degree from Milton College at Milton, Wisconsin, and his M.D. degree from the Physicians and Surgeons College at the University of Illinois in 1902. He came west after graduation and practiced at both Hoquiam and Clarkston until the building of the Lewiston Clinic, in which he was one of the owners, in 1918. He married Lura Burdick in 1903. She died in 1932.

Dr. Johnson became interested in X-ray and radium, but continued his general practice while studying them. This included a six month's course in X-ray and radiology in Vienna in 1935. He also married Alyce J. Peterson on March 6, 1935.

The doctor suffered a serious heart attack in the winter of 1945, but the great need for competent physicians during World War II kept him at his work beyond his strength. When he died, his brother, Ewing M. Johnson of Clarkston, said, "He was truly a war casualty."

He had three daughters, Elizabeth Green of Milton, Wisconsin, Marjorie Day of Washington, D.C., and Helen Johnson.

DR. JAMES S. NEWTON

Dr. Newton was born February 11, 1905, in Concord, Illinois, and went to grade school in Chambersburg, Illinois; high school, Sigourney, Iowa, and pre-med at the University of Iowa.

He received his M.D. degree from the University of Iowa Medical College in 1931 and had a rotating internship at Cleveland City Hospital; two year residency in general surgery. During 1942-43, he was surgery instructor at L.S.U., New Orleans. In 1948 he located in Lewiston for general practice and surgery. He was on the staff at St. Joseph's Hospital.

From 1943-46 he was in the U.S. Army where he was staff plastic surgeon with the 85th Field Hospital, E.T.O. He was also at Cushing General Hospital, Boston.

During the war he married Major Gertrude E. Premeau, who outranked him. They had no children.

DR. DAVID W. HEUSINKVELD

The son of a Cincinnati doctor, born on December 22, 1927, Dr. Heusinkveld came to Lewiston in 1959. He was educated at Dartmouth College and received his A.B. degree in 1948 and medical school, 1947–49. From 1949–51 he attended Harvard Medical School and graduated with his M.D. His internship was at the Salt Lake County General Hospital from 1951–52 and general surgery residency, 1954–59. He served as a captain in the U.S. Air Force, 1952–54; flight surgeon and squadron commander with the Utah Air National Guard from 1954–58. He has two sons and one daughter. He is staff member of St. Joseph's Hospital and served as treasurer in 1961; member of North Idaho District Medical Society and served as secretary-treasurer in 1961.

DR. D. K. WORDEN

Dr. Worden was born in Nebraska in 1900. His father was a railway engineer. He attended the universities of Wyoming and Nebraska. For three years he was at the Murray Hospital, Butte, Montana, on the board of oto-laryngology.

He practiced in Butte and Lewistown, Montana and moved to Lewiston in 1937. He was past president of the Idaho State Medical Society and alternate delegate to American Medical Association.

He was a private in World War I; served as mayor of Lewiston; and was active in civic affairs. As a physician, he sponsored the pre-payment plan.

The Wordens had two sons and two daughters.

DR. RICHARD F. STACK

Dr. Stack was born August 4, 1921, at Marshfield (Coos Bay), Oregon. His father was a mechanical and structural engineer, and a patent attorney. His brother, Dr. Roger Stack, practiced in Redmond, Oregon, and his cousin, Dr. Thomas J. Stack, in Portland.

He received his B.S. from Oregon State College in 1945, and M.D. from University of Oregon Medical School in 1948. He interned at Sacred Heart Hospital, Spokane, 1948–49, and had a urology residency at the V.A. Hospital San Francisco, 1953–56. He moved to Lewiston in 1956. He was on the staff at St. Joseph Hospital in Lewiston and Tri

State Memorial Hospital, Clarkston. From 1951–53 he was a captain in the U.S.A.F. stationed at Lanson A.F.B. at Moses Lake, Washington. He, and his wife, Marie, had one son and one daughter.

DR. R. C. COLBURN

The son of a Spokane attorney, Dr. Colburn was born on December 12, 1925. He attended the University of Minnesota and the University of Washington Medical School. Internship was at Ancker Hospital in St. Paul and surgical residency at Mercy Hospital in Janesville, Wisconsin. He spent three and one-half years at the University of Washington in orthopedic residency. He practiced in Clarkston, 1954 through 1958, moving his practice to Lewiston in 1961. He had staff appointments at the University of Washington Hospital as an instructor of surgery; St. Joseph's in Lewiston and Tri-State Memorial Hospital in Clarkston.

DR. WALLACE STRAWN DOUGLAS

Dr. Strawn was born January 1, 1901 at Hillsboro, Illinois. His father, son, brother, and nephew were doctors.

He went through high school in Hillsboro and graduated from Virginia Military Institute, Lexington, Virginia, with a bachelor of science in 1922. He received his M.D. in 1927 from Northwestern University Medical School. He interned at Childrens Memorial Hospital, Chicago.

From 1928–33 he practiced in Hillsboro and served in the Army 1933–37. Dr. Douglas moved to Lewiston in 1937. He was on the staff at St. Joseph's Hospital and belonged to the North Idaho Medical Society. During World War II he was a colonel on active duty from 1941–46. He received the Bronze Star.

The Douglases had three daughters and a son.

CLEARWATER COUNTY

Lewis and Clark followed an old Indian trail between the North and Middle Forks of the Clearwater River in 1805, as the first white men to see this part of the country. At a point near the present site of Weippe, they met the Nez Perce Indians who befriended them. They built canoes where they established camp, now known as Canoe Camp, near Ahsahka. They left their horses with the Nez Perce and canoed down the river to join the Columbia.

Pierce City came into existence where E.D. Pierce succeeded in leading a small group of prospectors into the area in 1860 looking for gold. It is the oldest mining camp in Idaho. During the Nez Perce War of 1877, the settlers fled to Pierce City for protection.

Clearwater is timbered mountain country. The Bitterroot range forms the boundary between Montana and Idaho.

DR. JOHN IRVINE McKELWAY

Dr. John Irvine McKelway, sixty-six, superintendent of State Hospital North at Orofino for the previous fifteen years and rated one of the best psychiatrists in the nation, died the morning of April 7, 1941, of heart disease, at his cottage on the hospital grounds.

Extensive improvements in facilities and methods of caring for the mentally ill were made by Dr. McKelway during his service at Orofino. He was well-known in Lewiston, speaking there frequently, often urging a more common-sense view of mental illness. His service at the hospital was marked by his kindness in caring for patients, friends pointing out that restraints were seldom necessary for patients under his care. When restraints were used, they were more to protect a patient from injuring himself.

Dr. McKelway was responsible for the advanced design of the new Givens Hall, which was occupied last year and relieved over-crowding. At his suggestion, additional improvements were made, including the construction of a laundry, which made possible better quarters for other personnel by the resultant shifting; expansion of occupational therapy which keeps patients busy at useful work in the gardens and an art room, and enlargement of the medical and scientific program being carried on.

Dr. McKelway long urged the adoption of a voluntary commitment law which would permit patients to go to the hospital in a frame of mind that would make them more receptive to treatment and care, and saw such a bill adopted at the 1939 session of the Legislature.

His skill in caring for the mentally ill was evidenced by the many offers he received from larger eastern institutions. He told associates that he preferred to continue his work among his friends in Idaho. He had been employed by some large institutions before coming west.

Dr. McKelway contributed numerous articles to medical journals. He was a member of the American Psychiatric Association, the Idaho and American Medical associations, and the American Legion. He was born at Philadelphia, December 23, 1875, attended Rittenhouse Academy and was graduated as a doctor in 1897. During the next two and a half years, he extended his training as an intern in the Philadelphia Orthopedic Hospital and Infirmary for Nervous Disease, the Philadelphia General Hospital, and the Pennsylvania Hospital. He also had charge of Blockley Hospital for some time.

In 1902 he entered the service of New York State at the state hospital at Binghamton. He continued until 1914, and was at Kings Park Hospital on Long Island, and the Bureau of Deportation at New York City.

In 1914 he went to Eastern Oregon State Hospital at Pendleton, but was called into the Army in the spring of 1918 and stationed at Fort Riley, Kansas as first lieutenant. After his discharge in December, 1918, he entered the Indian service on the reservation at Pendleton, and then on February 1, 1921 was made assistant superintendent of the Western Washington State Hospital at Fort Steilacoom. From there he went to Orofino in May, 1926.

Dr. and Ruth Chesley McKelway had one son, John.

DR. MYRON L. McCUMBER

A native of Miami, Florida and the son of an engineer, Dr. McCumber began his education at Southern Missionary College in Tennessee. He graduated from Emmanual Missionary College in Michigan with a B.A. and attended Loma Linda University to earn his M.D. in 1953. He interned at Spartanburg County General Hospital in

Spartanburg, South Carolina in 1954 and surgical residency at the V.A. Hospital in Coral Gables, Florida in 1957. He practiced in Platteville, Wisconsin from 1957–61.

He located in Orofino, Idaho in 1961. He served as captain in the U.S. Air Force and was commander at the U.S.A.F. Hospital in Ardmore, Oklahoma. He is the father of two boys and one girl.

DR. ALBERT B. PAPPENHAGEN

Dr. Pappenhagen was born in Perrysburg, New York, February 2, 1894. His father was a master mechanic.

He was graduated from Allegheny College, Meadsville, Pennsylvania in 1917 with a B.S. degree. From 1917–19 he was in the U.S. Army. In 1927 he received his M.D. from Northwestern University. He interned at Norwegian American Hospital in Chicago 1927–28, and residency at the Shriners Hospital in Chicago 1928–29.

He practiced in Orofino for many years. While there he was consultant at State Hospital North, and chief of staff at Clearwater Valley Hospital from 1957–59. He was president of the Idaho State Medical Association in 1948, and of the Idaho Chapter, American College of Surgeons in 1951.

The Pappenhagens had three daughters and a son.

DR. MYRICK WHITING PULLEN, JR.

Dr. Pullen was born July 24, 1915 in Baltimore. His father was a professor. He grew up in Baltimore, and attended the Maryland Normal School at Towson. His undergraduate work was at Johns Hopkins, and he received his M.D. in 1941 from Johns Hopkins Medical School.

He moved to Orofino in 1956, and was superintendent of State Hospital North. He was involved in developing the program from a custodial one to a treatment program. He was on the staff at Clearwater Valley Memorial Hospital, Orofino. He belonged to the Intermountain Psychiatric Association, and was a member of the Committee on Public Information, American Psychiatric Association.

He was in the Army Reserves, on active duty July 1, 1942 as a first lieutenant. He was assigned to the 282nd Medical Battalion, 2nd Engineer Special (Amphibian) Brigade, spending twenty-eight months in the Pacific. He received the Presidential Unit Citation and others. The Pullens have three daughters and three sons.

LEWIS COUNTY

Historic and stunning in its rugged beauty is Lawyers Canyon (named for Nez Perce Chief Lawyer), one of several deeply gashed canyon running through Lewis County. The county itself is named for Captain Meriwether Lewis who, with Captain Clark, spent the month of May, 1806, in the valley near the present town of Kamiah on their return trek from the Pacific coast.

Rich timberlands cover the southern part, with small agricultural communities dotting the Nez Perce prairie which encompasses almost half of the county. Lovely little Winchester Lake is a favorite fishing spot for many and the Kamiah Valley attracts the Sunday drivers and scene-seekers.

Doctors were attracted to Lewis County because of the variety of opportunities to provide medical service to the hardy lumbermen, hard-working farm people, and for its beauty.

DR. ELTON BANE ROGERS

The young Pennsylvania doctor who had been physician for one year at Deer Lodge, Montana, had heard of Winchester, Idaho, and accepted the offer of Craig Mountain Lumber Company in 1911 to become its surgeon and take charge of the hospital. He also engaged in general practice.

He was born May 27, 1877, at Bloomington, Illinois, where he lived until about fourteen and accompanied his parents to a farm at Bagley, Iowa. Dr. Rogers came from noted ancestry, being a descendant of John Rogers, who was born in 1500 and died in London in 1555 as a Christian martyr. Another ancestor was George Rogers Clark, American general and frontiersman who made the conquest of the Northwest Territory for the colonies. His parents were Lucius and Lucille Freeman Rogers.

In 1898, Dr. Rogers enlisted in Company U of the Forty-ninth Iowa Volunteer Infantry, for action in both the Spanish-American War and the Cuban campaign. His twin brother was a member of the Fifty-first Iowa Infantry and served in the Philippine Islands. Dr. Rogers returned to Iowa and studied for a bachelor of arts degree at Simpson

College, Indianola. By then he was determined to become a doctor and was graduated in 1907 with an M.D. from the medical department of Northwestern University, Chicago. Through employment in the circulation departments of several large newspapers in Chicago, he earned his way through Northwestern.

He interned at Cook County Hospital, Chicago, and at McKeesport, Pennsylvania, where he was physician for the U.S. Steel Company. His next medical work was at Deer Lodge and then to Winchester. In college he joined Phi Beta Pi and the medical honorary Alpha Omega Alpha.

At Gap, Pennsylvania, November 7, 1911, he married Catherine Shertz, daughter of Mr. and Mrs. Cyrus Shertz.

DR. K. H. COLLINS

In April of 1935, Lewis County Commissioners in session at Nez Perce, appointed Dr. K.H. Collins of Craigmont as county physician and health officer. He succeeds **Dr. Eli Taylor**, who resigned. Dr. Collins' territory will include all but the Kamiah highway district which will be under the charge of **Dr. C.H. Bryan**, on a contract basis.

DR. WILBUR F. McMAHAN

A representative member of the medical profession in Lewis, Nez Perce and Idaho counties was Dr. Wilbur McMahan. He had a large practice, with residence and professional headquarters in the attractive little town of Kamiah, but he served as physician for Lewis County.

Dr. McMahan was born at Sparta, Dearborn County, Indiana, on October 1, 1873, a son of John and Nancy J. (Cannon) McMahan. The father was a farmer. In Indiana the doctor attended public schools and Moore's Hill College. After four years as a teacher in the schools of Indiana, he went to Cincinnati, Ohio, and worked for nearly four years. He went to St. Louis, Missouri, to enter the medical department of St. Louis University, in which he was graduated as a member of the class of 1904, receiving the degree of Doctor of Medicine. He interned in St. Louis City Hospital, and then engaged in general practice there. On December 15, 1906, he came to Stites. About two years later he transferred his residence to Elk City, then moved to Kamiah.

He was an active member of the Idaho State and

American Medical associations, and served as physician of Lewis County. Kamiah is near the boundary line between Nez Perce and Idaho counties, and the doctor's practice extended over a considerable territory in each of these counties.

Dr. McMahan was a Republican, and while in Elk City he served on the Republican central committee of Idaho County. He was also a member of the board of education in his hometown. He was affiliated with the Masons, Odd Fellows, a member of Our Club, Kamiah, and the Baptist Church. Mrs. McMahan was a member of the Congregational Church.

In Chicago, on July 29, 1906, Dr. McMahan was married to Miss Lillie P. Findlow, daughter of James W. Findlow. Dr. and Mrs. McMahan had two daughters, Lillie Jane and Marian Ruth.

DR. DALE BASKETT

Dr. L. Dale Baskett was born to Leslie and Mamie Baskett, who lived at Nez Perce for many years, and attended the schools there. His father was music director for the school system for nearly a quarter century. Dr. Baskett spent most of his medical life practicing on Thousand Oaks Boulevard in Conejo, California, going there when both he and the town were young. He and his wife had been in the San Fernando Valley and wanted to get away from the traffic, smog and crowds. Thousand Oaks was then, 1953, a sleepy little town of 2,000 and in the intervening years had boomed to 60,000. In 1978, with their children, David and Leslie, they moved to the northern California town of Auburn.

Describing his life in Conejo, he said, "I need a change of pace, my wife is deathly afraid of earthquakes, and I want to build my own home to be heated with solar power, and I want to travel. I have been working fifty to sixty hours a week and there wasn't a nearby hospital for years, I made a lot of house calls. People don't change," he said, "but medicine has. We didn't have good tranquilizers nor treatment for hypertension. When I look back at the charts of twenty-five years ago, I just didn't have the tools I do now. But the patients were wonderful, they were so easy to deal with."

DR. ELMER G. BRADDOCK

As with most early-day doctors, Elmer Braddock is remembered for the people he treated and the lives he saved, but the one memory Lewistonians keep fresh in their minds is the day he shot the elephant.

A large circus had arrived for its annual show; a parade preceded it. Leading the parade were three big elephants chained together. "Mary," not the largest, but perhaps the strongest, broke the chains holding her to the other two and went on a rampage, apparently searching for the water from the Clearwater River just a block away. Swinging her trunk as a battering ram, "Mary" shattered several plate glass windows and overturned cars, then chased two of the town's best-known teachers, Lillian McSorley and Alberta Hibbard, down the street and to an alley, where they ducked into the Buick garage and up the stairs onto a balcony. In the meantime, the circus manager called Mayor-Doctor Braddock and said he had a rogue elephant on the loose and wondered if anyone in the town had an elephant gun. Dr. Braddock who often went big-game hunting in Canada, got his gun and went to the garage and killed "Mary," who had gone on such rampages previously.

Dr. Braddock was asked by Dr. John Alley to become the practicing physician for the Nez Perce Indians at Lapwai for several months while Dr. Alley took several young Nez Perce east to attend Carlisle University. Dr. Braddock agreed and he, his wife Nell, and baby daughter Sally lived in Lapwai for the several months Dr. Alley was absent, then moved to Lewiston upon his return. In Lewiston, they had a second daughter, Betty Lou, and a son, John R., who is a practicing physician in Lewiston now.

IDAHO COUNTY

Geographically, Idaho County is as interesting as its rich and colorful history. Its rough, mountainous area was cut by the deep canyons of the many rivers and tributaries of the Snake, the Salmon, the Selway, the Lochsa and the Clearwater. One of the world's largest primitive elk herds; some of the largest deer herds; a thousand miles of good fishing streams; more than two-hundred mountain lakes; large cattle and sheep ranches; excellent farming areas; and many deposits of gold, silver, copper, lead, zinc and other industrial minerals are all packaged within Idaho County.

When the size of Idaho County is considered, there is little wonder that it contains all this . . . and more. It is the largest of Idaho's forty-four counties, being larger than the entire state of Massachusetts, the state of New Jersey or the state of Connecticut. The county dwarfs the little state of Rhode Island by being seven times its size. If it were in Europe it could declare its intentions to become a country. If the residents remained of the same strength and character of those of Idaho County, my money would be on them to bring it about!

DR. A. F. WOHLENBERG

Dr. A.F. Wohlenberg was an early-day doctor in Kooskia. He also owned the principal pharmacy in the town. Carrying a full line of drugs, he also handled stationery, "talking machines," paints, school books, wall paper, photo supplies, sporting goods for hunting, fishing, baseball and football, Christmas and birthday gifts.

DR. JOHN EDWARD ROCKWELL, JR.

Dr. Rockwell was born March 26, 1924 in Los Angeles, and was graduated from San Mateo Junior College, College of the Pacific in Stockton, and Louisiana State University in New Orleans. He had rotating internship and residency at St. Mary's in San Francisco and Monterey County Hospital in Salinas from 1948–50.

Dr. Rockwell spent nearly two years in an interesting practice at the Stibnite antimony mining area as the only doctor. He had a well-equipped small hospital, and referred problem patients to Boise by air. A special problem was the effects of antimony on the noses of smelter workers, who found their septums being eaten away. The mine has since closed. The following two years, 1952–54, he was in the U.S. Air Force in Montgomery, Alabama, Fairchild A.F.B., Spokane; Randolph A.F.B., Texas, and bases in Tokyo and Fairfield, California. He was awarded the Bronze Star and other decorations.

He belonged to the Idaho Medical Society and was public relations chairman in 1961. He was chief of staff at the Grangeville hospital for several terms. He and Mrs. Rockwell moved to Grangeville in 1954. They have four boys and two girls.

DR. GEORGE S. STOCKTON

Dr. George S. Stockton arrived at then-Denver, Idaho in 1898, where he practiced for two years before moving to Grangeville. He was elected Idaho County physician and for several years his offices were in the hospital. When the Grabski Building was completed he obtained a suite there.

He was a graduate of Toronto School of Medicine in 1887, and took a graduate course in New York, while serving an internship at Mount Sinai Hospital. He practiced in Michigan four years before moving to Idaho.

DR. WILSON A. FOSKETT

Along that stretch of Idaho's Highway 95, between White Bird and Riggins is a small parking strip where many travelers pull off the road to read the words on a bronze plaque imbedded in a cement monument:

Dedicated to the Memory of
Wilson A. Foskett, M.D.
July 8, 1870–April 14, 1924
Devoted in Life and
In Death to the
Salmon River People
"No Greater Love Hath a Man
Than to Lay Down His Life
For His Fellowmen"

No one could say that Dr. Foskett did not know every stretch and curve of the road alongside the racing Salmon River as it made its onrush to join the Snake at the foot of the Camas Mountains. He had ridden horseback, driven horse and buggy, and later his automobile through Box

Canyon, both before and after the road was completed in 1921. He had traversed that rugged country in all kinds of weather at all times of day and night to care for the Salmon River People mentioned on the memorial.

There is a creek that empties into the Salmon River five miles above the mouth of Slate Creek. It is named John Day for a man who freighted for the U.S. Government while Fort Colville was being established. A way station was built there in the early 1860s and used as a stopping place for those on their way to the Salmon River mining diggings. A fresh mount was kept at John Day for Dr. Foskett, to use whenever he rode into that country to see a patient.

At age fifty-four, and at the peak of his medical and mental powers, his friends long mourned his untimely death; they sorely missed their doctor-friend. He had kept a long and steady pace for several days and nights and likely fell asleep from exhaustion the night of April 14, 1924, when his car plunged into the turbulent Salmon River. He was found with his back broken. He had

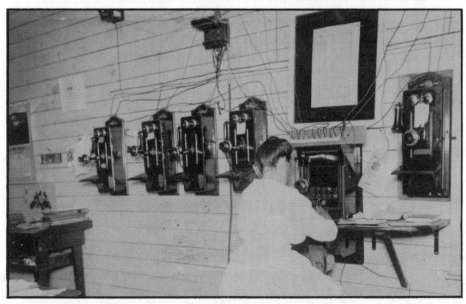

This switchboard was set up by the people of the Salmon River country in the vicinity of the Whitebird Canyon to keep in contact with Dr. Foskett and one another. When she was old enough, the switchboard became the responsibility of the doctor's daughter, Erna.

(Courtesy Erna Bentz)

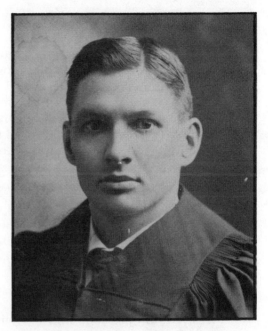

Erna Bentz of Grangeville, daughter of Dr. Wilson Foskett, says that theirs was a "very extended family, because father was in other people's homes almost more than our own." The doctor was killed when his car overturned into the Salmon River as he drove home from an all-night medical case. Erna describes his practice as a "community effort" as people kept spare horses and provided shelter for him. Operators of the river ferry met him at any hour to transport him to a patient.
(Courtesy Erna Bentz)

answered a call from his home in Whitebird, made the visit and was on his way home.

Friends found his car when daybreak came. In erecting the statue, those friends were joined by many admirers of the man who devoted his life to humanity without thought of personal gain. Whenever he was called, he went.

The first memorial was built by a Catholic priest from Grangeville, of native stone and topped with a cross, and dedicated in 1937. It was vandalized by the thoughtless and witless who broke off the cross and dislodged stones. A new memorial was erected in May of 1939 and was made of reinforced concrete in the shape of a pyramid. A bronze cross was mounted on the top. The cross has been bent and edges of the pyramid chipped away, but the marker with its loving message remains. Tourists by the thousands have now joined Idahoans who like to make a stop at the spot and contemplate the kind of a man who gave his life for his fellowmen just as surely as had he been killed in battle.

Dr. Foskett's daughter, Mrs. Frank McGrane, makes her home in Grangeville.

DR. JOHN H. POWELL

In the early months of 1863, Idaho was still a part of Washington Territory and the gold rush had started. There was an influx of families planning homes and crops as well as the miners with picks and shovels. John H. Powell arrived, homesteaded, planted and built a substantial home in which he had his medical office. A **Dr. John B. Morris** came from the St. Louis Medical College to Mount Idaho in 1875. No other information could be found on either doctor.

DR. SAMUEL E. BIBBY

Dr. Samuel E. Bibby had been diagnosed as having but a few months to live after he returned to his native New York from an arduous postgraduate course in medicine at Edinburgh, Scotland, and additional courses at Howard University and the University of New York. In the late 1870s, Bibby diagnosed his own case as being advanced tuberculosis, and believed that an outdoor setting in the west could cure him, and left within a week on a train for Fort Lapwai, Idaho. He had secured a commission as surgeon in the U.S. Army, assigned to the fort, and after presenting himself to the commandant, he set out to heal the Indians and the whites for miles around. He walked, he rode horseback and he drove a buggy. He rode a hundred miles on horseback to set the limb of a Nez Perce Indian who had broken it in a fall from his horse.

The rugged outdoor life brought him health and strength. He tired of the monotony at Fort Lapwai, and moved to Grangeville, built up a large horse and cattle industry on a ranch at Whitebird on the Salmon River, where he bred Hereford and Durhams and Hambletonian horses. He owned and operated a drugstore along with his medical practice at Grangeville. On Christmas day, 1889, he married Adelaide, first daughter of William C. and Balla Pearson, among the oldest pioneers on the prairie, and built for them a large home in Grangeville. He described himself as "a bookworm," and had one of the most extensive libraries in Idaho.

During the St. Louis Exposition, Dr. Bibby was elected vice president of the International Society of Army and Navy Surgeons, and was awarded a gold medal after giving a learned talk on diseases. He was named surgeon-in-chief of the Idaho National Guard by Governor N.B. Willey, 1891–92, which ranked him a lieutenant-colonel on the governor's staff.

He was born May 24, 1847 in Glens Falls, New York, the son, grandson and on up to great-great-grandson of physicians, coming from Scotland. At an age when his classmates were still in primary grades, Bibby was pouring over medical books and soon sent to Scotland to study. He returned to New York for eleven years of practice and became assistant or principal demonstrator at clinics held for students at Bellevue Hospital. This was followed by the postgraduate studies and the breakdown of his health.

DR. DONALD JACK SOLTMAN

Dr. Jack Soltman is a native of the town in which he has practiced medicine since 1946, Grangeville. He was born March 3, 1917 and attended grade and high schools in Grangeville and received his bachelor of science degree from the University of Idaho in 1937. His M.D. degree is from the University of Oregon Medical School in 1941, and he became a member of A.T.O. and Theta Kappa Psi fraternities. His internship and residency were at Ancker Hospital in St. Paul, Minnesota. He served as a captain in the U.S. Army infantry in the European theatre from 1942–46 during World War II.

While Dr. Soltman does not consider himself an "old time doctor" in the mode of **Dr. Wesley Orr, Dr. Slusser, Doctors Shinnick, Weber, and Chipman**, who are among those who preceded him at Grangeville, he has had two occasions to ride horseback into the back country to the scene of hunting accidents. He also remembers that his dad used to "drive buggy for old Doc Slusser when he was too tired to drive himself."

About five o'clock one morning he was called by neighbors to the Whitebird area to see a patient who had no phone. She lived on the other side of Whitebird Creek and the bridge had washed out in the spring flood. He drove to the place where the bridge had been, took his medical bag and walked up the creek until he found a place he could wade across. Another half-mile of walking took him to the house. After knocking and letting himself in, he found the patient in bed with her three children.

"Asking what kind of trouble she was having," the doctor said, "she told me that she was very nervous about the bridge being out and was 'kind of wondering' what she would do if she or one of the children got sick. I told her she would have to call a doctor in that case, and I returned to Grangeville."

Dr. Soltman is married to Mary Fran Marshall and they have two sons and two daughters. One son, Donald J. Jr., has gone into the medical administration and is vice-president of the Kootenai Medical Center in Coeur d'Alene, where he has been for ten years.

DR. WILLIAM H. CONE

Dr. Cone was born in Whitebird, Idaho June 27, 1922. His father was a farmer. He went through high school in Grangeville, then attended the University of Idaho for one year. He worked in Alaska one year, and spent three years in the armed forces as a paratrooper.

From 1946-47 he went to the University of Idaho; in 1951 he received his M.D. degree from the University of Oregon Medical School. 1951-52 he interned at William Beaumont Army Hospital. From 1953-63 he practiced in Grangeville. In 1963-64 he was in residency at Mental Health Institute, Cherokee, Iowa. He returned to central Idaho to practice psychiatry, and also practiced in Lewiston and Coeur d'Alene.

He was on the staff at Grangeville General Hospital. As coroner of Idaho County he had harrowing trips into Idaho wilderness regions by jet boat up Salmon River, and by airplane and helicopter.

He was a first lieutenant in the U.S. Army Medical Corp and received both the Bronze Star and the Purple Heart.

The Cones had three daughters and two sons.

CHAPTER
11

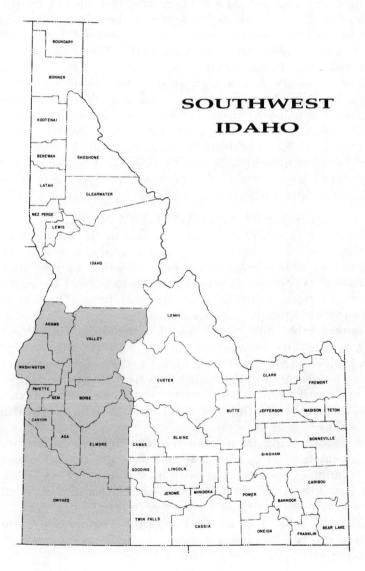

**SOUTHWEST
IDAHO**

VALLEY COUNTY

The last Indian war in the state was fought in Valley County. Settlers along the South Fork of the Salmon had been terrorized by a band of raiding Sheepeaters with ranchers killed, farms burned and cattle stolen. U.S. troops were sent from Fort Boise in the spring of 1879 but could not find the hideout. The soldiers were ambushed by the Indians and retreated to Vinegar (all they had to drink) Hill to wait for reinforcements which arrived from Fort Lapwai, Fort Boise, and Fort Walla Walla. The Indians were captured and taken to Vancouver.

Valley County has a sign post a few hundred yards north of New Meadows that proclaims the driver has reached the half-way distance between the North and the South Poles. It is a wildly beautiful area, with the white-water Payette River and the South and Middle Forks of the Salmon rocketing through it. The Boise and Salmon River Mountain Ranges tower over the green valleys, many lakes and caves, cliffs, and creeks.

DRS. JOHN AND MARGERY MOSER

The Moser medical team has worked in the small town of Cascade and served the Idaho mountainous back country for many years. They have traveled by dog sled, snowmobile, private aircraft and automobile to reach people in need of emergency medical help. They have become true legends in their lifetimes.

Coming from their World War II experiences, they knew they wanted to become physicians and practice where people needed them the most. John was also the victim of severe hay fever, and antihistamines had not yet appeared. He had worked with the Indian Service in New Mexico and Arizona before the war and found that hay fever did not bother him in the west.

After graduating from Case Western Reserve University in Cleveland in 1955, they traveled west for a place where they could set up a practice with little funding. They heard that Cascade's Dr. Dale Patterson was ailing and they went to help him. When Dr. Patterson recovered he moved to Boise, and sold his ten-bed hospital, equipment, and medical records for $250, a bargain.

Practicing in the primitive area, the Mosers soon realized that they must have some kind of communications system through which they could be contacted when people needed help. John had learned to fly in the war, and as soon as he could, he bought his own plane. They applied for a grant that no one thought they could possibly get, but, as a banker said, "We thought it was impossible, but the Mosers pulled it off, and their legend began."

They called it Wilderness Medical Service and communications stations, equipped with radios, were set up throughout the back country for several hundred miles radius. Lives were saved, broken bones were patched together, babies delivered, and all occurred in every type of weather imaginable.

In time, an inspector drove up from Boise to take a look at the old hospital. "He said, 'This is a fire trap,' and closed it down," Dr. John said. It was apparent to the community that something had to be done to maintain a community hospital. The people formed a local hospital district and contributions started coming in, primarily from the community, including the back country folk, mining prospectors, and ranchers.

When they had reached $35,000 they were sure it would be enough, but found they were $25,000 short if they were going to set up the twenty beds they needed. They knew the community couldn't put up anymore and federal funds were not available. The Mosers wrote out a check for the amount. One Cascade resident said, "That's the kind of people they were, always willing to walk the extra mile or fly the extra fifty miles, whatever it takes to take care of the sick people around here."

Both the Mosers were active in community affairs, she as church pianist, member of the Valley County Welfare Council and the National Study of Local Schools. Dr. John was a layman in the Episcopal Church, member of the Cascade Zoning Commission and a member of the school board for several terms. *The Sunday Statesman* featured them in Portrait of a Distinguished Citizen with a pencil sketch of the couple.

DR. ORLANDO J. HAWKINS

Dr. Orlando J. Hawkins died at age sixty-six on November 27, 1963, in Meridian. Born in Smith Center, Kansas on November 20, 1897, he graduated from Wesleyan University and received his M.D. degree from the University of Nebraska College of Medicine in 1933. In 1934, he received Idaho Medical License No. 1,433 to practice medicine and surgery. He practiced in Parma in 1934; was contract surgeon for the Civilian Conservation Corps in 1935-36.

He practiced in McCall from 1936-39 and then joined the Army Medical Corps, where he attained the rank of major. He returned to McCall where he practiced until his retirement in 1949 and then located in Meridian. He was a former Valley County Coroner and a member of the Southwestern Idaho District Medical Society and Idaho State Medical Association.

DR. A. EUGENE PFLUG

Dr. Pflug was born in North Dakota, moved to Idaho with his family, attended the Universities of Idaho and Oregon, before entering Oregon Medical School in 1948-52. He received his M.D. and practiced for a number of years at McCall.

He traveled by plane and helicopter to bring injured firefighters from the primitive area to the hospital. His practice included much walking to get to and from the patients and back to the plane. He once skied into the back country to treat a patient injured during a blizzard. There was no electricity and he had kerosene lamps by which to work There was no hospital at McCall for the first five years and patients were taken to the Council hospital, forty miles away.

Dr. Pflug was in the Naval Air Corps as a lieutenant j.g. from 1943-47. He and his wife, Margaret, had two boys and three girls.

ADAMS COUNTY

The county seat of Council in Adams received its name because the valley in which it is located was the meeting place for the Indian Councils of the Nez Perce and Shoshoni tribes. Another spot of historic interest is the Packer John Cabin in Old Meadows, where the first Democratic convention of Idaho Territory met. The Seven Devils Mountains make up twenty percent of Adams County and the rugged beauty of the area has become an attraction for travelers and campers. From the Devils, one can look down upon the Grand Canyon of the Snake River. Cattle raising is prominent in the county.

DR. WILLIAM M. BROWN

Dr. Brown was a physician of Cuprum, high in the hills of Idaho near the Seven Devils Mountains, where he moved in June, 1899. He was born in Preble County, Ohio, on November 18, 1860. His ancestors were early settlers of South Carolina, and his grandfather, James Brown, was born in Due West, South Carolina. James Scott Brown, the doctor's father, was a native of Preble County, and spent his entire life near the old homestead where he was born.

Dr. Brown was the eldest of nine children. He attended the public schools of the Buckeye State; he continued studies at the University of Oxford, Ohio, and at Monmouth College, Monmouth, Illinois. He was graduated from the Miami College of Cincinnati, Ohio, 1888, having completed a course in medicine. He engaged in the practice of medicine in Omaha, Nebraska, until June, 1892, when he went to Salubria, Idaho. Building a home, he lived there for seven years, and his practice constantly extended throughout the valley. In June, 1899, he moved to Cuprum, Idaho, where in connection with his practice, he conducted a drug store.

He was married on October 2, 1889, to Miss Emma L. Sherman, of New York. They had two daughters, Winifred and Mildred. Dr. Brown was a valued member of the Independent Order of Odd Fellows, and a Republican. He served as coroner of Washington County.

DR. JOHN ALBERT EDWARDS

Dr. John Edwards was born in Washington, D.C., April 14, 1919. His father was an attorney.

He received a B.A. degree in 1940 from George Washington University, Washington, D.C. In 1943, he received his medical degree from the George Washington University Medical School. He interned at the university from 1943–44. In 1944 he had a residency at the same university for ten months. He started his practice in Council on April 1, 1947.

The doctor was chief of staff, at the Community Hospital, Council. He was a past president of the Chamber of Commerce, and in 1963 received "Man of the Year." For several years he was a member of School District B-13 School Board. Dr. Edwards was in the U. S. Army Medical Corps, and served in the Philippines and Japan as captain. The Edwards have five sons and one daughter.

WASHINGTON COUNTY

Named for the first President of the United States, Washington County was first visited by white men in 1811 when Donald McKenzie and his companions stopped on their war to Astoria. He returned in 1818 to trap along the Weiser River and its tributaries. Pioneers began settling in the county in the 1860s and Thomas Galloway built a log cabin in what was to become Weiser. The first settlement was Weiser Bridge and in 1863 R.P. Olds built and operated a ferry across the Snake. The first flour mill was erected at Weiser in 1869, and the Union Pacific Railway reached the town in 1895.

The Snake River forms the western boundary of the county and several ranges of rolling hills and mountains run through the central section of the valley.

DR. M. S. McGRATH

Dr. McGrath was born July 12, 1908, at Star, Idaho. His father was a farmer. Before entering medical school he had a B.S. degree as a pharmacist.

In 1933 he was graduated from the Southern Branch of University of Idaho, Pocatello. He received his medical degree at Washington University Medical School, St. Louis, Missouri in 1937. He interned at St. Louis City Hospital. In 1939, he moved to Weiser and began his private practice.

DR. CHARLES ERNEST SCHMITZ

Charles Ernest Schmitz went to Cambridge in 1904, one year after he graduated from Barnes Medical College of St. Louis.

He was born October 22, 1879, at Fort Scott, Kansas, the son of John and Christinia (Bauer) Schmitz. Both parents were born in Germany. His father came in the early 1850s, settling in Wisconsin, then moving to Kansas after the Civil War.

Dr. Schmitz was the fifth of eight children, and was educated in Fort Scott, graduating from high school in 1897. He studied at the College of Physicians and Surgeons at Keokuk, Iowa for two years and Barnes Medical College, St. Louis to earn his M.D. in 1903. He interned in City Hospital, St. Louis. In 1907, after he spent one year in study in Germany, he stopped in Chicago, on his return, for a postgraduate course. He returned to Cambridge in 1908.

He was a member of the State and American Medical associations. He belonged to Woodmen of the World; Modern Woodmen of America; the Roman Catholic Church, being one of the instigators in the building of the new church; and a member of the Idaho militia. Dr. Schmitz was connected with the Cambridge Publishing Company and a sheep shearing plant. He owned two and a quarter sections of land in the county and a seven acre tract in town, and five city lots.

May 25, 1904, Dr. Schmitz married Myrtle M. McClain, daughter of John McClain, Shell City, Missouri. They had three sons and one daughter.

DR. SIMEON HOPPER

Dr. Simeon Hopper was born in an old log cabin in Middle Valley, two miles across the Weiser River from the present town of Midvale in Idaho Territory. It was March 4, 1886, and he grew up in the valley. When he was three his father, Moses Hopper, bought a relinquishment on a farm where Cambridge was later built, and the Hoppers farmed.

Dr. Hopper remembered the old Concord stages carrying mail and passengers from Weiser through Middle Valley to the now-extinct town of Salubria, on to Council and Old Meadows. Horses were changed at the stage station near the foot of the north side of Middle Valley Hill. The driver used four horses, which were changed for fresh animals at each of the five stations along the route.

During high school vacation, Simeon was running an edger in the sawmill and stepped on a saw, cutting a gash in his left foot. He was hauled in a wagon for twenty miles to Dr. C.C. Schmitz in Cambridge. He stayed there, walking on crutches every day for six weeks to the doctor. As his foot improved, he visited more with the doctor, who induced him to take up the study of medicine.

That fall, he entered Barnes University at St. Louis, Missouri, for two years before transferring to St. Louis University. Each vacation at home he studied medicine under Dr. Schmitz and accompanied him on horse-and-buggy home calls. After getting his M.D. degree, he returned to Cambridge, bought a team, "found a cheap buggy without a top," and was ready to practice. He bought a large umbrella to serve as the buggy top. He said, "It wasn't so bad during the summer but terrible during the winter, especially during an Idaho blizzard."

When the United States became involved in World War I, Dr. Hopper took entry exams with Lieutenant Colonel Wood, retired Army medical officer in Boise, and returned to Cambridge to await his call. It did not come until March 1918, when he was ordered to Hoboken, New Jersey to board one of fifteen troop ships, guarded by one battleship and four destroyers, for Liverpool, England. He had three weeks of physical training at Blackpool before being sent to Leeds University for bedside training on treatment of battle wounds. The chief surgeon for the Royal Family appeared twice a week to lecture.

Soon they set sail for France and the front and were assigned to the British Expeditionary Forces units to replace doctors who had been killed. Dr. Hopper was with the 80th American Division, as was **Dr. William Passer** of Twin Falls. After three months with an ambulance unit, he was wounded by shrapnel and evacuated to England for hospitalization.

Four months before an order to leave the 111th Field Ambulance Unit and proceed to Brest to sail for home, he was promoted to captain. He was discharged April 25, 1919, at Trenton, New Jersey, and went to New York, where his wife was waiting. After visiting New York and Washington, they returned to Cambridge. He found a new practice in Homedale and moved there in January 1920, where he became the Owyhee County doctor. In February 1929, Dr. Berry moved from Hazelton and Dr. Hopper was asked to take over his practice, which he did. The Idaho State Medical Association awarded him a certificate in 1960, commemorating his fifty years of practice.

DR. WILLIAM R. HAMILTON

Dr. William R. Hamilton was born on July 10, 1866, in Ontario, Canada, the son of William and Jane (Reid) Hamilton, natives of Glasgow and Aberdeen, Scotland, respectively. (The father was born in 1830 and came to Canada in 1851, where he was a pioneer farmer in Ontario. He died in 1868.)

Dr. Hamilton attended the schools of Brantford, Ontario, and his higher education was received at the Toronto School of Medicine, graduating in 1892. Soon thereafter he made his way to Payette, Idaho where he practiced medicine between the years of 1893 and 1898. In 1898, he moved from Payette to Silver City, where he lived until 1909. In February, 1910, he established himself in Weiser. While there he was named to the Idaho State Board of Health.

Dr. Hamilton was a Master Mason and a Shriner. He reached the second degree in the Knights Templar. In 1908 and 1909, he served as Grand Master of the Masonic Lodge in Idaho.

The doctor served as the Owyhee County physician for two years. He was a Democrat.

On September 28, 1898, Dr. Hamilton was married to Emma Coughanour, daughter of William A. Coughanour, Payette. They had two daughters, Marjorie and Dorothy.

DR. CHARLES B. SHIRLEY

Dr. Charles B. Shirley of Weiser was a member of an old Virginia family. Both of his parents, Charles B. Shirley (1819-1902), and Sarah Burchell Shirley (1821-1902), were born in Virginia. Dr. Shirley's father was born at Harper's Ferry, but lived at Alexandria, Virginia, the greater part of his life. He worked in government work for many years in Washington, D.C. The doctor was the eldest of eleven children. He was born in Alexandria September 14, 1848.

Private schools of Alexandria provided his education and he went to the District of Columbia, where he was a bookkeeper. His tendencies were scientific and professional, and he decided to study medicine.

He entered Howard University in 1876. Three years later he was graduated with the degree of doctor of medicine. Dr. Shirley's early practice was in Washington, D.C. After seven years there, Dr. Shirley wanted to change climate for the sake of Mrs. Shirley's health. They moved to Silver City, New Mexico, and were there from 1886-91. When they moved to Weiser, Idaho, it contained six buildings. He was the third physician to take up practice in that community.

Dr. Shirley was a leader in both the Idaho and Southern Idaho Medical organizations, and was one of the organizers of the latter. He was connected with the Ancient Order of United Workmen, and was one of the organizers in Silver City. He held all the chairs in the Knights of Pythias, and Grand Chancellor. He was a charter member in Weiser of Myrtle Lodge No. 26. To him was given chief credit for the erection of Castle Hall, built by the lodge in 1903 and 1904. His zeal and enthusiasm in this society have led to his being affectionately called, by his official brother Knights, "the Grand Old Man of our Lodge." Dr. Shirley was an Episcopalian, and a Republican.

Mrs. Shirley was August Van Swearingen. Her parents were Charles and Mary Van Swearingen. They had two children, Charles, born in 1890 and Marguerite born in 1896.

DOCTORS CONANT, THREE GENERATIONS

Dr. Jesse L. Conant was born May 31, 1831, in Essex County, New York, and after practicing medicine in Michigan, Nebraska, and South Dakota for a number of years before moving to Genesee. He had a basement and two-story building, with an adjoining drugstore, built for his practice. In 1900, he moved to Weiser, bought a drugstore, and practiced medicine for several years. He died in 1911 from a stroke after practicing medicine thirty years.

Dr. Conant Jr. was born in Michigan, attended Detroit Medical School and practiced for a few years in Herman, Nebraska. He then moved to Genesee to practice with his father before enlisting in the Spanish-American War, serving as surgeon to the First Regiment in the Philippine Islands. After the war, he moved to Weiser. He was appointed to the Board of Medical Examiners. He died May 3, 1910 from a stroke.

Dr. Carroll C. Conant was born June 20, 1884 in Hermon, Nebraska and moved with his family to Genesee, where he graduated from grade and high schools. He studied at the Detroit College of Medicine and interned at the Harper Hospital there.

He was appointed physician for the Northern Pacific Railway, but resigned in 1910 to take over his father's practice in Weiser, where he continued until 1932. He died from myocarditis at Letterman General Hospital that year.

DR. FRANK ALBERT SCHMITZ

Dr. Schmitz was born March 17, 1885 in Mapleton, Kansas, and worked on the family farm as a boy. After graduating *cum laude* as a physician and surgeon from the Barnes Medical College in St. Louis, Missouri in 1909, he came to Midvale, Idaho, and practiced for three years before moving to Weiser where he practiced for more than forty years. A brother, Dr. C.E. Schmitz practiced at Cambridge, Idaho.

He began his practice with horse and buggy, using a cutter in the winter. Sometimes it took him two days to complete calls in the isolated areas, where the same calls now could be made in a few hours. He was chief of staff at the Weiser Hospital. He and his wife had one daughter and two sons, eight grandchildren, and one great-grandchild.

DR. GEORGE M. WATERHOUSE

The Sunnyside Orchard Company in Washington County, which owned and operated a tract of several hundred acres of fruit-bearing property, was organized and promoted by its first president, Dr. George M. Waterhouse. Dr. Waterhouse was born in New London, Ohio, October 7, 1860, the son of I. L. and Hannah (Stow) Waterhouse.

His father served as mayor of New London at one time. He died in 1897, when he was seventy-eight years of age. His mother's family were early American citizens, several being soldiers in the Colonial Army during the Revolutionary War. His great grandmother was a half sister of the showman, P.T. Barnum. His mother died in 1905, at the age of seventy-seven. Dr. George M. was the fourth of seven children.

The doctor attended the public schools of Huron County, Ohio, and was graduated from Fitchville High School in 1880. He entered Eclectic Medical College, Cincinnati, where he was graduated in 1885. He then studied in Barnes Medical College.

In 1886, he began active practice in Weiser, where in

1910, at the time of his retirement, he was the sixth oldest practicing physician in Idaho.

In 1910, he became president of the Sunnyside Orchard Company. He was an organizer of the Weiser National Bank, of which he was president for five years. He was a Republican, and served as treasurer of Washington County for four years. In 1891, he became a member of the board of regents of the University of Idaho, serving for one-half a term; was president of the State Board of Medical Examiners for two years, and was on the board until he retired in 1910.

He was a member of the Shrine Blue Lodge, Red Cross of Constancy, and the Eastern Star, in which he held official positions.

Dr. Waterhouse lived at 407 W. Main Street, and had a forty acre orchard joining Weiser on the south. He was married October 22, 1889, at Fairfield, Nebraska to Annie M. Beswick, a native of Ohio. They had two children, Georgiana, born December 3, 1894, and Frederick, October 1, 1896.

DR. ERNEST O. FINNEY

Gifted with a love for medicine, Dr. Ernest O. Finney won the confidence of Weiser, Idaho, beginning in 1910. The doctor was one of the most skilled practitioners in his part of the state.

Dr. Finney was born July 27, 1879, at Rankin, Illinois, the son of Frank A. and Viola (Stalmaker) Finney. On the paternal side, Dr. Finney traced his ancestry back to the time of Charles of England. The American progenitor of the family came in the Mayflower. His father, a native of Indiana, moved to Illinois and resided at Rankin where he was a merchant. The oldest of four children, Dr. Finney secured his early education in the public and high schools of Rankin, graduating in 1896. He began clerking in the Rankin store, soon opening a general merchandise business of his own. By 1902 he had accumulated enough money to pursue his medical studies and entered the College of Physicians and Surgeons in Chicago, graduating with an M.D. in 1906.

In the following eighteen months he served as an extern in the various Chicago hospitals, and four months as an intern. He went to Europe for a year at the University of

Vienna and in Vienna hospitals. He returned to the United States in the fall of 1908 and became surgical assistant to the noted Dr. Edward H. Ochsner at Augustana Hospital in Chicago.

In 1910, he came to Weiser and engaged in general practice. His success with a number of complicated cases established the confidence of the people there. He was a member of the Chicago Medical Association, the Illinois State Medical Society, the Masonic Blue Lodge in Rankin, and the Royal Arch Masons of Weiser. Politically he was a Republican.

DR. HYDEN HANCHER

Hyden Hancher was born April 20, 1901 in Valley Center, Kansas, where his father was a Methodist Episcopal minister. He attended grade school in several Colorado towns and graduated from Central High School in Pueblo in 1919. He graduated from the University of Denver with a B.A. in 1922; his B.S. in 1924 from Northwestern University Medical School and his M.D. in 1924. His internship was at the Grace Hospital in Detroit from 1926–27 and an O.B. internship at the Chicago Lying-In Hospital from August 1927 until February 1928. He practiced in Salt Lake City and Brigham Canyon, Utah and West Yellowstone from 1928–29. He then went to Potlatch, Idaho until 1931. In May of 1931, he relocated to Weiser, Idaho and remained there except for service in 1941–46 in the U.S. Army Medical Corps where he served as a captain. Three of those five years were spent stationed in Lidwalls, England.

During his early practice he did a rib resection for a victim of emphysema following pneumonia. He also repaired massive scalp lacerations in an eighty-five-year-old man. The most unusual means of transportation was a wagon box on runners across the snow for twenty miles. He experienced a severe diphtheria epidemic in 1931–32. He was chief of staff at the Memorial Hospital in Weiser several times. He had two daughters, each of whom had five children.

PAYETTE COUNTY

A part of Ada and Canyon counties for fifty-three years before it came into its own, the name of Payette came from an early French trapper, Francis Payette, who rebuilt Fort Boise as a fur-trading post for the Hudson Bay Company. David Bivens established a stage station in 1862 with the first buildings in the county. Nathan Falk opened a store in 1876 and the settlement then became known as Falk's Store, developing into a busy trading center. When the Union Pacific built a railroad camp and supply house in 1883, it was called Boomerang, later becoming Payette.

DR. OLIVER H. AVEY

In 1902, Dr. Oliver H. Avey settled in Payette, Idaho, where he established his medical practice. Previous to locating in Payette, he had taught school fifteen years, principally in the west, and had been in medical practice for one year in Cedar City, Utah. He had cherished a desire to enter the medical field for years.

Dr. Avey was born in Logan, Ohio, on December 31, 1857, the son of George L. and Mary (Fox) Avey. The father, a native of Maryland, was born March 13, 1830, and moved to Iowa in 1850. He was a saddle and harness maker. (The senior Aveys also lived in Payette, where Mr. Avey died on April 19, 1912.) Dr. Avey's mother was a native-born German, who came to America with her parents at the age of seven. They settled in Ohio. There she later met and married her husband.

Dr. Avey was educated in the public schools, and later at Penn College, Oskaloosa, Iowa. He graduated in 1881 with an A.B. degree, following which he was an assistant postmaster for four years at the post office of Oskaloosa. He then was principal of the Oskaloosa High School for a number of years. In 1891 he moved to Salt Lake City, and for nine years was principal of Washington School. He was a prominent factor in the organization of the free public school system under the Mormon regime. When he severed his connection with education, it was to finally realize his ambition to enter the medical profession. In 1901, he was graduated from Rush Medical College with an M.D. degree.

In October 1902, he settled in Payette, Idaho, and continued to practice. In 1904, Dr. Avey attended the Chicago Post Graduate College, and kept abreast with the advances made in the medical field. He was a member of the Idaho State and the American Medical associations and the Northwest Rush Medical College Alumni Association.

Dr. Avey became identified with some of the leading financial and industrial concerns in the city, and was president of the Payette National Bank, since its organization in 1906. He was also president of the Payette Valley Land and Orchard Company, and owned property in the south of the city. Politically, Dr. Avey was a Republican; president of the Board of Education in Payette, a post which he had held since 1904.

Dr. Avey was a member of the Masonic Fraternity, Blue Lodge; Commandery in the Knights Templar; and the Ancient Arabic Order of the Nobles of the Mystic Shrine; Past Master of the Blue Lodge; and was a member of the Payette Commercial Club.

On July 6, 1886, Dr. Avey was married to Lorie Pomeroy, daughter of Stephen and Elizabeth Pomeroy, of Iowa. No children were born to Dr. and Mrs. Avey; they adopted a child, Irene Avey.

DR. GEORGE E. DAVIS

George Davis was born October 28, 1907, Auburn, Maine. When he was a child the family moved to Oregon Slope (between Payette & Weiser), where his father was a farmer. He attended a country grade school, and graduated from Payette High School. He took his pre-med at College of Idaho, 1925–28. He got his M.D. degree at the University of Oregon Medical School, Portland, 1932. He interned at French Hospital, San Francisco, 1932–33, and passed the state boards of California in 1933. From 1933–35 he practiced in Pasadena.

In 1935 he began practice in Parma for two years, then moved to New Plymouth. He was on the staff of Holy Rosary Hospital, Ontario, Oregon, and adjacent hospitals. He belonged to the American Medical Association, Idaho State Medical Society, and Southwest Idaho District Medical Society. The Davises had two daughters.

GEM COUNTY

Gem County, with Emmett as its seat, was established in 1915. The mountain peaks are in the panhandle section north of Ola. In the lowlands lying to the south is the upper Payette River Valley, most often simply called the Emmett Valley. Formed from an ancient lake bed, the valley opened to the north end where the rapid Payette River made its way to join the mighty Snake River just below the settlement of Payette. A good four-season climate makes for the bountiful growing of fruit, vegetables, hay, grain, sheep, and cattle.

Indian raids, cattle and horse thievery, heroic vigilantes protecting the settlers from desperadoes, and the important trading post known as Falks Store (now in Payette County) create a spell-binding and romantic history.

With the exception of Indian and home-grown remedies, the settlers depended upon doctors from Boise and Caldwell until 1891. It was in the 1870s that Dr. Ephraim Smith of Boise was the first doctor to make regular trips to the Emmett Valley to see patients. In 1882, when the railroad came to Caldwell, Dr. Charles Lee of Caldwell was usually called, as it was a shorter trip by train from Caldwell than by horse and buggy from Boise.

Soon Dr. Alfred F. Isham from Vermont settled in Caldwell, followed by Dr. W.C. Maxey. All four of the doctors made many trips to Emmett Valley, many of them hazardous, particularly during the snowy winter months. When a rider was sent at the fastest possible speed to call upon the doctor, he would often return by fast horseback, or by horse and buggy.

DR. WILLIAM BURGE

In 1864, Dr. William Burge of Mount Pleasant, Iowa, settled at Emmett with his family. In a fully equipped wagon train of twenty-eight of his own Conestogas and a large number of loose stock, in a train of 100 wagons, he brought a supply of drugs and medicines and opened a drugstore in his home. Many early-day doctors served both as pharmacists and practitioners.

Dr. Burge had gone to California from Iowa in 1848 and back to Mount Pleasant a few years later. He never "got the west out of his system," and having learned much about crossing the plains, he and his entourage started for Idaho on May 1, 1864. As they neared Emmett Valley, Dr. Burge took his fastest riding horse and carefully scouted out Freezeout Hill, which was a difficult bit of terrain to overcome, as well as the Boise, Emmett, and Payette valleys. He made a decision to locate two miles west of Emmett and not far from the old Block House on the Basin Trail. An elder daughter and her husband, John Patterson, who had accompanied the Burge train, decided to make their home in the Boise Valley near Eagle.

DRS. CALEB NORTH, DAVIS, AND DAVID GOODRICH

In the early 1870s, a Dr. Caleb North from Boston traveled through the Boise, Emmett and Payette valleys, selling homeopathic medicines. He must have been successful as it was said that every family kept a bottle of "North's White Liniment," one dollar a bottle, on hand.

In 1875, Dr. Davis (first name unknown) located at the home of James Bennett, an uncle of John and Price Bane who lived across the Payette River on the north bench. Dr. Davis stayed for only a few months.

For seven years, 1881 to 1888, Dr. David Goodrich practiced in Emmett Valley. He and his family came from Indiana. He was a druggist who built a store near the home he bought from William Fuller. The home was later the site of the Emmett Meat Company. He had a goodly supply of drugs and also practiced medicine. In 1888, the Goodrichs returned to Indiana.

DR. CLYDE CLYMER AND OTHERS

Dr. Clyde Clymer arrived from Portland, Oregon in 1892 and remained for a number of years, when he was forced to retire through ill health.

The first woman doctor, a Dr. McCahey, located in Emmett in 1893. She remained but a few months.

Doctors Burr and Roundville were partners in practice, arriving in 1904. They, too, remained a short time.

Dr. Ell Parish doctored the ill and ailing for nearly sixty years, from 1892 through 1950.

Among others were Doctors Skippen, arriving in 1902; Green, Parkinson, Carver, Rawlinson, Bullock, Chipman,

Goodwin, Newcombe; Fairchild, arriving from Placerville in 1907; Cummings, 1904; Moses Stevens, 1907; Dr. Reynolds, from 1907 through 1950; and a Dr. Clark.

DR. JAMES LEMMON REYNOLDS

Among the eminent physicians and surgeons of southwest Idaho was Dr. James Lemmon Reynolds of Emmett. Dr. Reynolds was born at Chatham, Virginia February 3, 1878, son of John B. and Telith (Mahan) Reynolds. His father had enlisted in the Confederate Army during the Civil War, and served four years under General Wise, fighting until the fall of Richmond, then returning to his mercantile business in Chatham. The Reynolds became parents of nine children, of whom Dr. Reynolds was the sixth.

Dr. Reynolds received his early education in the public and high schools of Chatham, following which he went to work in the tobacco fields, where he earned money to pursue his studies. He enrolled in science at the College of William and Mary, Williamsburg, which, next to Harvard, is the oldest college in America. His resources were about exhausted and he was obliged to contract a loan from his father, and entered Richmond College, beginning the study of medicine and surgery.

Dr. Reynolds finished his course there, but his health gave way under the pressure of studies, and he came west. His medical education was completed at the University of Denver in 1904. He interned at St. Anthony Hospital, Denver, following which he came to Albion, Idaho.

After two years he moved to Emmett, in 1907. He practiced in Emmett and the surrounding area, and became an examiner for a number of old line insurance companies. He was a member of the Southern Idaho, Idaho State, and the American Medical associations. He became deputy physician of Canyon County, which then included Emmett, and surgeon for the Idaho Northern Railway.

He was a member of the Butte Lodge No. 37, A.F.& A.M, in Emmett, El Korah Shrine Temple in Boise, the Emmett Kiwanis Club, Odd Fellows, Woodmen of the World, and was a Democrat. With Mrs. Reynolds, he attended the Baptist Church of Emmett.

Dr. Reynolds was married in Albion, Idaho, June 6, 1907,

to Miss Gladys Kossman, who was born in Cassia County, daughter of Fred Kossman, an early settler of that county. They had three daughters, Mrs. Lois Congdon, Boise; Mrs. Mary Randall, Salem, Oregon; and Ruth Reynolds of Emmett. Dr. Reynolds died at his home on March 24, 1954.

DR. BERT O. CLARK

Dr. Clark was born March 9, 1877, in Nodaway County, Missouri, the son of William H. and Judith M. (North) Clark. He attended public school in Missouri, and in 1896 entered Ensworth College, at St. Joseph, from which he was graduated with his M.D. degree. In 1907, he came to Idaho, and after spending six months in Boise, moved to Emmett. Dr. Clark possessed a large and valuable library. He held membership in the Idaho State and the American Medical associations.

On May 26, 1897, Dr. Clark was married in Gage County, Nebraska, to Anna Heaston, daughter of Lewis and Mary (Teter) Heaston, well-known farming people of Gage County. They had two boys.

Fraternally Dr. Clark was connected with the Masonic Order, the Shrine; Fellow of the Woodmen of the World, and Modern Woodmen of America. He was medical examiner for Mutual Life Insurance, Banker's Reserve Insurance of Des Moines, and the Idaho State Life Insurance Company.

In politics, a Wilson Democrat, he served efficiently as a member of the school board.

The doctor was fond of all out-door sports, hunting, fishing, and automobiling being his favorites. It was his belief that Idaho was destined to become the leading state in the northwest.

DR. ROBERT NEWTON CUMMINGS

Dr. Cummings, physician and surgeon at Emmett and surrounding area, arrived there in 1904 and remained for many years. He was born at Hindsville, Arkansas, July 18, 1874, to Ross Kinyard and Margaret Garrett Cummings, both of Tennessee. Robert had two sisters and one brother. His father, a farmer, died when Robert was four years old. Robert continued to live in Arkansas, attending grade and high schools and was graduated from the University of Arkansas with a bachelor of arts degree in 1898.

He became a member of Kappa Alpha fraternity. From 1898 until 1901, he studied medicine at Washington University in St. Louis. He completed his professional training at the University of Denver, with an M.D. degree in 1903. After a year of interning in St. Anthony Hospital in Denver, he came to Idaho. After investigating several cities, he chose to locate in Emmett.

On February 19, 1906, in Boston, Dr. Cummings was married to Harriet Reynolds of Brownsville, Texas. Her father, Captain S.W. Reynolds was an officer of the Union Army during the Civil War, and afterward bought a drug store. Dr. and Mrs. Cummings had two children, Margaret, born November 25, 1907 and Florence, May 20, 1910. A son, Robert Edward, born March 10, 1914, died at age five.

ASSIST DOCTOR STORK

The baby-transporting stork was assisted by a number of midwives in those early days. Mrs. Lick was there in the 1870s; Mrs. Charles Oakes from 1880–90; a nurse, Mrs. Minerva Kelly in 1880; and Mrs. J.O.R. Will for the entire decade of 1880. Ten dollars was the regular fee charged by all of them and it was reported that not one of them lost a mother nor a baby. All of them are buried in the Emmett bench cemetery with a lovely view of the valley.

THE DOCTORS JEWELL

Most medical doctors have enough unusual experiences to last a lifetime. When a doctor father is followed by a doctor son they can add up happenings enough to last four lifetimes. Leo Edward Jewell, who practiced in Meridian, and his son, William Bracken Jewell, who practiced in Emmett, lived enough episodes of life to fill a lengthy book.

These range from Dr. Leo being sent as a reserve officer with an Army division to the Mexican border in 1918 to capture the chubby Mexican revolutionary general Pancho Villa to Dr. Bill being told by a brand-new mother awakening from a too-little injection of anesthesia, "You sonofabee, that HURT!"

Dr. Leo was born October 16, 1897, in Oklahoma, where his father had staked out farm land in Oklahoma Territory. Leo had decided to go into teaching and went to Peru, Nebraska for his training. While there he met Susan Dobbs, who also received her teaching certificate and they were engaged to be married. World War I intervened and Leo was with the Army expedition headed by Brigadier General John J. Pershing and sent to Mexico by President Woodrow Wilson with orders to capture the renegade Pancho Villa. The Mexican general of an "irregular" army had executed sixteen U.S. citizens and done other dastardly deeds. The mission failed. Bill Jewell was told by his father that the U.S. was fearful of the powers which might be manipulating Pancha Villa and had no stomach for another world war. Leo was then sent to Washington, D.C., to serve in the military's chemical warfare division.

In the meantime, Susan Dobbs and her sister, Fannie, had gone from Nebraska to Notus, Idaho to teach. So, when the war was over, Leo immediately left for Idaho and married Susan. He had taught a short time at Notus when offered the principal job at St. Anthony. He spent one year there. From there, he went to the Albion Normal School and taught math and science. Their son, who was to become the doctor, William Bracken, was born on July 27, 1923 at Rupert.

The next move was to Casper, Wyoming, where Leo was high school principal. Another son, James Leo, was born there. Through all of these moves, Leo had in the back of his mind that "one day, I will study to become a doctor." It was often a topic discussed in the home. "In 1929, he and mom just pulled up stakes, took Jim and me and moved to Omaha where Dad entered the medical college at the University of Nebraska. They rented a large house in Peony Park and took in other medical students to room and board, which paid a big part of the expenses," Bill reported.

Leo received his M.D. degree in 1933 in the midst of the Great Depression and so took a six months job as doctor with the Civilian Conservation Corps near Russellville, Kansas. One day, Leo received a letter from Jim Rice, pharmacist in Meridian, telling him that Meridian sorely needed another doctor and to come on out. He went out and looked over the situation, finding that Dr. Joe Thomas had moved to Boise and Dr. John Brunn was preparing to leave. He went back to Arkansas, collected his family and belongings and moved to Idaho for the rest of his life.

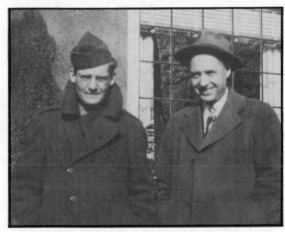

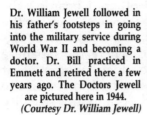

Dr. William Jewell followed in his father's footsteps in going into the military service during World War II and becoming a doctor. Dr. Bill practiced in Emmett and retired there a few years ago. The Doctors Jewell are pictured here in 1944.
(Courtesy Dr. William Jewell)

Among the difficult cases Dr. Leo received was when Jerry Everett was involved in an accident in which his neck was gashed so deeply as to sever the carotid (which carries blood to the head) artery. Dr. Jewell was successful in stopping the bleeding long enough to get Jerry to Boise for a life-saving operation.

As the only doctor in Meridian during WWII, Dr. Leo worked so hard and put in such long hours that he suffered a heart attack and was forced to retire. "Dad felt that a doctor's life was a hard one," Bill said, "and did what he could to discourage me from becoming one."

Dr. Leo went so far in discouraging a similar career for his son that he accompanied him to Moscow when Bill enrolled at the University of Idaho in 1941. His dad talked Bill into taking mining engineering. "By the end of the first semester, I knew that wasn't for me," Bill said, "so I switched to business administration. It probably wouldn't have made a lot of difference what I was taking as the war was hanging over all our heads. My brother Jim had already gone into the service and was in England. The more I thought about it, the more I knew I should be in pre-med, so that summer I switched.

"I had a good friend in political science, Professor Boyd Martin, and he called me in to talk to me about what I was doing and what I could do to get into medicine in the Army. I was sent for a technician training course of four months to Fitzsimmons General Hospital in Denver, where all the Army's surgical, medical, dental and lab technicians were taught. Then I went to Camp Barkeley in Abilene, Texas for bivouac and two months field training before going to the China-Burma-India theater.

"In January 1945, along with 5,999 others I boarded the Admiral W.S. Benson troopship in Los Angeles and for the next thirty-four days, without military escort, we zig-zagged all the way across the Pacific, where the Japanese subs were working double-duty, to dock unharmed at Melbourne, Australia. We were not permitted to get off the ship. There were too many of us to drop into any size city for a visit."

From Melbourne, the ship sailed the Indian Ocean with two small Canadian corvette destroyer escorts into Bombay. The troops were then divided and sent to Burma, China, or India. For fifteen months Bill was assigned to a B-24 airbase seventy-five miles north of Calcutta where the Burmese border fighting was taking place. The war came to an end in August of 1945. As no additional lab technicians were needed, Bill worked on the war wounded at the 30th Station Hospital, U.S. Army.

"It was like a Mash unit," Bill said, "a precursor of the Mash, but was then called a Portable Surgical hospital. Men injured in the raids over Burma were brought in for stabilizing treatment before being sent to the general hospital in Calcutta. We treated malaria and dysentery, and had an entire ward for venereal diseased patients."

Bill was reassigned as a lab technician to the 181st General Hospital, U.S. Army, in Karachi, India (now the capital of Pakistan). One of his experiences was to take care of a soldier who had become drunk and wandered into the desert. But, first he had to find him. The soldier's nickname was "Schnapps," which gave Bill an inkling of what kind of a guy he was looking for. He found him out on the desert, where he had wandered in a haze, brought him back and doctored him.

As another experience-giving action, Bill reassigned out of the medical corps to transportation and operated a boat on one of the big tributaries of the Ganges River. He had a crew of two Indian men and they patrolled up and down the river each day to check the big Army barges which were docked and carrying the remnants of aviation gasoline.

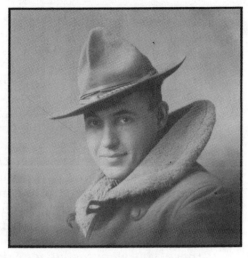

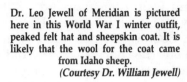

Dr. Leo Jewell of Meridian is pictured here in this World War I winter outfit, peaked felt hat and sheepskin coat. It is likely that the wool for the coat came from Idaho sheep.
(Courtesy Dr. William Jewell)

In June of 1946, Bill sailed home to America and Meridian, Idaho. He enrolled in pre-med physics at Boise Junior College (now B.S.U.) and in the autumn went back to the University of Idaho, from where he completed his pre-med degree in 1948. He then studied at Hahnemann Medical College at the University of Philadelphia from which he received his doctor of medicine degree in 1950. That summer he returned to Idaho to marry Norma Reynolds, whom he had met the previous year.

They moved to Ogden, Utah, where he served a one year internship and one year of general practice residency at the Thomas D. Dee Memorial Hospital, completing in 1954. Son, Paul, now a professor of geology at the University of Utah, was born in Ogden. They moved to Emmett and he immediately opened his practice. Their daughter, Ann (now Mrs. Dennis Woody of Baton Rouge, Louisiana), and son, Gary, a graduate of the Mennonite Seminary in Elkhart, Indiana, and Whitworth College in Spokane, Washington, were born in 1955 and 1958, respectively.

In the early days of practice, Dr. Bill was faced with a difficult case when an eight-year-old boy who had shot himself through the head was brought to him. The boy was in shock and Bill got him stabilized as well as possible, cleaning the bone fragments and chips from around the wound. He then telephoned the only neurosurgeon in Boise, Dr. Keefer, planning to take the lad to Boise for further treatment. He told Dr. Keefer that the boy had been playing with his father's .38 automatic pistol when it went off and the bullet evidently went through the frontal part of the brain and exited.

Dr. Keefer's advice was, "You might as well keep him in the hospital there. Now that the fragments, bone chips and brain matter have been removed from around the wound, all you can do is watch him and keep him hydrated." Bill said he did just that and the boy eventually recovered.

Sadness is a part of being a doctor. Bill delivered twin cretin children who had lacked the necessary thyroid. They weighed about two pounds each. "The nurses stayed with them and cared for them night and day, until their parents took them home," he said. Thinking that must have been a horrendous expense, as well as experience for the parents, the doctor reported that hospital rooms in those days were costing nine dollars a day.

In a birthing case, the baby's umbilical cord had come down before the head. "I called Dr. Harmon Holverson and he arrived immediately and pushed the head back and said, 'We've got to get this baby delivered NOW!' I decided the only way was to perform a Caesarean (cutting through the abdomen and uterus to remove the baby, which is the way Caesar was supposedly born) and as the anesthetist had not yet arrived, I injected a little novacaine right into the line in the skin where the incision was made. The anesthetist arrived and finished the job, but when that mother awakened was when I heard from a patient for the only time, 'You sonofabee, that HURT!' The baby boy is now a college graduate and doing real well in life."

Dr. William Jewell retired from practice on August 1, 1989. Not for the same reasons of his father, Bill also would not recommend to young people to become doctors. The way he explains it is, "The dealing with government, third parties, lawyers, and the interference with medical decisions has become intolerable. In one case where I remained several hours with a patient who was having chest pains, I was threatened with a $1,000 fine and one year in jail if I did not refund an 'extended care' charge of sixty dollars.

"In one six-week period, three lawyers asked for patients' records. They were supplied, but not one of them filed a charge. It just isn't worth it anymore." (A general comment from many of the retiring physicians and surgeons.)

BOISE COUNTY

No other Idaho county has a more dashing history than Boise. When gold was discovered in Boise Basin, August 1862, the beginnings of a great western state were made, for the basin was regarded as the richest and most extensive in the northwest. People flocked in to mine, establish shops and businesses, provide transportation and to practice medicine. Many of the doctors also practiced in Boise, Valley, and Elmore counties and some finally made their homes there.

Boise County was created February 4, 1864 by the first session of Idaho Territorial Legislature. Rugged and energetic Idaho City was named the county seat. Doctors came to Idaho City, Placerville, Centerville and rode horses to see the ill or crippled at Horseshoe Bend, Garden Valley, Crouch, Jerusalem, and Lowman. Those horseback rides through mountain grandeur, seeing elk and deer, brought forth many a letter to "the folks back home," and added to the influx of new residents.

DR. WILLIAM J. ROTHWELL

William J. Rothwell, born in 1840 in the eastern United States, first came to the Boise Basin to teach school. He fell in love with a beautiful fifteen-year old pupil, Clara Galbraith, and left the basin and school teaching with two goals in mind. He was going to become a doctor and come back to Idaho and marry Clara. He did both.

Graduating from Jefferson Medical School, Philadelphia, with an M.D. degree in 1874, he returned and married Clara. He became and remained for years the leading physician in the basin. Dr. and Mrs. Rothwell had one daughter and four sons. All the sons became doctors. After her children were established, Mrs. Rothwell also studied medicine. Mrs. Drysdale, wife of a Dr. Drysdale, said that the Rothwells made up a notable family.

Mrs. Sam Davis told of Dr. Rothwell riding horseback from Placerville to Cascade in Long Valley to set a broken leg for her father, Carroll Baird. Years later, Dr. Rothwell examined the leg and found perfect results. Dr. Allison remembered that a hand-quilted bed cover and pieces of rough lumber were used to immobilize the broken limb.

A yellowed and tattered news clipping, with no date nor name of publication, shows Dr. Rothwell to be a handsome man with wavy hair, mutton chop sideburns and a full mustache. A small item beside the picture is headed:

Rothwell Was Teacher

Other teachers in our school were Miss Leonard (later Mrs. Corbus) and P.D. Rothwell (may have been relative), quite a gay blade who later became a well-known physician in Denver. The Rothwells were a family of physicians, for in two generations there were seven or eight doctors. Dr. William Rothwell was the leading physician in the basin for many years. Like Dr. Dafoe, he journeyed over the great summits in storms to help those in distress. On one occasion while riding on horseback with another man, he lost his horse. They had stopped to cinch one horse and the other ran up the mountainside before they could catch him. So the two men rode "ride and hie" for six miles. It was good they did, for twin boys were born shortly after the doctor's arrival at the patient's home.

Dr. Rothwell died in Murray, Utah in 1931 at age ninety-one.

In her book, *All Along the River,* the late Nellie Ireton Mills wrote of a Dr. Rothwell being called from Placerville to attend a boy, Jim Ballantyne, who had been shot through his body by an Indian. Jim had been riding along upper Squaw Creek near Centerville checking the family's cattle. He was badly wounded, but managed to return home. A neighbor, Zeke Sweet, fastened a silk handkerchief to a ramrod and ran it through the boy's body to clean out the wound.

Dr. Rothwell was the nearest doctor, forty-five miles away, a day's ride to him with the news, and another day or two for him to arrive. The doctor had little, if any, hope that the boy would recover. His mother was a praying woman and combined that with good nursing to see her son recover and live a full life.

Dr. Rothwell never sent a bill, and years later Jim and his brothers learned of it and sent the aged doctor a liberal check. Jim's brother told the story years later. "All Jim got out of the shooting was an Indian bow and arrow he picked up at Indian camp. It was a dandy and the arrow so sharp we could shoot fish under water."

CANYON COUNTY

The route through today's Canyon County was the one most used by the early explorers and traders. Wilson Price Hunt and his party came through enroute to Astoria. In 1813, John Reed and his crew were murdered near the mouth of the Boise River; John McKenzie built a trading post for the Northwest Fur Company here in 1820. Thomas McKay built a better one to compete with Fort Hall, and Francis Payette was the kindly manager and cook who provided the good white bread and fresh vegetables that wagon train travelers hadn't eaten since they left home. The second Fort Boise was in Canyon County.

The Union Pacific strung its line across the county in 1882, making Canyon one of the fastest growing areas in the state. C.A. Caldwell platted the site of Caldwell in 1883 and it became a city in 1889. Nampa, largest city in Canyon, was incorporated in 1890. The College of Idaho (now Albertson College) was founded in Caldwell in 1890.

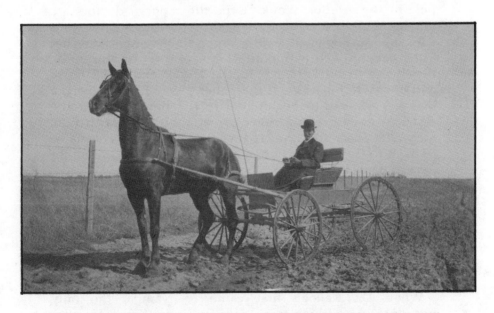

Dr. George O.A. Kellogg of Nampa and his favorite driving buggy and horse, Mingo (1905).
Dr. Kellogg became a legend in his own lifetime and it has grown since then.

(Courtesy Mrs. George Kellogg Jr.)

DR. GEORGE O. A. KELLOGG

George Kellogg's friends were legion, and he will not be forgotten for many years, as stories about him will be handed down for generations. He was born in Quincy, Kansas, March 29, 1879 and grew up in Colorado, where he received his medical degree from the Colorado University School of Medicine in 1903.

He came to Nampa, Idaho in the latter part of the horse and buggy era, and had a beautiful horse, Mingo, which he used in buggy riding, and a livery team which he used for forty-mile trips into the country. For greater distances he boarded Wells-Fargo or a privately owned stagecoach. He kept his heavy mountain buggy packed with sterile supplies and equipment, by which he meant his fishing tackle, shotgun, and rifle. He added surgical and obstetrical bags and a medicine case. The manager of the telephone company, in appreciation for the doctor letting the company know when any of its lines were down along the roads he traveled, gave him a repair kit, climbers and test set, so the doctor could get Central from any telephone pole in the interior. (Look at the fun modern doctors are missing with their cellular phones!)

He had arrangements with livery stable employees that if the patient lived within a distance of three or four miles, they were to hitch Mingo to the buggy and bring horse and buggy to his office. If the patient were further away, a livery team was to be hitched to the buggy, and if the distance grew great, a relief driver was to go with him. Stage stations were contacted to have fresh teams available to dash to the next station and they also placed orders for food to be picked up when the horses were changed.

When calls came, he notified Central where he would be, and was on his way. He said that there were two publications found in every ranch home, *The Doctor Book*, in the parlor; *Montgomery Ward* catalog in the "Chic Sales four holer." He said of Dr. Gunn's chapter, "What to Do Until the Doctor Comes," "That chapter is invaluable, the rest of the book, a damned nuisance."

When Dr. Kellogg first came to Nampa, the only hospitals in southwestern Idaho were in Boise. He performed eighty percent of his operations in the homes. Dr. Kellogg was ingenuous as an inventor. He was on a goose hunt on Snake River when called to a ranch, where a middle-aged woman was bleeding profusely from a submucous fibroid. He designed a Sims speculum from a stirring spoon, a Burnay packer from the bail of a lard pail, tore narrow strips from an old linen table-cloth for sponges and packing, added two pillow cases for drapes, and boiled everything on the kitchen stove. She was placed on a table and with a little care he packed the uterus, loaded her, mattress and all, in the back of a spring wagon and started the family to St. Alphonsus, with a note to Dr. McCalla. "I was back in my blind for the afternoon shoot," he said.

When Dr. Kellogg died at age eighty-two, after a short illness, he was mourned by hundreds. His only son, George E. and his wife, still live in Nampa.

DR. EUGENE HAROLD HOLSINGER

The son of a physician, Dr. Holsinger was born in Nampa, September 6, 1930 and lived there until age seven, when his father entered medical school in Portland. Dr. Holsinger's father later returned to Wendell to set up practice.

As a youth, Dr. Holsinger was active in band, basketball, and softball and graduated as salutatorian of his class. He remained active in extra-curricular activities in college and was twice selected for *Who's Who among Students in American Colleges and Universities.* He graduated from the College of Idaho in Caldwell with a B.A., *summa cum laude,* and continued on to medical school at the University of Oregon from 1953 until 1957 graduation. His internship and residency were served at Sacramento County Hospital.

Dr. Holsinger was certified by the National Board of Medical Examiners with an honorable mention for Part I, and among the top ten in Part II out of 2,500 medical students. Staff appointments were at Cottage Hospital and Cassia Memorial Hospital where he was chairman of the Medical Records Committee. He lived in Burley with his wife and two sons.

DR. ROBERT E. HAY

A native of Goshen, Indiana, born November 25, 1931, Dr. Hay came to Nampa in July 1961, after completing his residency at the University of Washington Affiliated

Hospitals in internal medicine and with a Fellowship in cardiology. He earned his B.A. at Wabash College in Crawfordsville, Indiana from 1949–53 and belonged to Beta Theta Pi and Phi Beta Kappa. His medical degree is from Indiana University Medical School, 1957, where he was a member Nu Sigma Nu and Alpha Omega Alpha.

Dr. Hay has two sons, Bruce Andrew and Jonathan Russell. His father was a dentist, and his father-in-law was Dr. Russell A. Sage from Indianapolis.

DR. THOMAS H. CALLOWAY

Dr. Calloway, husband of Dr. Mary Allen Calloway, was graduated from medical school at St. Joe, Missouri, in 1852 and after ten years in California, moved to Idaho City in 1862. It was at that time the most bustling city in the territory. He later went to Texas, arriving back in Caldwell in 1883, where he practiced for the next thirty-five years.

Dr. Calloway was an ordained minister in the Christian Church and spent the last years of his life as a minister. The Calloways had one son who practiced in Oklahoma for many years. The doctors Calloway organized the Christian Church in Caldwell. He died in Boise in November 1905, at eighty years.

DR. JOHN BENSEN CLAUSER

A former captain in the U.S.A.F., Dr. Clauser maintains an interest in photography and astronomy. He was born September 13, 1930 in Muncie, Indiana where his father, E.H. Clausen, was a physician. His training was obtained at Indiana University from 1948–51, where he earned his B.A. and Indiana University School of Medicine from 1951–56. He belonged to the Theta Chi Fraternity and the medical fraternity Nu Sigma Nu. He continued with an internship at Indianapolis General Hospital and residency was served at the V.A. Hospital in Denver. His staff appointments were at Mercy and Samaritan hospitals in Nampa, as an anesthesiologist.

DR. WILBUR LLOYD WATERMAN

Born on May 28, 1924, in Caldwell, Dr. Waterman attended College of Idaho before graduating from Johns Hopkins University in 1948. He completed an internship at Iowa Methodist Hospital in Des Moines from 1948–49, then a pediatric residency at Methodist Hospital in Memphis from 1949–50, and finally a pediatric residency at Baptist Hospital in Memphis from 1950–51.

He began practice in Caldwell in 1951, left to serve as a captain in the U.S. Army from 1953–55 and then returned to his practice in Caldwell. He was a staff member at Caldwell Memorial Hospital as well as Nampa State School. He was a member of the Idaho State Medical Association, the American Medical Association and the North Pacific Pediatric Society. He and his wife had four children.

DR. JOHN W. GUE

Dr. John W. Gue practiced medicine in Caldwell. He became president of the Idaho State Medical Society. Dr. Gue was born at Tulon, Illinois, July 25, 1870, son of George W. and Anna (Roberts) Gue.

His father, George W., was born in Ohio in 1844, and early in life became a minister of the Methodist Episcopal faith. When still a young man he was called to a pastorate in Illinois, where he was married. He eventually went to Portland, where he was in charge of the Methodist Episcopal Church. He died in 1909, at the age of sixty-five. The doctor's mother was a native of the Prairie state, and died in Portland at sixty-six years of age. They had six children; Dr. John W. Gue was the third.

His early education in the public schools of Tulon was followed by the Rock Island High School, from which he graduated in 1890. Subsequently, he went to the Columbia Medical School, graduating in 1894. He went to Portland, Oregon to intern in the Portland Hospital for one year. He went to Hailey, Idaho, and in 1895 entered active practice of medicine. After one year he moved to Custer, and for six months acted in the capacity of company physician. At that time Dr. Gue went to Mackay, in the same county, and became physician for the White Knob Copper Company, a position he continued to hold for eight years. In 1905 he went to Caldwell.

Dr. Gue was president of the Idaho State Medical Society, and for two years was physician of Canyon County. One of the foremost boosters of Caldwell, he was president of the Commercial Club, and a director of the Caldwell Building & Loan Association. Fraternally he was identified with Odd-fellowship, and was a trustee of the lodge.

On June 3, 1906, Dr. Gue was married to Miss Emma Harris, at Hailey, Idaho. She was the daughter of Mr. and Mrs. A. P. Harris, of Delhi, Iowa. They had no children. Dr. and Mrs. Gue were members of the Methodist Episcopal Church.

DR. OSEA BYRON BELLER

Few members of the Canyon County medical profession have overcome life's obstacles as did Dr. Osea Byron Beller of Nampa. The son of an agriculturist who intended him to become a tiller of the soil, in his ambition to enter professional life he met with stern parental opposition. He was finally compelled to educate himself without assistance and to work out his own career. Probably the necessity for hard and industrious effort during his youth served as a spur to stimulate his energies and achieve success.

Dr. Beller was born in Vinton, Iowa, September 17, 1873, son of David and Carrie (Barton) Beller. His father, a native of Ohio, moved to Iowa in 1854, farming and stock raising in Benton County where his death occurred in 1906. He was seventy-two years of age. Mrs. Beller was a native of Illinois and moved to Iowa with her parents in 1855. She survived her husband and made her home with Dr. Beller in Nampa.

Dr. Beller attended the public schools of Vinton, Iowa, and graduated from high school in 1892. From earliest youth he cherished the ambition to become a physician, but his father desired him to continue in the line in which the elder man had gained such success. The youth finally left the parental home and started working his way through Tilford Academy. He graduated and entered the Cedar Rapids Business College, earning his tuition by working at whatever job he found, and eventually was able to attend Cornell College for two years.

He then began to prepare for a medical career, entering Rush Medical College, where he was graduated in 1907. Following his graduation, Dr. Beller became an intern in the Presbyterian Hospital, and later in the Lying-In Hospital, both in Chicago. He returned to Vinton and opened his practice. Three years later he moved to Garrison, but after a like period returned to Vinton for four years.

Dr. Beller came to Idaho in February, 1908, and located in Nampa. He also invested heavily in lands. He served as examining physician for the following insurance companies: New York Life, Michigan Mutual Life, Bankers Life of Des Moines, Bankers Reserve and the Modern Woodmen of America; and assistant examiner for Idaho Life Insurance Company. His office was in the Smallwood Building, and his residence at N. 909 Third Street.

Dr. Beller took an active interest in the work of the Canyon County and Idaho State Medical societies and the American Medical Association. His affiliations were with the Knights of Pythias in Vinton, Iowa, and the Modern Woodmen of America at Nampa and the Republican party. He served in 1909 and 1910 as Canyon County physician. On December 30, 1902, Dr. Beller was married in Vinton to Elfreda Stoeker and they had one child, Elsie, on January 15, 1910. Dr. and Mrs. Beller also adopted the daughter of his widower brother, Vivian.

DR. H. P. ROSS

Dr. H.P. Ross was born in Ontario, Canada, March 9, 1875 to Donald A. and Clara (Naughton) Ross, the former a native of Canada and the latter of Boston. Donald Ross, for many years, was the proprietor of a planing lumber mill in Ontario. His mother had been a resident of Canada since her childhood. The three children of the family are: William, engineer, Doctor Ross, and Warren, a resident of Minnesota.

Educated in the high school at Clinton, Ontario, H.P. Ross entered Trinity Medical College, where he was graduated in 1899. In his native province he began practice and subsequently moved to the state of Minnesota which remained his home until 1904. That fall Dr. Ross established his office and residence in Nampa. He was a general practitioner, but specialized in surgery.

He was affiliated with the Modern Woodmen of America; member of the Episcopal Church; and a Democrat. After moving to Idaho he became financially interested in mineral resources, and was secretary of the productive Golden Crown Mine in Owyhee County.

On September 3, 1902, in Minnesota, Dr. Ross was married to Miss Claudia Cross, a daughter of Robert G. and Mary (Mace) Cross, of Minnesota. Her parents subsequently moved to Nampa, where they lived the rest of their lives. Dr. Ross and his wife had two children, Alice born in 1905; and Hugh Robert born August 22, 1912. He died January 13, 1913 in Nampa.

DR. A. F. ISHAM

Albert Franklin Isham came to Caldwell from Vermont in 1883. Caldwell was then a tent town, with even the post office in a tent. The first hotel was moved into town on rollers. He immediately became surgeon for the Oregon Short Line. In 1885 he married Lida Johnson, born March 23, 1864, one of the first white children born in Boise Valley. They had four children.

For years he was in general practice, spending many hours on horseback reaching his patients. Later he drove horse and buggy and was often called long distances and was gone for days to Jordan Valley, Rockville and other places. There was no telephone and people would come long distances at all hours of day or night to see the doctor. After thirty years, he retired from practice. Dr. Isham was active in Odd Fellowship and in the American and Idaho Medical associations. He died at age seventy-two.

DR. DONALD J. BARANCO

Before entering medicine, Dr. Baranco worked as a construction worker and had a dance orchestra. He played music with Louis Prima, Phil Harris, and Chick Webb. His father was a district manager with Southern Bell Telephone and Telegraph. He was born March 4, 1917 in Houma, Louisiana. He and his brother both became physicians. He attended the University of Southern Louisiana and L.S.U. Medical School. His internship was at the Charity Hospital at New Orleans in surgery for one year. He was an instructor at the School of Aviation Medicine at Randolph Field, Texas and had an orthopedic residency from 1946–49. He was charity chief from 1948–49. He practiced at the Lovelace Clinic in Albuquerque from 1949–53 and relocated to Caldwell in 1953.

Hospital staff appointments were in Albuquerque and

Canyon County. He belonged to the American Academy of Orthopaedic Surgeons, the American College of Surgeons, Western Orthopedic Association, and the North Pacific Orthopedic Society. His military career was from 1942-46 as a captain, M.C., at the School of Aviation Medicine as an instructor and an operation officer at the Air Evacuation Center. He enjoyed golf, fishing, hunting and sports cars and his family of four boys and one girl. His oldest son attended Arizona State University and hoped to go into medicine.

DR. HAL E. REYNOLDS
The late Dr. Reynolds was a native of Idaho, born in Boise August 11, 1923. His father was in radio repair and no other relatives were doctors. His childhood was spent in Boise and he began his college education at Boise Junior College from 1942-43. He went to New York University in 1944 and on to Biarritz American University in France in 1945. He returned to Idaho to complete his B.A. at the College of Idaho from 1946-48. He then attended the University of Washington Medical School form 1948-50. His internship was at Buffalo General Hospital where he completed a rotating internship, 1952-53.

All of his general practice was in Caldwell, after his return in 1953. He was a staff member of Caldwell Memorial Hospital. He was a member of the A.M.A. of Southwest Idaho. His military service was in the Army with the Engineer Corps from 1943-46 in the European theater. He and his wife, Dorothy, became the parents of six children.

DR. ERLAND ROBERT CARLSSON
Dr. Carlsson was born July 22, 1919, at Marquette, Kansas. His uncle Dr. Edward Carlsson practiced in LaCrosse, Wisconsin.

While still in grade school, the family moved to Jamestown, New York, where Erland finished grade and high school. He returned to Kansas to go to a church school, founded by a great-uncle, Bethany College, Lindsborg, Kansas, and was graduated in 1941 with a B.S. degree. From 1944-45 he interned at California Hospital, Los Angeles, and from 1945-47 had a residency at the University of Kansas, in internal medicine.

From 1947–51 he practiced in Coeur d'Alene. He spent two years in the Air Force at Valdosta, Georgia. He practiced in Boise from 1953–55, and moved to Nampa in 1955. While in Coeur d'Alene, during the winter of 1948, he waded in snow up to his waist while trying to get to Post Falls on a call. The town plow had to pull him out.

He was secretary of Mercy Hospital staff; on the staff of Samaritan Hospital. For two years he was captain and flight surgeon with U.S. Air Force. He was a major for three years in the Idaho Air National Guard.

He and his wife had three girls and two boys.

DR. FARBER JACK RUSSELL

A native of Payette, Idaho, born November 9, 1919, Dr. Russell completed his high school education in just three years. He then went to the University of Idaho and completed his bachelor of science degree in chemistry. In 1940 he began his medical school education and graduated in 1944 with his M.D. His internship was at the Medical Center in Jersey City from 1944–45. His residency in pediatrics was at the St. Louis Children's and Barnes Hospital of St. Louis from 1948–50. He attended Harvard Medical School during the same period.

Dr. Russell had a general practice for two years in Ontario, Oregon, from 1947–48 after he returned from his military duty as a captain in the U.S. Army stationed in Japan. After his additional residency, he began a pediatrics practice in Nampa in 1950. Early in his practice he experienced dealing with the polio epidemic while in Ontario and St. Louis. He served as chairman for the Polio Immunization Program and for the Cerebral Palsy Drive. He was a member of the Mercy and Samaritan hospitals in Nampa and the Caldwell Memorial Hospital. He was also a consultant at Baker, Oregon and McCall, Idaho.

He is married and has two daughters and one son.

DR. HAROLD W. BROWN

Dr. Brown was born May 10, 1927, in Alhambra, California. His father was a protestant minister.

From 1945–47 Dr. Brown was in the U.S. Army Quarter-master Corps. He was graduated from the College of Idaho in 1951 with a B.S. degree. In 1951–52 he did graduate work in biology at the University of Oregon. He received his

M.D. degree from the University of Washington School of Medicine in 1956. From 1956-57 he did an internship at Bellevue Hospital, New York City. He did his residency in internal medicine at the University of Washington Affiliated Hospitals from 1957-59. From 1959-61 he had a fellowship in neurology at the University of Washington Affiliated Hospitals. He was assistant in medicine at the University of Washington from 1957-61.

He moved to Nampa in 1951 and was associated with the Canyon Medical Center. He was on the staffs at Mercy and Community hospitals, Nampa. At Caldwell Memorial Hospital and Veterans Administration Hospital, Boise, he was a neurology consultant. His wife is Marguerite Spencer Brown, well-known Canyon County resident.

DR. S. DEVON COLONGE

Previous to 1908, before Dr. Colonge moved to Nampa, he taught school in Illinois and Idaho. He was a prominent educator, but felt drawn to the medical profession. He studied at the College of Physicians and Surgeons in Keokuk, Iowa and graduated in 1908. Nampa became his home and there he established his practice.

Born in Gregory, Missouri on October 24, 1878 as the seventh son of twelve children, Dr. Colonge served a two-year internship at St. Joseph's Hospital as an assistant to a Dr. C.E. Ruth, a general surgeon. He returned to Nampa as a general practioner. He was the medical examiner for several insurance companies and he was a surgeon for the Idaho Light and Power Company.

He married Lelia Heath from Salt Lake City and they had two daughters.

DR. J. R. MANN

Dr. Mann was born October 1, 1925 in Twin Falls. His father was a real estate broker. He went through high school in Jerome, pre-med at the University of Idaho. In 1949 he received a B.S. degree at the University of Idaho, and his M.D. degree from the University of Utah in 1952. He served in the armed service in the Aleutian Islands.

The doctor interned at the Deaconess Hospital, Spokane, and moved to Parma in January, 1954. In the Nyssa hospital he delivered Siamese twins. From 1960-61 he was chief of staff at Malheur Memorial and at Caldwell Memorial hospitals from 1963–64.

The Manns had two boys.

DR. WILLIAM M. MITCHELL

Dr. Mitchell described himself as being, "meanest kid in Pennsylvania and New York" as a boy. He was born November 24, 1878, Hornell, New York. His father was a physician practicing in Idaho. He attended University of Maryland, Baltimore, and Johns Hopkins Hospital. He practiced in Idaho from 1905–1963. He traveled by horse and buggy and when he went on an obstetric case in the hills he usually stayed over night.

For one year he was Canyon County physician. He and Mrs. Mitchell had three sons.

DR. J. H. MURRAY

Dr. J. H. Murray located at Nampa the year Idaho was admitted to the Union, 1890. He was born in northern Indiana, December 19, 1860. He spent his boyhood in Iowa, arriving there when one year old, and lived there until twenty-four. The doctor was educated in the public schools and in the Mitchellville Seminary. He entered the College of Physicians and Surgeons at Des Moines, and was graduated and began practice in 1884. His first office was in Arnold, Nebraska, where he remained six years. In 1890 he came out to the newly admitted state of Idaho, and settled in Nampa.

Dr. Murray identified himself closely with the interests and activities of his home city. He was director and vice president of the First National Bank. In politics he was a Progressive Republican, and was often called into public service. For two years he was mayor; served on the school board; in 1899 served in the house of the state legislature.

During his residence in Custer County, Nebraska, Dr. Murray, in 1889, married Miss Mary J. Robertson. She was an active member of the Presbyterian Church. They had two sons.

DR. ROBERT H. JENSEN

Born and raised in the Caldwell area on his parents' ranch, Robert Jensen returned after his training to practice in Caldwell. He was born on November 25, 1926, and attended Caldwell schools and the College of Idaho in 1946. He graduated with a B.S. in zoology in 1950 and went on to Stanford University and earned a degree in physical therapy in 1951. He returned to school at the University of Oregon Medical School in 1956 and earned his M.D. in 1956.

His internship was at the Good Samaritan Hospital in Portland, Oregon from July 1960 until July of 1961. He served as a Navy radioman third class from 1944–45. He was on the staff of the Caldwell Memorial Hospital and served as secretary-treasurer.

He and Mrs. Jensen had two sons and one daughter.

DR. CHARLES E. KERRICK

Dr. Kerrick was born November 13, 1923 in Parma, where his father was a bookkeeper. He attended one year of college at the University of Idaho and completed his B.A. at the University of Idaho, Southern Branch in 1944. He went on to Creighton University Medical School and earned his M.D. in 1948. His internship was at St. Joseph's Hospital in Omaha from 1948–49.

His Naval active duty was from 1949–50 and from 1953–54. At his discharge, his rank was lieutenant. Dr. Kerrick's practice was at Caldwell, starting in 1950. He was chief of staff at the Caldwell Memorial Hospital from 1960–61 and vice chief from 1959–60. He also served as secretary from 1957–58.

He is married and has three sons and two daughters.

DR. CHARLES EDWARD KRAUSE

Before completing his college degree, Dr. Krause served in the armed forces as a captain in the Medical Administrative Corps. He completed his B.S. degree in 1947 at Kansas State College and went on to Kansas University in 1951. His internship was at Kansas City General Hospital and was completed in 1952. He practiced in Caldwell (except for an eleven month bout with tuberculosis in 1953–54). He was on the Senior Medical Staff at the Caldwell Memorial Hospital and also served as a past president. Early in his career in 1952, he was the first to use a polyethylene catheter in the femoral vein.

He and his wife, the former Marjorie Kinsey, have three boys.

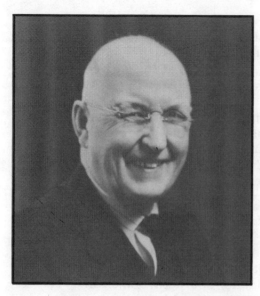

Dr. Fern M. Cole, an early-day physician in Caldwell, traveled many miles to outlying area to care for patients. His patients and friends honored him many times for his generosity to those who could not afford to pay him.
(Courtesy
Governor Robert E. Smylie)

DR. FERN MORTON COLE

Robert E. Smylie, former Governor and Attorney General of Idaho, was one of those who knew him best. A nephew of Dr. and Mrs. Cole of Caldwell, Smylie said "If it had not been for him, I would likely still be driving a bread truck in Iowa." Dr. and Mrs. Cole thought young Smylie should receive higher education and offered him room and board in their home, helped him to find a job in Caldwell, and encouraged his enrollment in the College of Idaho.

Dr. Cole began his medical practice in Caldwell in 1909, becoming president of the Idaho Medical Association and a member of the American Medical Association. For more than thirty years, he was the physician for the Odd Fellows Home and refused to take a penny for his services. Born into a Methodist family, he maintained activity in the church all of his life, including teaching Sunday School classes and acting as a trustee.

He was considered a statesman within the Republican party, urging talented and trustworthy people to seek office. He was a community worker, instrumental in organizing and he became the first president of the Caldwell Kiwanis Club. He was a member of the Elks, Odd Fellows, Caldwell and American Rose Society, and a thirty-second degree Mason. Because he provided much medical care to families of the Odd Fellows without charge, one year they surprised him with the gift of a new car. In 1939, a whispering and note-writing campaign went forward to surprise Dr. Cole with a note of thanks. He received about 4,000 letters, telegrams, and postcards of thanks.

Dr. Cole served the United States in both World War I and II. He served with the Sixth Division as captain with the Medical Corps in WWI, and in charge of Selective Service for Idaho doctors in WWII. For several years, he was a member of the Idaho National Guard. He received a Presidential Citation and decoration for his military service.

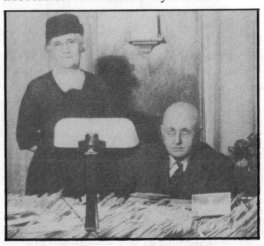

Dr. and Mrs. Cole were presented with a gift of a new car one year as a token of thanks and esteem. Several years later, they were inundated with about 4,000 written, telegraphed, and telephoned messages of gratitude. Here they are with some of the correspondence.
(Courtesy Governor Robert E. Smylie)

Born January 18, 1876, in Illinois, Dr. Cole attended grade and high school in Ida Grove, Iowa. He studied for two years at Grinnell College before studying medicine at Northwestern Medical School, receiving his degree in 1898. That year he was married to Leila Jane Smylie, whose Methodist minister father performed the ceremony. Dr. Cole practiced in Iowa until 1909, when he moved to Caldwell. For the next ten years he practiced alone, and then entered a partnership with Dr. Clifford M. Kaley, a lifetime friend.

They established the Caldwell Sanitorium, later donating the equipment to the Caldwell Memorial Hospital, which both had worked diligently to develop. The modern hospital was opened the week following the death of Dr. Cole on April 2, 1950.

DR. JOSEPH B. MARCUSEN

Joseph Marcusen was born June 14, 1921. He received his B.S. degree from the College of Idaho, and went to the University of Oregon Medical School for his M.D. He interned at St. Lukes Hospital, San Francisco, and had a O.B. residency at University of California Hospital, San Francisco, for one year.

He started his practice in Nampa July 1, 1949. He was secretary of the Idaho Chapter of American Academy General Practice. Also he was on the advisory board of the *Northwest Magazine* for Idaho Society. From 1951–53 he was in the Army, stationed in Korea.

The Marcusens have three daughters and one son.

DR. JOSEPH SALTZER

Born in London, England on November 11, 1909, Joseph Saltzer was reared in Montreal, Canada. He attended the McGill University in Montreal and earned a B.S. in 1927 and went on to attend the McGill University Medical School and graduated with an M.D. and C.M. degrees in 1935. He did a rotating internship at the Beth El Hospital in Brooklyn and completed his residency at the Montefiore Hospital, also in New York from 1937–38.

After completing his training, he located in Homedale from 1938–41 and then located in Nampa in 1941. He was chairman of the medical staff at Mercy Hospital for two years and at the Samaritan Hospital for one year.

He was active in local and regional medical societies and served as president of the Idaho Heart Association for one year.

DR. ALFRED H. ROSSOMANDO

Dr. Rossomando was born in New York City April 4, 1910, where his father was a grocer. After graduating from Rutgers in 1938, he worked for seven years with Western Electric and pharmaceutical houses before returning to medical school at the New York Medical College in 1942. He served his internship at the Flawers and Fifth Avenue Hospital in New York City in 1942–43. He took a urology residency at the Metropolitan Hospital from 1943–44. From 1944–46, he served as a captain in the U.S. Army Medical Corps and received several medals.

He worked with sulfa drugs during the experimental

stage from 1936–38 and participated in research on combinations of drugs and sulfa therapy from 1943–44.

He has held the position of attending urologist at the Mercy and Samaritan Community hospitals in Nampa and was a consultant in urology at the Union Pacific Railroad Employers Hospital Association.

He and his wife have one daughter.

DR. GEORGE W. MONTGOMERY

Before entering medical school, Dr. Montgomery was a school teacher in Oregon for three years. He had earned his B.A. from Dallas College (1907–11). Three years later he began working for his M.D. at the University of Oregon Medical School and graduated in 1918 with an M.D. His internship was at the Bremerton Naval Hospital from 1918–19. He returned to Caldwell and began his practice, and later became chief of staff at the Caldwell Memorial Hospital which opened in 1952.

He and his wife had one son who also became a doctor and is an American Board Surgeon.

Many of Dr. Montgomery's early confinement cases were in the home with deliveries by kerosene lamp light. The lighting was especially poor because the lanterns were often located in a doorway because of the fear of explosions from the combination of ether fumes and kerosene. Infections were rare due to the freely used lysol solutions. Often, the doctor did not see the patient until time for delivery.

DR. SAMUEL CLAYTON TAYLOR

Born in Langford, Kansas on April 1, 1923, Samuel Taylor spent his early life in St. Francis, Kansas. He left his hometown to attend Phillip University in Enid, Oklahoma in 1941 through 1943. He attended Tulane Medical School from 1943–47 when he received his M.D. degree. His rotating internship was at the Kansas City General Hospital in Missouri from 1947–48 where he also did a surgical residency from 1948–51. He completed another surgical residency at the Memorial Hospital of New York City and became a Diplomate of the American Board of Surgery in 1955. He also qualified to be a Fellow of the American College of Surgeons in 1957.

After serving two years in the Navy from 1951–53, he

spent from January to September 1954 as the chief of surgery at the V.A. Hospital in Hot Springs, South Dakota.

He began his practice of general surgery in Nampa in September 1954. He was a staff member of the Samaritan and the Mercy hospitals in Nampa. He also served as the past chief of surgery on the executive council of the Mercy Hospital.

Dr. Taylor married Jean Maan in 1949 and had three sons and two daughters.

DR. GRAYDON O. CROSS

Dr. Cross was born in Plainville, Kansas, January 10, 1923. He attended Bethany Nazarene College and East Texas State Teachers College. He completed pre-med at Louisiana State University and medical school at Southwestern Medical College, University of Texas. He interned at Baylor University Hospital, 1948-49, and completed a residency at Nun Fran's Memorial Hospital, Jacksonville, Texas.

Dr. Cross practiced in Eagle, Idaho. From 1943-46 he was in an Army specialized-training program; 1951-53, first lieutenant, Army Medical Corps, Korea.

In 1953 he started a medical practice in Nampa. He was on the staff at Samaritan Community and Mercy hospitals. Dr. Cross belonged to the American Medical Association, Idaho State Medical Society, Southwestern Idaho Medical Society, and A.A.G.P.

He and his wife, LaJuana, have three daughters and a son.

DR. JAMES HOWELL CUYKENDALL

The doctor was born July 21, 1918, at Fort Collins, Colorado. He received a B.S. degree from the University of Denver in 1941, and his M.D. in 1950 from the University of Colorado. For one year he interned at St. Joseph's Hospital in Denver, and a three years residency at the Denver Veterans Administration Hospital.

From 1954-55 he practiced at Albuquerque, New Mexico and in Detroit. He moved to Caldwell in 1957. He was a radiologist at Caldwell Memorial Hospital. Dr. Cuykendall was a member of the Idaho State Radiology Society. He served in the U.S. Army.

ADA COUNTY

Its geography ranging from foothills at the southern tip of the Boise Ridge to the mesa lands, and sixty-mile long Boise Valley, Ada County is marked by the mighty Snake River as its southern boundary. Called "home" by Indians, trappers, explorers, farmers, and ranchers, it has always been a governmental site. First, the federal government in 1868 set up a military post to face serious trouble with the Indians. It soon became a town and then capital of the new Idaho Territory. The capitol building at Boise is still the most widely visited tourist attraction in the state. The early-day doctors played a large role in the settling of the territory, and the later ones in influencing the developing culture.

DR. OLIVER P. HAMILTON

At the time of his death on a Sunday morning, March 19, 1950, Dr. Oliver P. Hamilton, sixty-eight, was Ada County physician and maintained his offices at the county hospital. He had been ill for two months previous to the heart attack which took his life.

A graduate of Northwestern University's Medical College in Chicago, Dr. Hamilton went to Mountain Home in 1920 to practice and moved to Boise in 1930 to set up offices in the downtown Eastman Building. He was born on June 5, 1882 at Lawrence, Massachusetts.

During World War I he served as a captain in the Army Medical Corps attached to Jefferson Barracks in Missouri.

Dr. Hamilton and his wife, Louise, had one son, O.B. Hamilton of Boise.

DR. JOHN CARL HILL

A general practitioner who, to a considerable extent, specialized in surgery and diagnosis, was Dr. John Carl Hill. He came to Boise in October, 1910, after three years as a member of the hospital staff of the Colorado Fuel and Iron Company in Pueblo.

He was born November 2, 1881 to John H. Cordelia Thomas Hill at Hannibal, Missouri. John's mother died when he was nine. He then moved with his father to Grand Junction, Colorado, where he received his grade and high school education. He spent seven years pursuing classical and professional courses at the University of Colorado. He received the Bachelor of Art in 1904, and the Medical Doctor degree in 1907. In 1912, he was married to Elizabeth Whitehill at Morgantown, West Virginia.

After three years in Boise, he took a sabbatical to do graduate work in the New York Polyclinic and the New York Lying-In Hospital, and returned to Boise in 1913. He held membership in the Idaho and American Medical associations; Physicians and Surgeons Club of Boise, which he served a term as president; Beta Theta Pi fraternity; the Commercial and Elks clubs of Boise.

Dr. and Mrs. Hill became the parents of two daughters, Jane and Elizabeth, and were members of the Methodist Episcopal Church.

DR. JOHN M. TAYLOR

An engineer before becoming a physician of forty-years practice in Boise, a tireless civic worker, husband, father and grandfather, whose life inspired grandson, Ted Walters, to become a doctor. All these were Dr. John Martin Taylor, who arrived in Idaho Falls in 1882. He was in business with his brother, Samuel, and Edward Henry in the cattle business for three years. In 1885, he worked as a civil engineer for the Union Pacific Railroad and in changing gauge divisions. His engineering for Union Pacific took him to Kansas City, Missouri for a time. He returned to Idaho 1889 and developed irrigation projects for canal companies, as well as laying out the townsite for Idaho Falls.

He realized his dream of becoming a doctor when he graduated in 1890 from the University of Pennsylvania Medical School and interned at Johns Hopkins, where he met Alice Witman, who was training to become a nurse. Her ancestry held a number of doctors, including Dr. Bodo Otto, a surgeon on the staff of General George Washington. They were married April 8, 1904.

Dr. Taylor moved to Boise in 1902 and resided there until his death in 1946. Mrs. Taylor died in 1966. The Taylors became the parents of John M. Jr., David Krause, Alice (Mrs. John Walters, mother of Dr. Ted Walters), Robert Simpson, and Mary (Mrs. Erwin Schwiebert).

Dr. Taylor was a dignified gentleman who always wore wingback collars. His bow ties were made by Mrs. Taylor.

His office secretary was a well-known Boisean, Clara Wood, daughter of Colonel Wood.

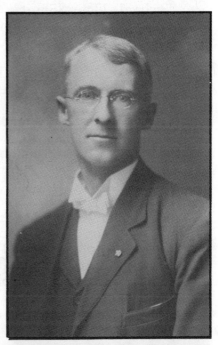

Dr. John Martin Taylor and his wife, Alice W. Taylor, were early-day residents of Idaho. He was a civil engineer when he arrived in the Idaho Falls area in 1882. He worked on irrigation and railroad projects. Within a few years he entered medical school in Pennsylvania and graduated in 1900. He returned to Idaho in 1901 and married a nurse. Mrs. Taylor began keeping records for a history of Ada County doctors and wives, which her daughters loaned to Mrs. Ralph (Irene) Jones who had planned to prepare a book for the Idaho Territorial Centennial in 1963. All of that material and more is contained in this book. Note the old Idanha Hotel in the background of the snapshot of Dr. and Mrs. Taylor with their grandson, Ted Walters, who is a practicing physician in Boise.

(Courtesy Alice Taylor Walters)

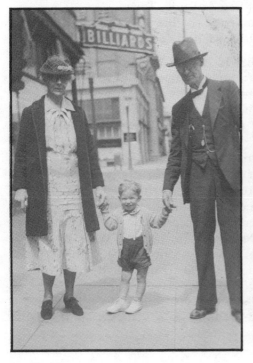

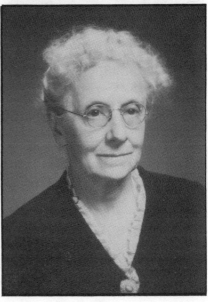

DR. RICHARD E. SHURTZ

Another hard-working-farmboy-turned-doctor was Richard Elmer Shurtz, youngest of two sons and a daughter born to Watson and Malinda Asher Shurtz on a farm in Champaign County, Illinois. While growing up and working on the farm, he kept thinking of how he might get to medical school. After schooling near the farm and reaching seventeen, he turned to teaching, which was not unusual for someone of his age at that time. He saved money for pre-med and medical study at Illinois State University in Champaign.

In 1893, Richard entered Rush Medical School, Chicago, graduating in 1897. He practiced for years in Champaign, during which time he took advanced study at Johns Hopkins and Harvard Medical School.

The family moved to Boise in 1911, when he became the 630th doctor licensed to practice in Idaho. He became active in the Elks and Odd Fellows lodges and the Republican party. Dr. Shurtz took six months to serve as captain in the medical corps of the U.S. Regulars in World War I, and was stationed at San Antonio, Texas.

Upon graduation, he married Nellie Turn on June 5, 1892. They had two daughters, Malinda and Mary.

DR. JAMES L. STEWART

For many years one of the northwest's most eminent physicians, Dr. James L. Stewart of Boise was described by his colleagues as "one of the doctors largely responsible for the building of St. Lukes Hospital and for the close-knit medical society in Idaho." He was one of the founders of the American Board of Surgery and chairman of the Idaho Credentials Committee for that board for many years. He was one of three trustees for *Northwest Magazine*, president of the Idaho Medical Association and for more than twenty years chief of staff at St. Lukes.

Dr. Stewart was born December 16, 1874, at West Point, Iowa, and died in Boise at seventy-four on December 15, 1948. He was graduated in 1898 from Rush Medical College, Chicago, and worked for two years at Cook County Hospital. The next two years he was contract surgeon on the San Pedro-Chihuahua, Mexico, railroad project.

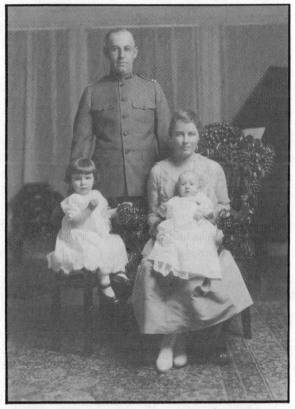

Dr. J.L. Stewart was one of Boise's leading physicians. He devoted himself to the practice of surgery and was well-known throughout the northwest. In this 1918 portrait, he is still wearing his World War I uniform. His wife, Modjeska Caldwell Stewart is holding the baby, Dorothy Stewart German of Westport, Connecticut. Beside her is Loma Jean (Mrs. Willard Burns) Stewart.
(Courtesy Loma Jean Burns)

He then moved to Boise and became an active member of the community. He was a member of Boise Lodge AF&AM, Masonic Council, Knight Templar and Shriner.

Dr. and Mrs. Stewart, who preceded him in death, had two daughters, Loma Jean Burns and Dorothy German and several grandchildren.

DR. ALFRED M. POPMA, F.A.C.R.

"Cash was scarce, but the living was good," Dr. Alfred Popma of Boise reminisced of early practice in the little town of New Plymouth, Idaho, population 600. "Those three years of practice were enhanced by an understanding wife, who became a good assistant at minor surgery, office work, bookkeeper, and wife and mother. Many patients paid bills with milk, cream, meat, butter and wood . . . the living was good."

Dr. Popma was born November 26, 1906 in Orange City,

Iowa. After grade school, he graduated in 1924 from Northwestern Classical Academy, later Northwestern College. The course included basics, four years of Latin and two of French. He graduated with a major in science from Hope College in Holland, Michigan, where he won letters in track and cross country. He was lab assistant in vertebrate zoology and comparative anatomy. His M.D. was received in 1932 from University of Iowa College of Medicine. He and Dorothy Wiersma were married September 7, 1928.

A fortuitous detour to Idaho on return to Iowa from Santa Clara County Hospital, San Jose, where he interned, resulted in a chance visit to New Plymouth. Dr. W. Drysdale had left after twenty-five years and his furnished office was for rent at twenty dollars per month. A two-bedroom house was available at fifteen dollars a month. After a superb sales talk by R.S. White, hardware merchant; a telephoned agreement by Dr. R. Nourse, chairman, Board of Medical Examiners, that Dr. Popma would be allowed to practice for the three months until the board met, "in order that New Plymouth might have medical care," the decision was made and Idaho was to be given a gift that would make a difference to cancer patients by the thousands.

Major surgical cases were in the Holy Rosary Hospital, Ontario, Oregon, fifteen miles distant. As the youngest member of the hospital staff, Dr. Popma was given assignment as "roentologist," with no salary and no other staff member wanted it. It changed his life by arousing an interest in that specialty. After three years in New Plymouth, he received a residency at the University of Nebraska, Omaha, learning radiology.

After residency, Dr. Popma received offers to remain in Omaha, to teach at Stanford or Duke, but they were rejected in favor of returning to Idaho, where there was no trained radiologist. He associated with Dr. Harold Stone and was appointed radiologist to St. Lukes Hospital. The department expanded greatly, and Dr. Popma was in demand as a consultant radiologist to many hospitals in Idaho, Montana, and Oregon. He is a Diplomat, American Board of Radiology, and has held virtually every position in the American Cancer Society, for which he was president in 1954; the Idaho Medical Association, and groups in the northwest; has written extensively for scientific publications; participated in scientific programs throughout the world; and received medals from state and national groups. Dr. Popma originated a film on self examination of the breast, "Life-saving Fingers," used by the American Cancer Society.

His vision, and that of others, brought about the Mountain States Tumor Institute.

Dr. and Mrs. Popma are active Presbyterians, and he has been an Elder since 1943. Both have been active in the advancement of education. They had two daughters, Ann Frances (Mrs. Richard Parsell) and Mary Louise, who died in 1955.

DR. JUNIUS WRIGHT

Dr. Junius Wright said that the two diseases most encountered during the gold rush days were malaria and typhoid. In 1865, he treated a man forty years old and a girl of eight for malaria, but later became convinced it was spotted fever. It was in the 1880s that Idaho doctors began to see what became called "Rocky Mountain Spotted Fever." It had been reported in Montana in 1873 and called "black fever." Numerous Idaho doctors contributed study and did experiments with living ticks to bring about knowledge necessary to prevent or treat the disease.

Dr. Wright was Idaho's first practicing physician, other than Army doctors, and lived to be well over 100 years. After he moved to Portland, he continued to subscribe to the Caldwell newspaper to keep up with the community he helped to build in his younger years. On his 102d birthday he was asked by a reporter how he accounted for his long life. In his usual wry way, he said, "Because I was born so long ago."

During that same interview, Dr. Wright strode to the middle of the room and said, "Congress is crazy!" Back of that statement was years of study of congressional law, and he continued, "They have buried all the country's gold in a hole in the ground in Kentucky. Let congress have it coined into ten-grain dollars. Every troy ounce would make forty-eight dollars and the total would be twenty-two billion. Let congress irrigate the arid plain states. Four years more, if they did that, our assets would be doubled and we'd be greater than any two nations in the world."

Dr. Wright first practiced in Iowa in 1860 and in 1861 he married Elizabeth Jones. In 1864, they learned of the gold rush in Idaho, started west in a covered wagon, reaching Boise in September. They started farming and selling produce to mining towns in Boise Basin and soon gave up any idea of returning to Iowa. He started his country practice and in 1876 opened a drugstore, which he sold ten years later to Dr. Ephraim Smith. They moved to Caldwell and he built another drugstore and became active in the canal projects. His interest in medicine returned toward the turn of the century and while in the legislature in 1896, he was active in the passage of one of the medical acts. It was not until he reached seventy-five that he gave up the practice of medicine.

DR. JAMES COUGHLIN

Dr. Coughlin was born in Boise on December 28, 1916, attended St. Joseph's grade and high schools and graduated from St. Teresa's Academy High School in 1934. He remembers many of the pioneer doctors and Dr. McCalla was the Coughlin family physician, as were Doctors Stewart and Pittenger in later years.

He attended the College of Idaho for two years, Gonzaga University for one year, and was admitted to St. Louis University School of Medicine in 1937, graduating in 1941 with a doctor of medicine degree. He was a member of Phi Chi medical fraternity.

Dr. Coughlin's internship was from July 1, 1941 to the same date in 1942 at St. Vincent's Hospital in Portland. He had a fellowship in orthopedic surgery at St. Louis University from May 1946 until October 1948, and received his master of science degree there in 1948.

Boise has been the only place Dr. Coughlin has practiced, beginning November 1, 1948, associating with Drs. Pittenger, Shaw and Mack until March 1951, when he opened his own office. In 1959, Dr. J. Gordon Daines and Dr. Coughlin became associated in orthopedic surgery, erecting a building at 1015 North Eighth Street for that purpose.

He has practiced at St. Lukes, St. Alphonsus, Elks Rehabilitation hospitals and as a consultant to the Veterans

Hospital in Boise. Dr. Coughlin held membership in the American, Idaho and Ada County Medical societies, Fellow of the American College of Surgeons, Diplomate of the American Board of Orthopedic Surgery, and member of the North Pacific and the Western Orthopedic societies.

Dr. Coughlin entered active military duty in the Army on July 1, 1942 and was discharged in 1946. He took a train to Carlyle Barracks, Pennsylvania, where about 1300 doctors, all out of their internship, had congregated for what was called the Thirteenth Refresher Class. After one month of training, 100 were chosen to leave for overseas duty, and Dr. Coughlin was one of them. He was sent to the South Pacific and landed at Brisbane, Australia, in September 1942. He was assigned to the 155th Station Hospital and remained there in orthopedic surgery. He was overseas forty months, traveling through Australia, New Guinea, East Indies and up to the Philippines. He was discharged with the rank of major and returned to St. Louis for his residency. Dr. and Mrs. Coughlin have three sons.

DR. CAROL LINCOLN SWEET

Perhaps the most influential of all Idaho doctors in establishing the Idaho Medical Association in 1893, was Dr. Sweet, called the "Father of Organized Medicine" in the state. It was also due to his enthusiasm and efforts that the Idaho Medical Practices Act was passed.

Dr. Sweet was born in Phoenix, New York, January 3, 1860, in a long line of medical men dating from Caleb Sweet, New York regimental surgeon on the staff of General George Washington. Carol was educated at Phoenix Academy and Cornell University and graduated in 1882 from University Medical College in New York.

Dr. Sweet arrived in Boise in 1890. There was no state medical organization, so he became active in establishing one and working on the passage of the Medical Practices Act. He served first as secretary and then president of the IMA, secretary to the Board of Medical Examiners, was surgeon general for the Idaho National Guard, assistant surgeon for the U.S. Army and post surgeon for Boise Barracks, 1898–1903.

Dr. Sweet moved to Nevada in 1906 and to California in 1913, where he practiced until retirement in 1930.

DR. CHARLES SANFORD ALLEN

Dr. Allen began his Idaho practice in Atlanta during the gold boom days when the I.W.W.s were conducting a reign of terror. He treated people who had been injured in bombings, homes burned, and other acts of terrorism. He delivered his first baby with basting spoons, as his surgical instruments had not yet arrived. He taught himself to shoot after observing several street shootings.

He was born in Cleveland, Ohio in 1884 and was graduated from medical school at Schenectady, New York. To get to Atlanta, the young doctor had a long, hard, horseback trip up the Middle Fork of the Boise River and found a group of wooden shacks. He watched many a poker game with ten and twenty dollar gold pieces used for chips. Blizzards, wild animals, and fires were additional hazards to his practice.

He left Atlanta in 1916 to practice in Boise and he left Boise to become superintendent of the state school and colony at Nampa in 1943. He married Madeline King in Salt Lake City in 1915, and she became active in various clubs in Boise and was president of the Ada County Republican Women's League.

DR. J. GORDON DAINES

Dr. Daines was born May 4, 1914 in Blackhawk, Utah, where his family had Daines Manufacturing Company. He attended several universities in pursuit of his medical career. He received his bachelor of science degree in 1936 from Utah State University; attended Washington University in St. Louis in 1937-38; George Washington University from 1940-43, and was granted his M.D. degree. He took his internship and residency from 1943-46 at the Central Dispatch and Emergency Hospital in Washington, D.C., and Northwestern University in 1958.

He moved to Boise in 1948 and he associated with Dr. J.K. Burton. He had his office at 2900 Overland from 1950-58, and from 1958 at 1015 North Eighth Street, in association with Dr. James Coughlin. He practiced at St. Lukes, St. Alphonsus and the Elks Convalescent hospitals and was president of the staff at St. Alphonsus. He was a member of the American, Idaho and Ada County Medical associations.

Dr. Daines spent two years as captain with the 1st Army at Staten Island Hospital. The Daines became parents of two girls, Hollis and Alison, and one son, J.G. "Pete" Jr.

Dr. Daines' widow, Lucy, has been an active member of the Idaho Medical Association Auxiliary and her article on southeastern Idaho medicine was incorporated in large part in this book.

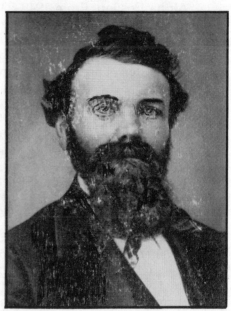

Dr. Ephraim Smith was one of the first medical men to come into the Territory of Idaho in 1863. There were 10,000 people in Placerville when he arrived there and opened a drug store. He was appointed to the first Territorial Legislature in the Council (Senate) and was named as the first treasurer of the Territory. He was credited (or blamed) as one of the men who "stole" the capital from Lewiston.
(Courtesy Idaho Historical Society)

DR. EPHRAIM SMITH

Another of the first doctors to arrived in Idaho Territory was Dr. Ephraim Smith of New York. He had followed the gold rush to California in 1850 and came to Placerville three years later. He started a drugstore when the town had more than 10,000 people. Dr. Smith was named to the first Territorial Legislature in the council (senate), and when he was appointed first treasurer of the Territory, he moved to Boise. He was one of those who helped in "stealing" the capitol from Lewiston.

Mrs. Smith was a charter member of the first Presbyterian Church on the present site of the Idanha Hotel and had trees planted on the parking. Dr. Smith carried water from their home at Eleventh and Grove to keep them alive.

DR. FRANK E. MATHER

Dr. Mather was born March 25, 1924 at Givens' Springs, Idaho, and lived on a ranch until five, when his family moved to Boise. He attended Boise schools, including Boise Junior College, 1941-43 when he enlisted in the Army. When he returned in 1946, he entered the University of Idaho, receiving a B.S. degree in 1948. He joined Sigma Alpha Epsilon. From 1949-53, he attended the University of Oregon Medical School, receiving his M.D. He joined Alpha Kappa Kappa.

Dr. Mather's internship was at Thomas D. Dee Hospital in Ogden and his residency at University of Oregon Medical School in Portland (1959). He practiced in Boise from 1954-57, and started again in 1959. He was an Army T/5 in Europe from 1943-46.

Dr. Mather comes from a medical family. Others who were doctors were John Boeck, grandfather; Albert Boeck, uncle; Edward Naugle, uncle; John A. Mather, brother; and two cousins, Jack Naugle and Marshall Sims, the latter two in Colorado.

Dr. and Mrs. Mather had two daughters and a son.

DR. SAMUEL POINDEXTER

When Samuel Marshall Poindexter of Boise tendered his resignation as chairman of the Idaho Board of Medicine to then-Governor Robert E. Smylie, he had served from 1949 through the early sixties by appointment of three Governors, Charles A. Robins, Len B. Jordan, and Smylie. The governor wrote, "I salute both personally and officially your distinguished service to the medical profession and to the people of Idaho in this responsible and difficult position."

Dr. Poindexter was born at and spent most of his life in Boise. His birth was July 19, 1902, and he attended grade and high schools in Boise before taking pre-medical studies at the University of Idaho in 1925. He pledged Delta Chi. He taught science in high schools at Arco, 1925-27, and Boise, 1927-30. He had saved enough money to enter and graduate from the University of Oregon Medical School in 1933, where he joined Alpha Kappa Kappa and Alpha Omega Alpha.

His internship was at King County Hospital in Seattle and he practiced from 1935-36 in Puyallup, before opening his office in Boise on November 1, 1936. He was an active staff member at St. Lukes, St. Alphonsus, and the Elks Rehabilitation hospitals.

Dr. Poindexter belonged to the American, Southwestern Idaho and Idaho Medical associations; Fellow, American College of Physicians; president Southwestern Idaho Association, North Pacific Society of Internal Medicine, Idaho State Board and Federation of State Medical Boards of the United States; vice-president, National Board of Medical Examiners; and consultant to Idaho Public Assistance Department.

Dr. and Mrs. Poindexter had a daughter and son. Marilyn Farneman, a graduate of Westminster Choir College in Princeton, New Jersey and minister of Music and Education, First Methodist Church, Alexander City, Alabama. Charles Wadsworth Poindexter is a graduate of the College of Idaho with a bachelor of science in 1961 and of the University of Oregon Medical School in Portland.

DR. REX BORUP

Dr. Rex Borup has been in medicine for many years in the city of his birth, Boise. He attended grade and high schools in Boise and studied at Brigham Young University in Utah for three years of pre-med. The last four years of medicine he attended the University of Utah. His internship was at the Thomas Dee Hospital in Ogden. Spare time and vacation activities include golf, swimming, tennis, hunting, fishing, and reading.

Dr. and Mrs. Borup have one daughter, Pamela; and three sons, David, Mark, and Jeffrey.

DR. WILLIAM T. DRYSDALE

Dr. Drysdale came to Boise in 1946 after practicing medicine for many years at New Plymouth. He was a veteran of World War I. Born July 27, 1882, in India, Dr. Drysdale received his medical degree in 1903 from the Denver and Groose College of Medicine. He served at Veteran's hospitals in Togus, Maine; Milwaukee, Wisconsin, and Des Moines, Iowa, before coming to Boise.

He was a certified member of the American Board of Psychiatry and Neurology. He and his wife, Ruth, had three sons and one daughter. Dr. Drysdale passed away on November 16, 1943.

DR. FRANK W. CROWE

Dr. Crowe was born July 2, 1919, in Boise. His father was an electrical engineer. He attended Boise schools and was graduated from the University of Idaho in 1941 with his B.S. degree.

During four years of World War II, from 1941–45, he was a Japanese prisoner of war in the South Pacific. Upon his return, in 1946 he went to the University of Oregon for one year, and was graduated from the Utah Medical School in 1949 with an M.D.

He interned at Ancker Hospital, St. Paul 1949–50. In 1950–51 he had a residency at University Hospital, Madison, Wisconsin, and University Hospital, Ann Arbor, 1951–53. He practiced in Boise from November 2, 1953 until his death.

Dr. Crowe was considered one of the few expert doctors on the disease of neurofibromastosis, and wrote a book on the subject, which was widely used in the medical profession.

He was active on the staffs at both St. Alphonsus and St. Lukes. From 1954–55 he was treasurer of Southwestern Idaho District Medical Society.

The Crowes had two daughters and a son.

DR. DALE D. CORNELL

Dr. Cornell was born October 12, 1909, Greenfield, Iowa where his father was a druggist. He grew up in Greenfield, and in 1935 received his M.D. degree from the University of Iowa. In 1951 he received his M.S. from the University of Colorado Medical School.

Dr. Cornell interned at the Robert B. Green Hospital, San Antonio, Texas. He had a residency at the University of Iowa in psychiatry in 1946, and University of Colorado, 1949–51. From 1936–41 he practiced in Greenfield. From 1941–45 he was a lieutenant colonel in the Army, 41st Infantry Division. He practiced in Sandpoint from 1947–49, and then moved to Boise in 1951.

He was on the staff of St. Alphonsus and St. Lukes hospitals, and a consultant at the V.A. Hospital. He belonged to the Intermountain Psychiatric Association and Mental Health Committee.

The Cornells had one daughter.

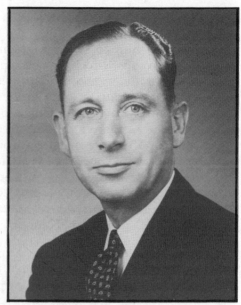

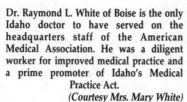

Dr. Raymond L. White of Boise is the only Idaho doctor to have served on the headquarters staff of the American Medical Association. He was a diligent worker for improved medical practice and a prime promoter of Idaho's Medical Practice Act.
(Courtesy Mrs. Mary White)

DR. RAYMOND L. WHITE

A cancer victim and yet an optimist, Dr. Raymond L. White suffered with leukemia for nearly a quarter of a century, yet gave hope to hundreds of others. During that time, he lived a life of such activity and accomplishment that those who were unaware that he had leukemia wondered how he could do so much. Those who observed him as chief of surgery at Hickam Field during the Japanese attack on Pearl Harbor, December 7, 1941, wondered the same thing as he worked around the clock. Many close to him knew what a special individual he was, and felt that it was precisely because he knew that his time on earth was limited that he put it to the highest possible use.

Born December 19, 1917, in the small town of New Plymouth, Idaho, to Roy Seymour and Lillian Van Sickle White, Raymond Leroy had the typical childhood of an Idahoan. While attending grade and high school and becoming an Eagle Scout, "Bud" (Raymond) worked for his father in White Hardware and Implements. He liked the outdoors and enjoyed fishing, pheasant and deer hunting, later adding golf, candy-making, and woodworking to his hobby list. He attended the College of Idaho.

During these formative years, the doctor who delivered him at birth, **Dr. William T. Drysdale**, encouraged and inspired him to study medicine. Raymond was graduated from Loyola School of Medicine, Chicago, 1939. Loyola kept track of his career and in 1964, he received the Alumni Citation for outstanding services in the field of medicine.

While studying in Chicago, he had time to meet and court an attractive nurse, Mary Ellen Barragree of Watseka, Illinois. They were married on Valentine's Day, 1940. The young couple went west to Idaho and Dr. White worked for several months as physician for the National Youth Administration, until being commissioned first lieutenant in the Army Air Corps. During the next year, he was stationed at Allen Hancock School of Aviation, Santa Maria, California, with two months out to attend the School of Flight Surgery at Randolph Field, Texas. From there, he was assigned to Hickam as chief of surgery.

While assigned to McCord Field at Tacoma, Washington, 1942–44, he was sent to attend the School of Tropical Medicine at Walter Reed Hospital, Washington, D.C.

In July, 1944, after several months at Letterman General Hospital in San Francisco, Dr. White was diagnosed as having a malignant giant cell follicular lymphoma. He was retired from the service as a major, whereupon he moved to Boise.

In Boise, he became associated with Dr. James Stewart, a brilliant and distinguished surgeon, in general surgery. Four years later, he was named president of the Southwest Idaho Medical Association. For ten years, he was chairman of the executive committee of the American Cancer Society, from which he received the bronze medal for outstanding service. During those same years, he was the first doctor to serve two terms as president of the doctor's staff at St. Luke's Hospital; a director of the Idaho Public Health Association; medical consultant to the Ford Foundation for Lockheed Missiles and Space; senator from Ada County in the Idaho Legislature, 1952–55, during which he chaired a committee to rewrite the Idaho Medical Practices Act and shepherded it through the Legislature.

Dr. White was the only doctor from Idaho to serve on the staff of the American Medical Association. He served as executive director of socio-economic activities of Environmental Medicine from 1961–66. Among the multitude of positions held were: appointment to the Air Defense Command, with special assignment to Aerospace Defenders; founder and executive director of the Idaho Foundation for Medicine and Biology; and he was featured as an Outstanding Idaho Citizen by the *Idaho Statesman* newspaper.

An Elk, Mason, Knight Templar, Kiwanian, country club member in both Boise and Chicago, Dr. White was not a "let George do it" Christian. He served as an elder and member of the Sessions in the First Presbyterian Church, Boise. He and Mrs. White were the parents of a daughter, Susan Eleanor White Newhouse, and adopted a son, Robert Martin White, when he was one day old.

After his death on December 18, 1968, Mrs. White found among his papers an article, "Life with Cancer," which he had written. "Because I felt he had a message for others living with cancer," Mary White said, "I sent a copy to Dr. John H. Talbott, editor of the Journal of the American Medical Association (JAMA) for him to evaluate. His response was to publish it in the Journal." It was also published by numerous other groups because of its timeless appeal. Here are excerpts:

> As a physician and a long-time cancer patient, I have faced the usual problems of cancer patients as well as the special problems of the physician as patient. No doubt my life would have been far different had I been able to maintain the state of average or better health I enjoyed until age thirty-one.
>
> As this is written (October, 1967), I lack six months of attaining my fifty-sixth birthday. I have had cancer for twenty-four years. This is over two-thirds of my adult life, representing all of my 'productive' years and nearly half of my entire life span. Twenty-four years with lymphoma characterized by serious exacerbations, remissions, and quiescent periods is a long time, and I hope it will be twenty-four years longer. Yet, as a doctor, I recognize that just as the pendulum swings in a shorter arc as the clock begins to stop, so do the recurrences come at more frequent intervals. . .
>
> I have always sought medical and surgical care like any other patient and have tried to follow the attending physician's or surgeon's advice . . . being a good

patient isn't easy for anyone, physician or not. In addition to cancer itself, many of my periods of hospitalization and inability to work arose from the complications of successful therapy; for example, skin grafting to an area severely damaged by X-ray therapy; and a long period of physiotherapy which followed a biopsy for tumor involving the left lower femur with a subsequent deep hemorrhage under the quadriceps muscle.

In many ways, I have been fortunate . . . I get well quite readily and have always been able to return to work of some kind . . . perhaps more important I was born at the right time in history and contracted my cancer coincidentally with the great discoveries in cancer treatment. Had my disease started five years earlier, I would have long since been dead for one reason or another. Medical research has produced a half dozen new therapeutic methods which were nonexistent when I first became ill. The 'cobalt' bomb for radiation therapy and other high energy radiation devices had not been invented. The Rh factor which has caused so many adverse reactions in blood transfusions was discovered at the precise moment I was developing severe reactions from weekly transfusions. The steroid hormones and the chemotherapeutic drugs were also developed in time to aid me. These, combined with surgical operations to remove diseased tissue, and conversely to repair damaged tissues, have brought me to the twenty-four year survival point.

The heartbreak of searching far and wide for 'miracle cures', combined with the economic loss and the burdens placed on families . . . is one of the recurring tragedies of our society. Following the advice of . . . own physician . . . is usually the best way of assuring continuity of care the patient needs.

The point is that even as a physician, I have followed my doctor's advice.

DR. CHARLES C. REGER

Charles C. Reger served as lieutenant colonel with the Marine Corps, U.S.A.R.; as assistant chief surgeon with the 6250th General Hospital; and staff surgeon with the 321st Engineer Combat Battalion's General Hospital during World War II.

On May 21, 1917, he was born in Leadville, Colorado,

where his father was an assayer, a mine superintendent and a businessman.

He was graduated with a Bachelor of Science in chemistry from the University of Colorado in 1938. He received his Medical Doctor degree from the same university in 1942. He was a member of Nu Sigma Nu and was named to the prestigious Phi Beta Kappa, America's oldest fraternity, established in 1776, and based on high scholarship.

Dr. Reger served his internship at the University of Colorado Hospital in Denver, 1942-43; and his residency at Strong Memorial Hospital in Rochester, New York, 1946-47; and was resident general surgeon at Provident General Hospital, 1947-48, and resident general surgeon at the Veterans Administration Hospital, 1950-51. The latter two are located in Seattle.

He began practice at Boise in 1948 and was assigned to the active staffs at Saint Alphonsus and St. Luke's hospitals. He also has been consultant in gastroscopy at the Boise Veterans Administration Hospital.

DR. LEWIS CAMPBELL BOWERS

Dr. and Mrs. Bowers were attracted to Boise when they made a short stop there in 1889 enroute to Pendleton, Oregon from Kansas, to open a new practice. They stayed in Oregon for one year and moved to Boise, remaining until his death November 14, 1928. Their only child, Helen Bowers Moore, was born in Boise on August 4, 1904. Dr. Bowers was Boise and Ada County physician and became well known for investigating the cause of an epidemic of typhoid in 1904. He served as Idaho Medical Society president and helped to draft legislation on admittance to practice in Idaho.

DR. ROLLIN S. GREGORY

Small wonder that Rollin S. Gregory wanted with all his heart to become a doctor. When the boy was seven years old, his father died from what is now thought to be appendicitis. When he was ten, his mother died from typhoid fever. Two sisters died within a few days of the same disease. The only survivors of that family was Rollin and his brother, Elmer, age thirteen. Rollin vowed to himself that if there was any way possible, he would become a doctor and save lives. There were to be a number of hurdles before the ten-year-old could reach his goal, but reach it he did.

Rollin was born June 7, 1864, in Niagara County, New York, to Harry and Sarah Albert Gregory, both New Englanders. They moved from Connecticut to New York, and subsequently to Marseilles, Illinois, when Rollin was five years old.

After the parents and sisters died, Rollin and Elmer went to Iowa to open up a farm on a piece of prairie land left them by their father. While they were doing this, they both continued their grade and high school educations in Mason City. One of Rollin's teachers was Mrs. Carrie Chapman Catt, president of the National Woman's Suffrage Association and considered one of the most brilliant women in America. He was graduated from Mason City High School in 1886. At that time, it was possible to teach with a high school diploma. As another step toward his goal of becoming a medical doctor, Rollin taught for three years, saving as much of his salary as he could for further schooling.

He then entered the medical college at Rochester, New York, during 1889–90, and he concentrated on learning all he could of electro-therapy. He spent several years in the practice of electro-therapeutics, first at Ashville, North Carolina, and later in Chicago, Hot Springs, North Carolina, and Trinidad, Colorado. In 1897, feeling there was much more to be learned he enrolled in the Denver Homeopathic Medical College where he received his M.D. degree in 1899.

Dr. Gregory moved immediately to Boise and opened his practice at 204-205 Sonna Building. During an epidemic of smallpox in the spring of 1900, he was put in charge of the city pesthouse.

He also established a residence at 1107 North Eighth Street. On February 12, 1902, he and A. Virginia Jessee were married in Boise. Mrs. Gregory was a native of Harrison County, Missouri, and moved to Idaho in 1886 with her parents. Children born to the marriage are: Sherman, Esther, Dorris, Glen, and Rollin Jr.

In 1913, the Gregory family moved to eastern Washington and settled near Newport. Dr. Gregory maintained a limited practice for the next five years, when he returned to Boise and reopened offices for a full-time practice.

While Dr. Gregory owned property in Iowa, Texas, and Idaho, he never held large financial interests, as he felt that his work was to be for the relief of ill and suffering people. In 1903, he was appointed a member of the Idaho Board of Medical Examiners, and served for six years. He was a member of the Republican party, but concentrated more heavily on never losing an opportunity to vote for the prohibition of the manufacture and sale of intoxicating liquor. He was a strong advocate of direct legislation, namely the initiative, referendum, and recall. He read broadly and continued research and investigation into matters medical all of his life. He was considered to have a powerful intellect.

Fraternal organizations to which he belonged included: Woodmen of the World, for which he was a council commander and medical examiner; Women of Woodcraft, for which he was manager and medical examiner; Knights of Pythias, Ivanhoe Lodge, of which he was chancellor commander in 1904, and later was director; State Lodge of the Independent Order of Odd Fellows. He was also a prominent member of the American Institution of Homeopathy.

His religious faith was that of the Unitarian Church.

DR. C. C. JOHNSON

A native Idahoan, Dr. C.C. "Cliff" Johnson was born November 9, 1916, in Oreana in one of the country's largest counties, Owyhee. He attended grade and high schools in the county and moved to Caldwell to attend the College of Idaho. He taught high school for two years to earn funding for medical school.

Summer school at the University of Southern California was followed by St. Louis University where he received his M.D. in 1943. After an internship in New Orleans he received a fellowship at Mayo Clinic for three and one-half years. That year, 1949, he received a Master of Science at the University of Minnesota. He served in the armed forces 1948–50 and began internal medicine practice in Boise in 1950. Dr. and Mrs. Johnson (Ruth Danielson) have three children, Jane, Carolyn, and Dan.

DR. JEROME K. BURTON

Born March 15, 1909 at Pittsburgh, Jerome Burton took pre-med at Johns Hopkins University, 1927–32; University of Maryland Medical School, 1932–36 for an M.D. After residency and internships at Baltimore Hospital for Women, he did orthopedics at Johns Hopkins, 1938–40. Two years of practice was followed by a move to Boise. He was on staffs at St. Alphonsus and St. Luke's; consulting at Mary Secor, Emmett, Mercy, Nampa, and Memorial, Weiser. He belonged to American, Idaho, Southwest, and Ada County Medical societies. Dr. and Mrs. Burton had two sons, one in medicine and the other in law. Dr. Burton played with the Boise Symphony.

DR. ADOLPH BLITZ

Moses Blitz, a merchant in Prussia and father of Adolph, died when his son was a small boy. Adolph was born February 10, 1845, and spent much of his first nineteen years reading and hearing of America. When he was nineteen he sailed to this country to enlist in the Union Army during the Civil War. He was one of the 60,000 men who followed General William Tecumseh Sherman on his "March to the Sea." It was the bloodshed and death he saw that compelled him to study medicine. He was graduated from the Cincinnati Medical College in 1873.

Dr. Blitz was a workaholic and twice during his teaching and practicing he was forced to take time away to recuperate. During one of those times he and Mrs. Blitz (Anna Wickes of Massachusetts) took a sea voyage to Alaska. They decided to take a train east upon their return, but when the train stopped in Boise they liked the looks of the town, and took a few days to meet Boise doctors. Because he was a specialist in eye, ear, nose, and throat and would fill a gap in the town, doctors urged him to return. He did so in 1900 and lived there until his death November 19, 1911.

DR. GLENN E. TALBOY

Dr. Talboy was born at Weiser, Idaho, August 13, 1921, and began his medical practice in Boise in 1954. He attended Boise Junior College (now Boise State University), 1939–41; College of Idaho, 1941–43; and St. Louis University, 1943–46, from which he received his M.D. degree.

His internship and residency training were at St. Louis City Hospital, St. Louis University Hospital; and in surgery at the State Cancer Hospital. Dr. Talboy worked long hours during the 1949 yellow fever epidemic in Panama, where he served in the military as a captain. He holds active staff appointments at St. Lukes, St. Alphonsus, and the Elks hospitals. He served as secretary of the Southwest Idaho Medical Society in 1957.

Dr. and Mrs. Talboy had five boys and one girl. He had two uncles and a cousin who were also doctors.

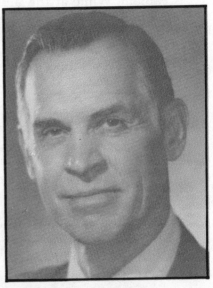

Dr. Quentin E. Howard completed a term as president of the medical and dental staff of St. Luke's Hospital, Boise, in February 1977, and said: "In the wake of the onslaught of governmental regulations which have spread a depressing pall upon us for some time, we have learned many lessons . . . to adjust, to communicate, to rebound after failure. We have used these experiences to serve us in the improvement of patient care."

DR. QUENTIN HOWARD

Dr. Howard was born at Emmett on May 9, 1919, and worked on the family farm until studying pre-med and medicine at Northwest Nazarene College in Nampa, University of Southern California, and George Washington University in Washington, D.C., from which he received his degree in 1947.

He served in the Army from 1943 through 1951 in this country and Guam, Iwo Jima and Okinawa. He practiced in Emmett from 1951 to July 1954, and after two years practicing in British Honduras, he moved to Boise in 1959. He and Mrs. Howard had four children, Quentin Jr., Marita, Joanne, and Ronald.

DR. H. A. P. MYERS III

"Hap," or Harvey Arlington Patrick Myers III, born on March 6, 1928, in Seattle, proved his ability to work hard while still a student. He attended grade, high school, and the University of Washington Medical School, Seattle. He was married and had an eighteen-month-old daughter when he started medical school.

In the interim he spent two and one-half years as a second and first lieutenant in the U.S. Marine Corps. When he resigned from the U.S.M.C. it was with the rank of captain. While at the university, he became affiliated with Alpha Delta Phi; was vice-president of the psych honorary Psi Chi; and was named to the honorary collegiate society based upon the highest scholarships, Phi Beta Kappa. At the medical school he became a member of Nu Sigma Nu. He was graduated in 1950.

Dr. Myers had one year of pediatric internship and one year of residency at Strong Memorial-Rochester Municipal Hospital in Rochester, New York. He served a one year residency at the Children's Orthopedic Hospital in Seattle. Boise is the only city in which he has practiced.

He served as secretary of the Ada County Medical Society in 1960–61. Dr. Myers is interested in church activities and has been a Sunday School teacher, a lay reader, men's group leader and Christian Education leader. He is also active in musical circles and has been a member of the Boise Philharmonic board of directors. Dr. and Mrs. Myers have one daughter and three sons.

DR. FRANKLIN BERNARDT JEPPESEN

Known to family and friends as "Jep," Dr. Franklin B. Jeppesen was born on June 7, 1905 in Emmettsburg, Iowa, where his father was a contractor. He received his early schooling there and took two years of pre-medical training at Iowa State College in Ames. For one year he studied at the University of Iowa in Iowa City, before entering medical school at State University of Iowa, receiving his M.D. in 1929.

Dr. Jeppesen interned for one year at University Hospital in Iowa City, before going to Cleveland, for the next four years. By that time, he knew that he wanted to establish a practice in Boise, where he arrived in 1934 and remained.

He served as active staff member at both St. Lukes and St. Alphonsus hospitals, and was chief of staff at St. Lukes. He was secretary of the Boise Valley chapter of the American College of Surgeons and the Idaho Medical Association. He was president of the Idaho, Southwest Idaho societies, Western American Urological Association, and the Boise Valley chapter of the American College of Surgeons. Dr. Jeppesen was a member of the Western Surgical Association and Governor of the American College of Surgeons.

He enjoyed fishing, hunting, boating, photography and gardening which he often shared with his wife, Dorothy, and daughter, Suzanne, and sons, Robert and Harold.

DR. ROY ESTEN FREEMAN

Roy Freeman was born in Valley County's mountain meadow village of Meadows on July 19, 1904. His father was a cattle rancher in the valley, and it was there that Roy attended grade school. The family had moved to Boise when he was ready for high school and he graduated with the class of 1923.

At the University of Idaho, from which he graduated in 1928, he became a member of Phi Gamma Delta. At Northwestern University's School of Medicine, from which he graduated with an M.D. degree in 1934, he joined Nu Sigma Nu. Special skin and cancer training from 1940 to 1942 in New York and internship at King County Hospital in Seattle January 1, 1934 until May 1935, prepared him for practice.

He married Beulah Brown of St. Maries in 1928. They had a daughter, Sally, and son, John Esten. In Port Alexander, Alaska in 1935, he performed an emergency appendectomy at the home of the patient. As hobbies, Dr. Freeman enjoyed fishing, photography and oil painting.

In addition to Alaska, he practiced in Longview, Washington from November 1935 until June of 1939. After a two-year sabbatical, he practiced in Boise, with offices in the Eastman Building, until his death in December, 1951.

Dr. Freeman's medical colleagues who were pallbearers included Doctors Roscoe C. Ward, Raymond L. White, S.M. Poindexter, Robert S. McKean, Donald J. Harrison and Harold E. Dedman. Honorary pallbearers included Doctors

F.B. Jeppesen, Fred A. Pittenger, Richard D. Simonton, M.B. Shaw, Ralph R. Jones, Everett N. Jones, Bruce C. Budge, and Alfred M. Popma.

DR. LOUIS FRANK LESSER

Louis Lesser was a quiet man who was born on November 13, 1903, in Ribnica, Yugoslavia. He came with his family to the United States at an early age and settled in Denver, Colorado. His father had mining interests near Denver. After grade and high schools, he entered Denver Business College, from which he graduated before entering the University of Colorado. He earned his B.A. degree in 1931, his M.D. from the Medical College in 1934. He was a member of Delta Sigma Phi.

Dr. Lesser took internship and residency training at the Thomas Dee Memorial in Ogden, Utah in 1934-35. He moved to Gooding, where he practiced from 1936 through 1938, going on to Mountain Home for the years 1939-49. He moved to Boise in 1950.

When his secretary asked the doctor to tell of any unusual experiences he had as a practitioner it was without result. She wrote, "I can't get him to talk!"

He became an avid rockhound and searched the hills in his area for Idaho's gems. He also enjoyed reading and playing duplicate bridge.

Dr. and Mrs. Lesser had two sons, Thomas Davidson, and Robert William.

DR. FRANK A. MINAS

Frank A. Minas was born, received all of his grade and high school education, and returned to practice medicine in Boise. He received his bachelor of science degree from the University of Idaho. His father was a Boise merchant.

He entered graduate school at the University of Wisconsin and received his M.D. at the University of Oregon Medical School. He belonged to Phi Delta Theta, Nu Sigma Nu and Alpha Omega Alpha. His internship was at Letterman General Hospital at the Presidio in San Francisco and residency at Station Hospital on Governor's Island in New York. He was named a colonel in the U.S. Army Medical Corps.

After practicing medicine for two and one-half years at Tripler General Hospital in Honolulu; one year at Letterman in San Francisco; two years at Billings General Hospital and one year at Fort Benjamin Harrison Station, both in Indianapolis; one year at O'Reilly General, Springfield, Missouri. He returned to Boise to open a general practice.

Dr. Minas was assistant chief of surgical services, Fort Jay, New York, and Tripler in Honolulu; chief of surgery in Billings, Fort Harrison; and chief of rehabilitation at O'Reilly General. He joined Ada County, Idaho, and American Medical associations. He and Mrs. Minas became the parents of two sons, James and Richard.

DR. ROBERT T. HOLDREN

Dr. Holdren and his wife, the late Dr. Mary Lou Holdren, came to Boise in 1959 and he has practiced in that city since. He was born July 13, 1918 at Philipsburg, Pennsylvania. His education was extensive, receiving a B.S. degree in chemical engineering from Penn State in 1939; his Ph.D. in organic chemistry from Iowa State in 1946; his M.D. from Tulane University in 1951. He became a member of Phi Sigma Kappa, Alpha Chi Sigma, and a Diplomate with the American Board of Surgery and the Board of Thoracic Surgery.

Dr. Holdren's internship was at Southern Pacific Hospital in San Francisco for one year, and resident in surgery for one year. He was a resident surgeon at Gorgas Hospital in the Panama Canal Zone for two years. He did thoracic surgery at the National Jewish Hospital in Denver for two years. He practiced at Madigan Army Hospital and was on the surgical staff from 1955-57, before settling in Boise.

The Doctors Holdren had a son, Glen Robert, and daughter, Barbara Louise. Dr. Holdren's hobbies include duplicate bridge, hunting, fishing and cooking. Even he admitted that his cheese cake is a specialty.

DR. EDWARD J. KIEFER

Born in Milwaukee, Wisconsin February 6, 1916, Edward J. Kiefer attended grade, high school, and college there. He was a student at Milwaukee State Teachers College, 1933-36; Marquette University's School of Medicine, 1936-40, where he received his M.D. in 1941. He became a member of Phi Beta Pi and A.O.A.

His internship and residency were at Milwaukee

Hospital and the Mayo Clinic (University of Minnesota graduate school) where he received an M.S. degree in neurosurgery in 1949. He practiced in Milwaukee, 1941–42 and again after his M.S. degree, 1949 to 1955, when he moved to Boise.

From 1942 until 1946, he served as lieutenant commander in the U.S. Naval Reserve.

Dr. Kiefer was associate staff member at the Milwaukee, St. Joseph's and Columbia hospitals in Milwaukee; neurosurgical consultant for the Veterans Administration Hospital in Wood, Wisconsin, and clinical instructor of neurosurgery at Marquette University School of Medicine. In Boise, he was on both St. Lukes and St. Alphonsus staffs; a consultant at the Veterans Administration Hospital and secretary to the Southwest Idaho Medical Society.

He was a member of the Elks Gleemen and enjoyed skiing, golf and hunting. He and his wife, Gretchen, had a daughter, Lynne, and son, Fritz.

DR. ROBERT S. McKEAN

When Robert V. Hansberger of Boise, then well and widely known president of Boise Cascade Corporation, sent out invitations in April of 1962 to the "Humanitarian Award" dinner honoring Dr. Robert S. McKean, it was in glowing terms. As well it should have been. Hansberger was chairman of the dinner committee and he noted that the previous year's winners were President and Mrs. Eisenhower.

The award to Dr. McKean was only the twelfth time that it had been given in the United States. "I know you will share my pride in having Dr. McKean, a citizen in our own Idaho, selected for this honor," Hansberger wrote.

It was co-sponsored by United Cerebral Palsy of Southwest Idaho and the Ada County Association for Retarded Children. Among those on Hansberger's committee were Mrs. Harry W. Morrison, sponsor of the Treasure Valley Auxiliary of the Nampa State School for the Retarded, and Dr. Terrell O. Carver, Idaho Administrator of Health. Keynote speaker at the dinner was Dr. Brewster S. Miller, medical advisor of United Cerebral Palsy, New York, and special guests included Dr. Tony Vaughn, director of special education at Greeley State College and Idaho Governor Robert E. Smylie, who presented the award.

Mrs. M.A. Bodahl was chairman of arrangements and working with her were Keith Jordan, Clarence Hettinger, John O'Toole, Bert Alden, Mrs. Ferd Koch, Mrs. Donald Lowry, Mrs. Dorothy Campbell, Mrs. J.B. Monette, and Mrs. M.S. Merrill.

Dr. McKean, pediatric neurologist, was then director of the neurological team in the Crippled Children's Service of the Idaho Department of Health. He held membership in the American Academy for Cerebral Palsy, American Academy of Neurology, and the American Association on Mental Deficiency. He was an active staff member of St. Alphonsus and St. Lukes hospitals, and the Idaho Elks Rehabilitation Center, as well as director of the Seizure Clinic of the Nampa State School.

Both co-sponsoring groups support classes and summer camps for handicapped children, provide speech therapy; workshops for teachers in special education, provide films and other educational materials on needs of the physically handicapped and mentally retarded.

Robert McKean was born January 11, 1906, at Wahpeton, North Dakota, where his father was a merchant. After grade and high schools, he attended Yankton College, receiving his B.A. degree in 1928, and the Medical School of Northwestern University with an M.D. degree in 1933. Internship and residency were at Iowa Methodist Hospital, 1932-33; Mayo Foundation Fellow in Pediatrics, 1934-35 and again from 1938 until 1941. He practiced in Murray, Iowa and Worland, Wyoming, before coming to Boise in 1941.

He became Lieutenant Commander McKean in the U.S. Naval Reserve during World War II. He served as secretary of the Idaho State Medical Association, 1951-55; and president in 1956 and 1957. Dr. and Mrs. McKean became the parents of two sons, Scott and Tom, and one daughter, Anne.

DR. HOWARD MICHAEL CHALOUPKA, F.A.C.S.

Dr. Chaloupka's birthplace was Wilber, Nebraska and he lived in Omaha until after he graduated from medical school. Dr. Chaloupka came to Boise in 1936 after completing his training at the Ancker Hospital in St. Paul, Minnesota and St. Lukes Hospital in San Francisco.

After his arrival in Boise, Dr. Chaloupka served as Dr. James L. Stewart's assistant for three years and then ventured into his own practice until serving as a Navy commander from 1942–46 where he distinguished himself with three air medals. Several years after his return from the Navy, Dr. Chaloupka served as chief of staff at St. Lukes in 1950 and chief of surgery in 1951. He was a Fellow of the College of Surgeons.

Dr. and Mrs. Chaloupka had a family of two girls and one boy.

DR. CARL MASON JOHNSTON

Born in Lillbourne, Missouri, Carl Mason Johnston received his lower and high school educations in that town. He entered Miami University in 1939 and received his Bachelor of Art degree in 1943. He studied at the University of Cincinnati College of Medicine from 1944 through 1948 and received his Medical Doctor degree. He became affiliated with the Phi Chi medical fraternity.

His internships and residency took place at Southern Pacific General Hospital and Hahnamen Hospital (general residency), both in San Francisco; and the Children's Hospital, East Bay, in Oakland.

Upon completing these facets of his medical career, he entered the military service as a captain, going from North Carolina to Japan and on to Korea. While in the service, he practiced medicine at Fort Bragg, North Carolina and Tokyo, Japan. Following military service he practiced in Boise.

Dr. and Mrs. Johnston became the parents of four boys and two girls.

DR. JAMES E. HOLLINGSWORTH

Born in Avon, South Dakota where his father was a physician, Doctor Hollingsworth attended the University of South Dakota in Vermillion, and went on to Yankton College. He also attended the University of Wisconsin in Madison where he graduated with a B.A. in 1933, and Northwestern University in Chicago to earn his M.D. degree in 1938. He was a member of the Psi Upsilon and Nu Sigma Nu. His internship was at Cook County Hospital, Chicago, from August 1, 1937 until January 1, 1939.

He began practicing in Atlanta, Idaho, in 1940 and moved to Boise, Idaho in late 1940 until December of 1961. He was an active staff member of St. Alphonsus Hospital and a member of the Public Health Committee and the Ada County Medical Society.

Dr. Hollingsworth served in the U.S. Army as a captain in the Medical Corps. He participated in the battles and campaigns in Normandy, northern France, Ardennes, Rhineland and central Europe. He was decorated with five Bronze stars and the Meritous Unit Service Badge for his part in the European-African-Middle Eastern Campaign.

He and his wife had four children.

DR. LUCIEN P. McCALLA

Entering the practice of medicine in Boise in 1898, Dr. McCalla specialized in surgery. He had received fine technical training in America and Europe, and was identified with the educational work of medicine. He participated in local interests, and associated with Martin Curran in ownership of one of the large sheep farms in Boise Valley, raising Shropshires and Hampshires.

Dr. McCalla was born in Alcom County, Mississippi, August 23, 1865. He was the son of James Moore and Anne Eliza (Irion) McCalla. James McCalla was a graduate in both schools of medicine and law, University of Virginia. He was a great admirer of President Lincoln. Anne did much to relieve suffering and distress during the Civil War, without discrimination toward those to whom she ministered.

Dr. Lucien McCalla was educated in the public schools of Mississipi, and a student for two years in Tulane University, New Orleans. He entered the medical department of Washington University, St. Louis, from which he was graduated in 1888 and received his M.D. degree. He later completed postgraduate courses in the medical department of John Hopkins University, Baltimore. He also studied in England, Austria, and Germany.

After his graduation, Dr. McCalla practiced in central Texas for five years; in professional work for two years at Trinidad, Colorado; and for an equal period in Salt Lake City. In April, 1898 he established his residence in Boise and specialized in surgery. The doctor was a member of the Ada County, Idaho, and the Southern Idaho Medical societies, and of the Board of Pension Examining Surgeons for Ada County. He was president of the Idaho Medical Society and the Board of Pension Examiners. He was a member of the Republican party, Elks Lodge, and the Catholic Church.

At Taylor, Texas, on August 23, 1894 Dr. McCalla married Cecelia McDonald of Pennsylvania. Dr. and Mrs. McCalla had two children, Randolph, who studied at Georgetown University, and Eileen, who attended St. Theresa's Academy in Boise.

DR. WILLIAM R. TREGONING

Dr. Tregoning was born in Havre, Minnesota, December 25, 1920. His father was a bookkeeper. He went through twelve years of school in Yakima, Washington, played high school football, and got his B.S. degree in 1942 from the College of Puget Sound, Tacoma. From 1942–45 he went to Northwestern University, Chicago, Illinois and received his medical degree.

He interned at Mare Island Naval Hospital, California while in the Army, 1945–46. During that time he received a good conduct medal. From 1948–50 he had a residency at Hines, Illinois V.A. Hospital. He had a residency at Children's Orthopedic Hospital, Seattle, Washington, 1951–52.

He moved to Boise in 1952. He was on the staff at St. Lukes and St. Alphonsus, secretary-treasurer of the latter in 1958. He was a consultant at the V.A. Hospital, and the Elks Rehabilitation Center.

The Tregonings had two daughters and a son.

DR. MANLEY B. SHAW

Manley B. Shaw traded the title of doctor for that of commander, U.S. Naval Reserve (a title he held from 1936 through 1953) during World War II. He was on active duty from 1942–45 at the U.S. Naval Base Hospital No. 2 in the New Hebrides of the South Pacific, and the U.S. Naval Hospital amputation center on Mare Island.

Back in medical practice in Boise, he was equally as active as president of the Saint Alphonsus Hospital staff; medical director for the Idaho State Elks Rehabilitation Center; served as president for both the Southwest Idaho

Medical Society and the Idaho State Medical Society. In his "spare time," he painted in oils, did sculpturing and worked in ceramic art.

He was born in Wahpeton, North Dakota, where his father was a farmer and an abstracter. The family moved west and Manley attended grade, high school, and received his Bachelor of Science degree from the College of Idaho, all in Caldwell. He graduated in 1925 and from Johns Hopkins Medical School in 1931. He became a member of the medical fraternity Alpha Kappa Kappa.

Dr. Shaw had one year of general surgery and a three year residency in orthopedics at Johns Hopkins Hospital in Baltimore, Maryland. He opened his practice in Boise and, with the exception of the years of his military service, he practiced there. He and Mrs. Shaw have a son, Bradford, and a daughter, Diane.

DR. J. WAYNE TYLER

Dr. Tyler was born May 7, 1922, Pullman, Washington. His father was a college professor, and his brother a doctor in Los Angeles, California. Dr. Tyler went to high school in Cheney, Washington. In 1943 he got his B.S. degree from Washington State College. He was graduated from the University of Oregon in 1946 with his medical degree. For fifteen months he interned at San Bernardino County Hospital. He had an eye residency for three years at the U.S. Veterans Administration Hospital, Long Beach.

In 1947-49 he was a general practitioner in the Army Medical Corps. From 1949-51 he practiced at Oakridge, Oregon. He was an eye doctor from 1954-55 in Caldwell, and moved to Jones Clinic, Boise, 1955.

The Tylers had three daughters and one son.

DR. HENRY GOODFRIEND

Henry Goodfriend made eight different trips to Europe to continue his medical education after receiving two degrees in New York and interning in Lebanon Hospital and Trudeau Sanitarium at Saranac Lake, New York. He practiced two years in Cleveland, Ohio, before arriving in Idaho in 1907. On his European stays he took special courses in Vienna, Berlin, and Heidelberg.

Born in New York City on January 28, 1876, he was one of a family of seven sons and three daughters born to John

Jacob and Esther Title Goodfriend. The parents were born, reared, and married in Austria, sailing across the Atlantic to settle in New York City in the early 1870s. Three of the brothers, Henry, Edward, and Nathan all became doctors.

Henry received the Bachelor of Arts degree from City College of New York in 1897; and medical degree from Columbia University in 1902, before his interning and practice brought him to Idaho. From 1907 until 1912, he practiced at Albion before moving to Boise to establish his home and medical service.

In 1907, Dr. Goodfriend married Matilda Iverson, who died within a few months. In September 1912, he wed Lois Little of Boise. They were members of the Congregational Church and he was a Knight Templar Mason. He also belonged to the Mystic Shrine, the Knights of Pythias, a member of the Country Club and the Boise Commercial Club. He was a Democrat, but had no desire to hold a political office.

DR. CHARLES B. CALLARD

A prominent Boise doctor, Charles B. Callard, was born in London, province of Ontario, Canada, on January 19, 1883. His parents, John and Emily (White) Callard had a drugstore in London for thirty-five years.

Charles attended the public schools of London and entered the Western University's School of Medicine there, graduating in 1903. For the next nine months he served an internship at Guelph Sanitarium, Ontario. Moving to the neighboring United States, he began his practice that autumn at Campbell, Nebraska. On the day after Christmas, 1906, Dr. Callard married Mabel Barber, daughter of Frank Barber, pioneer banker and land owner in Franklin, Nebraska. The young Callards lived at Campbell until March 1907.

They then moved to Idaho and the mining town of Placerville for the next two years. In the fall of 1909, they moved into Boise. Dr. Callard joined another physician, Dr. Ross, in practice. They had five well-equipped medical rooms in the McCarthy Building in downtown Boise. Dr. Callard was a specialist in skin and blood diseases and was most successful.

Dr. Callard became an active member of the Republican

party; the Benevolent and Protective Order of Elks, Fraternal Order of Eagles and the Masonic order. With the Masons, he was also a member of the Knights Templar and Shrine.

Dr. and Mrs. Callard had no children.

DR. ROBERT H. WILKINSON

Dr. Wilkinson arrived in Boise in 1957 to open an office at 403 Idaho. He was born and reared at Syracuse, New York, and studied at Cornell University in 1944 and 1945; received his B.A. in 1947 from Wesleyan University and his M.D. in 1951 from Cornell University Medical College.

A rotating internship at Rochester, New York, General Hospital for one year; at Denver Children's Hospital for two years; and training in pediatric cardiology for one year at the University of Colorado Medical Center completed his training.

In 1954, Dr. Venning had the experience of working with the Vietnam Refugee Evacuation operation. He held the rank of lieutenant with the Marine Corps, USNR. His staff appointments include clinical instructor in pediatrics at Upstate Medical Center, Syracuse; St. Lukes and St. Alphonsus in Boise; as secretary-treasurer at St. Lukes in 1961; scientific program chairman for Ada County in 1960 and 1961; Fellow of the American Academy of Pediatrics; American Heart Association board of directors.

Along with H. Swan and S.G. Blount, Dr. Wilkinson had writings on "Repair of Aortic Stenosis Under Hypothermia" (Thoracic Surgery) published in February of 1958.

Dr. Wilkinson was married to Marilyn Clark, a Wells College graduate, who was also graduated from the Harvard-Radcliffe program of business administration in 1954. They became the parents of three daughters, Karen, Randa, and Holly.

DR. RICHARD G. GARDNER

Dr. Gardner was born August 20, 1924, at Payette. His father was a pharmacist. From 1942–43 he went to the University of Idaho and College of Idaho, 1946–49, and received his M.D. degree in 1953 from the University of Oregon Medical School. He had residencies in several hospitals before moving to Boise in 1958. He was on the staffs at St. Lukes and St. Alphonsus. Dr. Gardner was a member of the American, Ada County, and Idaho Medical societies.

From 1943–46 he was in the Navy and took boot camp at Farragut, Idaho. He was in the South Pacific, New Caledonia, and Philippines.

The Gardners had twin girls and a son.

DR. WILLIAM LUCAS VENNING

Dr. Venning arrived in Boise to begin his practice in 1955, coming from Charlotte and Winston-Salem, North Carolina, where he practiced. Born August 14, 1914, he first secured an A.B. degree in 1935 from Duke University, where he joined Sigma Chi fraternity. He attended Harvard Medical School in 1940 and Duke, where he received his M.D. degree. He was a member of the medical fraternity A.O.A.

Internship was at Duke, 1939–40, with the following two years at Baltimore City Hospital, and back to Duke for the years 1941 and 1942. His residency was at the Bowman Gray School of Medicine until 1945. Dr. Venning practiced in Winston Salem and Charlotte, North Carolina from 1943 until 1955, when he moved to Boise.

Dr. Venning had staff appointments at all hospitals in Winston Salem, Charlotte, and Boise. He was chief of podiatrics at three hospitals in Charlotte, and North Carolina chairman for podiatrics.

He and Mrs. Venning are the parents of four sons and three daughters.

DR. NORMAN C. HEDEMARK

The tornado of 1939 in Anoka, Minnesota gave Dr. Hedemark active experience in first-aid during his residency. He came to Boise in 1941 to live, except for a brief period in the Army, a lieutenant colonel from 1942–46; Chief of Eye Service in the Air Corps, Big Spring, Texas and White Sulphur Springs General Hospital in West Virginia. He was named Diplomate of the American Board of Otolaryngology, 1942; American Board of Ophthalmology, 1946; active member of the executive board at St. Alphonsus; secretary and chief of staff in 1954.

The doctor was an April Fool's Day baby born in 1911 at St. Paul, Minnesota Dr. Hedemark's family has a number of doctors. His two brothers, Truman and Homer, practiced in

Ortonville, Minnesota and his uncles, Albert and Adolph Aherens in St. Paul. His son is carrying on the tradition and studied pre-med at the College of Idaho.

DR. TERRELL O. CARVER

Dr. Carver was born July 21, 1921 at Preston, Idaho. His father was an attorney. He attended schools in Preston, Pocatello, and Boise, including Boise Junior College.

In 1943 Dr. Carver received his B.S. from the University of Idaho, and in 1945 his M.D. from the University of Oregon Medical School. He went to Tulane University in Louisiana from 1948–49. He interned at the U.S. Marine Hospital, San Francisco, from 1945–46.

Dr. Carver was not in private practice, but he was elected a Diplomate by the American Board of Preventive Medicine. He served as Idaho's chief medical health officer as director of the Department of Health. He was a consultant for St. Lukes and St. Alphonsus hospitals in Boise.

The Carvers had two boys.

DR. O. H. PARKER

When twelve years of age, the boy who was to become Dr. O.H. Parker of Boise, moved with his parents from New York City to Arkansas City, Kansas in 1885. He was born in New York, March 15, 1872. When eighteen, he entered the department of pharmacy at the University of Kansas, graduating in 1894.

He entered Kansas City Medical College, graduating in 1897. Moving across the line to Kansas City, Missouri, he spent fifteen years in practice. During 1899–1901 he was in charge of the Kansas City General Hospital. He also served as Jackson County, Missouri's coroner from 1904 until 1908.

In 1901, Dr. Parker was married in Kansas City to Mrs. Pauline St. John. He was another young doctor who heeded the call to "Go west, young man, go west," and he and Mrs. Parker arrived in Boise in 1912 and opened an office. He was a constant reader and kept in touch with the trends of science.

Dr. Parker was a member of Masons, Elks, Knights of Pythias, Modern Woodmen of America, and Boise Physicians Club.

DR. FARRAR W. SKILLERN

Farrar Skillern had many talents, even before he took up the study of medicine. He also knew the pain that patients felt, for in 1918 he was caught in a terrible hotel fire in Tishomingo, Oklahoma, and barely escaped with his life. Jumping to safety, he suffered eighteen fractures.

He was born in Hamilton County, Tennessee, July 19, 1851. His boyhood was on the family farm and he attended a country school until fourteen. College prep was at Pikeville, followed by Vanderbilt University and medical, literary and scientific courses at the same time.

He taught at Rockdale, Texas, and in 1883 returned to Tennessee to practice medicine. His elder brother, John, had moved to Idaho and became one of the most prominent sheepmen in the state.

Turning to another profession, Dr. Skillern went to Texas and Oklahoma, where he became a large oil operator. On February 9, 1874, in Belton, Texas, he married Alice Williams of Tennessee. They had two daughters, Martha and Kathryn. Dr. Skillern and his family moved to Boise to be near his brother John. He was an active member of the Methodist Church and a Master Mason. The Skillern home was one of the most beautiful in Boise as a result of the wealth earned in oil.

DR. WILLIAM S. TITUS

Born in Tracy, Lyon County, Minnesota, September 20, 1879, Dr. Titus was the son of Henry Harland Titus. He graduated from high school in the class of 1899 and then entered the University of Minnesota and graduated with an M.D. in 1904. After a one year internship at St. Mary's Hospital in Duluth, Minnesota, he opened and operated a hospital in Mora, Minnesota specializing in surgery. After four years, he sold his successful hospital and relocated to Boise where he became an associate of Dr. W.H. Tukey, who was for many years the head surgeon of Fort Boise.

As his practice grew, he continued to keep abreast of new changes in the medical field. He also pursued his interest in writing and published a book on the history of Minnesota. He married and had two daughters. He and his wife, Frances, enjoyed hunting and fishing trips. Recognizing the potential, he invested in real estate in Boise.

ELMORE COUNTY

The Union Pacific Railway built its first mainline across the Elmore area in 1833 and permanent settlement followed. Farming and cattle raising began to replace mining as a major industry and by 1889 the county was established. Mountain Home became the county seat. Mountain Home remains the site of a Strategic Air Command Wing.

Three of Idaho's best known mountain ranges (Sawtooths, Trinity, and Soldier) dominate the land. The county is rich in histories of gold and silver mining, early railroading, overland stages, and rugged, colorful characters who built the area.

DR. F. S. WRIGHT

Dr. Wright was born in Hamilton, Canada, of Scotch-Irish parentage, and married Miss Anna Edward.

He was graduated from Portland Medical School in 1887, following which he practiced in Centerville, Oregon, for one year. The next three years he spent in Rocky Bar, Idaho. From that time he practiced medicine in Lemhi County, following his appointment as Government Doctor to the Lemhi Indian Agency, at which post he remained five years.

In 1899 he was elected State Senator, and was active in obtaining passage of the State Medical Law. He served as U. S. Examiner for enlisted men for the Spanish War, and the World War, and was county physician many times. He was examiner for the pension department, and the civil service department, as well as coroner at Rocky Bar in 1889.

DR. WILLIAM F. SMITH

A physician and surgeon of Mountain Home, county seat of Elmore County, Idaho, Dr. Smith maintained his residence there since 1889. He was born in Richmond, Virginia, August 11, 1863.

The doctor's grandfather, Hiram M. Smith, and his father, Isaac T. Smith, were manufacturers in Richmond. During the Civil War they manufactured arms and munitions for the Confederate Army. The doctor's father was a native of the old capital city on the James River, where he was reared and educated. He married Miss Philomena Clew, a native of New York. They had seven children. William F. Smith was the eldest son, and he grew to maturity in his native city, where he received his early education. He completed his literary training in Richmond College, after which he pursued his medical studies in Richmond Medical College, in the local hospitals, where he secured clinical work.

In 1887, Dr. Smith left his home and journeyed to Pendleton, Oregon, where he began the practice of medicine. After a short interval he came to Mountain Home, where he practiced. When he arrived there was no doctor in the town, and he received the heartiest of welcomes. The doctor took a postgraduate course at the New York Polyclinic in 1895.

Dr. Smith was a member of the Idaho State Medical Society; American Medical Association; local physician and surgeon of the Oregon Short Line Railroad, having also the railway practice at Glenn's Ferry. He served as coroner of Elmore County for several years, and was physician to the county poor.

He was a Democrat, and was one of the electors of Idaho during William Jennings Bryan's campaign, and took to the national capital the results of the election in Idaho. He was a member of the Idaho Legislature in 1889, and in the same year a member of the Mountain Home baseball team. He was past chancellor commander of the Knights of Pythias; passed the chairs in the Independent Order of Odd Fellows, and he represented his lodge in the grand lodge of the state; member of the Ancient Order of United Workmen and of the Masonic fraternity; was a master of the lodge, and the Mystic Shrine.

Dr. Smith had a well-equipped office in Mountain Home, and owned other property in the little city.

DR. MALONE W. KOELSCH

Born October 8, 1924, and raised in Boise, Dr. Koelsch was the son of an attorney who was a clerk of the Supreme Court of Idaho. Dr. Koelsch has practiced in Mountain Home, Idaho since 1952. He went to college at the University of Idaho from 1942–43 and then to the University of Idaho Southern Branch, Navy V-12 1943–44.

He entered the University of Oregon Medical School in 1944 and graduated in 1948. His rotating internship was at the San Bernadino County Hospital from 1948–49 and continued there in a general practice residency in 1949–50. He was recalled to the Navy as a lieutenant during the Korean War from 1950–52. During his practice in Mountain Home, he served as chief of staff at Elmore Memorial Hospital. He enjoys outdoor activities such as hunting, fishing, and gardening, and has five sons.

DR. ORRIS W. HALL

Dr. Hall was born in 1860 in Vermont and studied as a medical apprentice to a Dr. Bromley in Richard, Vermont, and did some study at the University of Vermont, after which he was granted an M.D. in 1883.

He then married Ollie Bostwick and they moved to Ketchum, Idaho. The village had no hospital and surgery was done in the homes and was limited to amputations. His first delivery case was in a hotel in Ketchum. They moved to Atlanta, Idaho, where he was the only doctor and mine surgeon.

After four years he moved to Mountain Home for a few months and on to Star, where he maintained his home, even when practicing in Boise. He was one of the first members of the Idaho Medical Society and remained active. He was sent to Idaho Legislature from Ada County in 1898. He was licensed first in 1897, and again in 1899. He was a brother of Mrs. Frank Martin Sr. of Boise.

OWYHEE COUNTY

In 1863, the beginning of the legend of the Blue Bucket Mine in Owyhee County began a stampede of miners over the Snake River to get a share of the supposedly fabulous gold strike. Owyhee is believed to be a corruption of the word, "Hawaii," used by several Sandwich Islanders who were members of the Astoria party and killed by Indians.

Although sparsely settled, the county is one of the nation's largest at 7,648 square miles, and home of a "wild horse" herd that has stirred the imaginations of thousands. The county lies south of the Snake River and the Oregon Trail was the prehistoric Indian and buffalo trail for thousands of years before trappers and immigrants ever rode over it.

Silver City, now a ghost town visited by many, was the most flourishing of the mining towns. The famed Poorman Mine was discovered in 1865 and the content of its gold-silver ore won the quality prize at the 1886 Paris Exposition. Bruneau Canyon, the steepest of canyons in the country, is only one of the many scenic wonders of Owyhee.

DR. BELKNAP

The mention of an Owyhee County Doctor Belknap is contained in this colorful article from an October, 1881, issue of the *Owyhee Avalanche*:

FIRST AND ONLY LEGAL HANGING IN
OWYHEE COUNTY

The morning of Friday, October 15, 1881, the day appointed for the execution of Henry McDonald, dawned dark and disagreeable, a heavy snow storm prevailing, as if nature was angry that man, created in the image of God, should fall so low as to make capital punishment a necessity. All preparations for the execution had been completed by Sheriff Springer, and at one o'clock p.m. the prisoner was taken from his cell, and in company with the sheriff and deputy, walked down to Jordan Street, where a wagon was in waiting to carry him to the gallows and the grave. He showed no sign of emotion; walked very erect, and got in the wagon, in company with the sheriff, deputy, and Father Nattini, and was driven to the place of execution, at the old Ruby City cemetery, which has been unused for many years. About 300 people gathered about the scaffold, many having come in from adjacent valleys. At seventeen minutes past one o'clock the prisoner firmly ascended the scaffold, and until 1:45 remained in consultation with Father Nattini, at which time Sheriff Springer read the death warrant. McDonald shook hands with those who had guarded him while in jail here and the priest, bidding them goodby, but had nothing else to say.

James T. Griffin pinioned his hands and feet, and Father Nattini adjusted the black cap. At six minutes before 2 o'clock the sheriff sprung the trap, and thus without a sign of emotion or a word of complaint the bloodstained soul of Henry McDonald was ushered into eternity. In fourteen minutes life was pronounced extinct by Dr. Belknap, and the remains were buried within a few yards of the scaffold.

The evidence in this case is well known and the law has been vindicated. Not only should the youths of this place remember, but those men who are ready to draw the deadly knife and revolver, that "He who sheds man's blood, by man shall his blood be shed." This is the first execution by law in this county; may we hope that another will never be required.

DR. JOHN N. WESTON

Arriving in Silver City in 1889, Dr. John N. Weston became county coroner and physician. He was also named surgeon of the Miner's Union Hospital. He was born in New York City in 1860 and after attending the public schools entered Phillips Exeter Academy and Harvard University. He studied medicine and was graduated from the College of Physicians, and Bellevue Hospital in New York.

The year after arriving in Silver City, he married Minnie Grete on February 26, 1890. He was a member and Worthy Matron of the Masonic Lodge, Silver City No. 13, A.F. and A.M.

DR. R. GEORGE WOLFF

Originally from Cardston, Alberta, Canada, R. George Wolff was in the implement business and pool hall and bowling alley business from 1935-37. He was born in Irvine, Alberta on December 7, 1915 where his father was in the implement business. He did not attend a college but did attend the University of Alberta Medical School in Edmonton, Alberta and did a rotating internship in the University of Alberta's hospital. He was a member of the Canadian Army Medical Corp from 1943-46 where he served in the European theatre as a captain. He practiced in Bellow, Alberta, Canada from 1946-51 and then relocated to Homedale, Idaho from 1951-64. During the severe winters in Canada he traveled by horse and cart and spent lots of time shoveling snow, especially to get out of his garage. He was on the staff of Caldwell Memorial Hospital and Mercy Hospital; and was a past president of the medical staff at each hospital. He was active in the local and regional medical societies.

CHAPTER
12

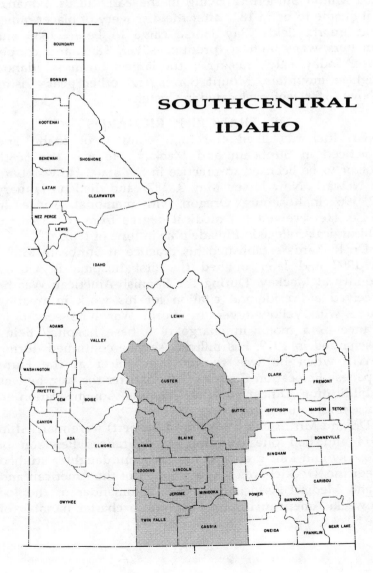

SOUTHCENTRAL
IDAHO

CUSTER COUNTY

Established in 1881 in some of Idaho's most rugged mountain country, Custer County was visited years previously by traders in search of valuable furs. It is known that Nathaniel Wyeth, Jedediah Smith, and Alexander Ross trapped there in 1824, with Alexander Ross and Milton Sublette arriving in the early 1830s. Bonanza City came to be in 1877 after the discovery of placer mines and quartz fields. Bay Horse came to be in 1880 and smelters were built to produce silver, lead, and copper ores. Today, cattle raising is the largest business. Idaho's highest mountain, Mount Borah, and other peaks rising above 10,000 feet are located in Custer.

DR. FRANCIS P. RICHARDS

Dr. Richards liked the high country of Idaho and practiced in Sunbeam and Mackay. He was the 568th doctor to be licensed to practice in the state. He was born in Newark, New Jersey May 3, 1877 and died on January 12, 1962 in Roseburg, Oregon, with memorial services in Boise. He received his medical degree from the Medico-Chirurgical College in Philadelphia in June of 1902.

Dr. Richards established his practice at Sunbeam Mines in 1909 and later opened the first hospital in Custer County at Mackay. During the Spanish-American War he received a Presidential citation for his work in treating those with yellow fever. In World War I he served in France as a major in charge of a base hospital, being discharged in 1919. His military service continued during WWII, when he was the medical officer at the Hunt Japanese Relocation Center in Idaho. After the war, he was Adjudication Officer for the Veterans Administration in Boise until retiring in 1953.

Dr. and Mrs. Richards (Mildred Burnett) were married in 1914 and had one daughter, Mrs. Frances Peterson of Moscow and four grandchildren. A granddaughter studied medicine. Dr. Richards was a member of the American and Idaho Medical Associations, past commander of the Joe Nowacki American Legion Post, and a charter member of the 50 et 8.

BUTTE COUNTY

In 1823 Antoine Godin and his French fur traders were the first white men to visit the Lost River country, which was to become Butte County, and named what we know as Lost River, Godin River. Nearly fifty years later, Jack Hood drove the first wagon into the area.

A suspension bridge was built across Big Lost River at old Arco (the only crossing in high water), the direct wagon route to Oregon and the Northwest. Cattle, sheep, and horses were trailed through this important stage junction. In modern times, the National Reactor Testing Station, the largest such installation in the world, is near Arco. The lava beds containing the national monument, Craters of the Moon, are located in the heart of the desert area and is visited by geologists from all over the world.

DR. JACK CHESTER REINES

Doctor Reines spent his medical career caring for the citizens of Arco, Idaho. The son of a semi-skilled factory worker, Jack was born on January 8, 1922 in Meyersdale, Pennsylvania. He graduated from the University of Toledo in 1943 with a B.S. degree and went into the U.S. Army as a sergeant for three years. Returning to Toledo, he graduated with another B.S. degree in 1949 and went to the University of Louisville, Kentucky for his medical degree.

After a rotating internship at St. Marks Hospital in Salt Lake City, he moved to Arco in 1950. He was an active staff member of the Lost River Hospital in Arco and was chief of staff from 1960 to 1963.

DR. FRANK MULLEN CANNON

Dr. Cannon relates this story common to his first years in practice in the Arco area. "For quite a time I was the only physician in Butte County, and like many another country doctor in those days, my experiences in sagebrush surgery were wide and varied. With a pressure sterilizer on the kitchen stove, the instruments were boiled up, a nice old lady opened and passed the sterile bundles, the abdomen was painted with iodine, a drunken dentist gave the ether, I asked my God for wisdom and drew the blade down the midline.

"Getting in is easy, but getting out is not. Single-handed

and alone, to hold back the intestines with one hand and stitch with the other is no easy task with an abdomen heaving under an ether anesthetic. We had no wonder drugs, nor intravenous supportive therapy for post operative treatment, but these were a tough breed of people familiar with hardships and poverty."

Dr. Cannon was born November 24, 1889 in Cherokee, California and reared on an Arizona cattle ranch. He attended the University of Arizona, and later Valparaiso University in Indiana. He graduated from Chicago College of Medicine and Surgery in 1917. He interned at Illinois Central Railroad Hospital in Chicago until ordered to duty in the U.S. Navy during World War I.

Dr. Cannon began practice in Arco in October 1919, moved to Point Reyes, California from 1924–33; San Rafael from 1933–40; served in the U.S. Navy Medical Corps from 1940–54 when he retired as a captain.

During World War II Dr. Cannon commanded a Medical Company attached to the First Raider Battalion of the U.S. Marine Corps in the Solomon Island landing. In the darkness of the early morning of August 7, 1942, the Japanese attacked, and he and his men were ordered to cease first aid and help defend the command post. They did, and with minor casualties, held the Island of Tulagi.

DR. ROBERT FULTON BARTER

Dr. Barter of Arco learned of the great Idaho distances when he delivered his first baby eighty miles up the Salmon River near Warren. He quickly learned of the hardship caused by Idaho winters in 1950, when he flew from Mackay to Howe in a plane equipped with skis, landed in a sheep field and walked to a home to deliver another baby. Dr. Barter practiced in Arco until 1964, providing medical service to patients in faraway Challis and Mackay.

He was born June 15, 1919, in Mt. Vernon, Indiana, attended Indiana University between 1937 and 1947, taking time away from his studies to serve in the U.S. Navy. While at Indiana University, he was a member of Nu Sigma Nu and Delta Tau Delta. He completed his internship at the U.S. Navy Hospital in San Diego.

He served as a pharmacists mate, 1st class in the Navy Medical Corps, 1942–44 and later lieutenant, JG, 1947–48. Dr. Barter was married and the father of three children.

BLAINE COUNTY

Alexander Ross led an expedition into the area of what was to become the wealthiest of Idaho's counties, Alturas, in 1824. Blaine was organized from a remnant of Alturas. Known as the Gold Belt, mining claims were filed as early as 1865. After driving out the Indians, settlers came in 1879. The first farming was along Spring Creek, with a fine cattle and sheep industry following.

Blaine was a "first" county, with the first electric light plant in the Territory, first town with electric lights, and second earliest paper, the *Wood River Daily Times*, first all-year holiday resort built by Union Pacific at Sun Valley in 1937. The jagged and gorgeous Sawtooth Mountains attract artists and writers, movie makers and sportsmen. Ernest Hemingway made Ketchum his home and there wrote some of his best works.

DR. ROBERT HENRY WRIGHT

Dr. Robert Henry Wright was the first doctor on the scene during the 1917 avalanche at the North Star Mine north of Hailey when fifteen were killed and seventeen injured. He married Cynthia Beamer, June 30, 1906 in Bellevue, shortly after he graduated from the American College in St. Louis, Missouri. They returned to Missouri, where he practiced for six months, and returned to Hailey and remained until his death, November 20, 1970.

Dr. Wright was in partnership with Dr. J.J. Plummer for three years before opening his own practice which continued until he retired in March 1967. He traveled by horse and buggy, changing to a sled in the winter, to reach his patients. He performed surgery in the homes before a hospital was built. Mrs. Wright often accompanied him and served as nurse and assistant. He was county health officer for thirty years and coroner for thirty-five.

Dr. Wright was past master of Hailey Masonic Lodge, past patron of Bethany chapter of Eastern Star, member of the Shrine, fifty-year Scottish Rite bodies. The Wrights had one son and a daughter.

DR. JAMES D. McCURDY

In the character and work of Dr. James Darwin McCurdy, were many characteristics of Scotland. Perseverance, energy, and determination gained success for Dr. McCurdy and when he retired from the practice of medicine in Blaine County, he stayed actively interested in mining, and was owner of a group of mines in Wood River Valley.

Dr. McCurdy was born in Kentucky, March 22, 1820. The family originated in Scotland. The doctor's father, James Darwin McCurdy, Sr., an only son, was born in Virginia. He married Livenia Sharp, and Dr. McCurdy was one of eleven children, only two of whom reached maturity. The father died at the age of sixty-three; and the mother at the age of eighty-seven.

The doctor was educated in Kentucky and in 1848, the degree of M.D. was conferred upon him by the University of New York. Returning to Kentucky, he began the practice of medicine, but after a short time moved to Missouri, and in 1852 crossed the plains to Oregon, with an emigrant train filled with many stricken with the dread disease, cholera. The services of Dr. McCurdy were in great demand by the sufferers and, keeping two horses ready for use, he treated the emigrants in trains both ten miles in advance and ten miles in the rear of his own train. It was arduous doctoring, but was gratefully received.

In 1853, Dr. McCurdy was commissioned surgeon-general of the Oregon forces raised to suppress an outbreak of the Rogue River Indians. When the Indians began to exhibit hostilities, the white settlers asked for help from the governor, George L. Curry, who responded with a call for volunteers. With promptness, they came forward. The governor appointed as commander General Joseph Lane, who was later elected one of the first two United States senators from Oregon. Dr. McCurdy served as surgeon general of the army until peace was restored.

When Dr. McCurdy arrived in Salem, he engaged in practice until 1857, when he returned to Kentucky and on to Weston, Missouri, where on September 2, 1858, he married Mrs. James H. Baldwin, formerly Susan B. Thornton. They moved to St. Joseph, where he ran a drug store for seven years. He sold it and moved to Denver to open a drug store and practice medicine. They also lived in Salem and Walla Walla. In 1882, hearing of mining excitement in the Wood River Valley of Idaho, the doctor made a trip and invested in mines, purchased land and built a home in Bellevue. He continued to practice his profession to 1896, when he retired to take care of mining and other property. He was part owner of seven silver and lead and two gold mines located in the Camas District, No. 2, of the Gold Belt.

He became a Mason in 1850, and belonged to the Templars' Society.

DR. JOHN RAAF

In a letter to Gretchen and Don Fraser of Sun Valley, Dr. John F. Raaf, physician and surgeon in Portland, Oregon, wrote of his father, a Blaine County doctor of many years ago, and recalled the county and happenings there. The doctor's letter related, in part:

"I well remember the old Blaine County Courthouse. Gordon Gray was my constant companion when we were little boys and he lived in back of the courthouse, and ran around through the courthouse constantly. Why nobody threw us out, I do not know. I remember some of my father's battles in Hailey. Dad graduated from medical school just before 1900 and started practice in a little town on the banks of the Mississippi River in Missouri. He got malaria to such an extent that he knew he could not live in that country any longer. He came to Idaho and looked all over for a place to settle.

"Dr. Robert Nourse was already practicing in Hailey and was secretary or president of the Board of Health which licensed physicians. He frankly told my father that he would not pass the State Boards if he was going to practice in Hailey, but if he wanted to practice anywhere else in Idaho, he could pass. Over the next few years, Dad took the boards three times and failed three times. In the meantime, he continued to practice in Hailey without a license. Every now and then he would be arrested and stand trial for practicing without a license. Each time the jury would bring in the verdict 'not guilty', and he continued to practice.

"When I was about eight, my father got into another altercation. There was a half-witted day laborer around Hailey who had cut his hand and my father sewed it up. He asked how much and my father said, two dollars, and he complained that was too much. My father then said the fee would be nothing. Not satisfied, the man kept arguing. Dad chased him out of the office. A few days later, Dad was standing on the street corner and out of the corner of his eyes saw the fellow coming down the street, but paid little attention. He jumped on Dad's back, threw him to the pavement, and the revolver Dad carried fell out of his pocket. One of the onlookers picked it up so nobody was too badly hurt, but my father got a broken nose.

"The next day or so, Dad took the train for Salt Lake to get his nose fixed. While Dad was away I remember sitting in our living room with my mother. The loaded revolver was always on the dining room table but the man didn't come around while Dad was gone. The man was tried for assault. The jury verdict was 'not guilty', so you can see the Hailey juries were always fair regardless of the actual facts in the case."

DR. JOHN R. MORITZ

Dr. Moritz practiced medicine in Beatrice, Nebraska for six years before coming to Sun Valley in 1939. A brother, Alan, was also a doctor in Cleveland. Dr. Moritz was born at Blue Hill, Nebraska, May 31, 1905 and made his home in Ketchum. He was graduated from Seward (Nebraska) High School, and the University of Nebraska at Lincoln with a bachelor of science degree. He interned at Lakeside Hospital in Cleveland in 1929 and was surgical resident there until 1933. Dr. Moritz was navy commander in the Medical Corps 1942–45. He and his wife had a daughter, Derry Ann, who became a nurse; and two sons, Alan Fisher and Edmund D.

DR. J. J. PLUMMER

Dr. J. J. Plummer was born on April 8, 1860 in Missouri. He attended the Birmingham Academy in Iowa. He graduated from the Starling Medical School in Columbus, Ohio in 1882 and then opened a medical practice in Bonaparte, Iowa. After two years he relocated to Kansas for six years before moving to Baker City, Oregon. In 1890 he moved to De Lamar to become the physician and surgeon for the De Lamar Mining Company. He also engaged in general practice and ran the only drug store in the town of Hailey.

He married Margaret C. DeQuette, the daughter of a Boise basin pioneer.

GOODING COUNTY

In the early 1860s, Ben Halladay ran his famous stages through what is now Gooding County. Relics of a station can still be seen at Uhrlaub's Crossing, and Horse Heaven, where the horses were fed and rested is nearby. The mainline of the Union Pacific was punched through in 1883, with a stop at Bliss. An abundance of water from springs for agriculture use, gold in Snake River sands, a treasure in fossil remains, and the silent City of Rocks, worked together to build a county of beauty, farms and cattle ranches, and scientific research. Medicine men and doctors aided in the building.

DR. HAROLD FRANKLIN HOLSINGER

Giving that "little extra" was not uncommon for Dr. Holsinger. During the winter of 1948–49 he found he was the only available doctor at St. Valentines Hospital for several days. During that time, another doctor's patient needed a Caesarian section because of a hydrocephalic baby. This was done with help of the Sisters nursing at the hospital.

Dr. Holsinger was born in Flora, Indiana in 1906 and grew up on a Nampa farm, and graduated from high school. He taught school eleven years in Boise Valley before entering medical study. Studies included summers at U.S.C. and Colorado State Teachers College; pre-med, College of Idaho; and University of Oregon Medical School, Portland. His internship was at Tacoma General Hospital. Dr. Holsinger began practice in Wendell on July 6, 1942.

He served as chief of staff at St. Valentines, St. Benedicts and Gooding County Memorial Hospital. He was president of South Central Medical Society, Medical Director of Idaho State Cancer Society for twelve years, and on numerous committees for the Idaho Medical Association. Dr. Holsinger was a school board member, on the College of Idaho Board, and involved in many church related activities.

Dr. Holsinger and his wife, the former Mary Campbell of Nampa, had two children; Dr. Eugene Holsinger of Burley and Mrs. Rosemary Beal of Castro Valley, California.

DR. MARION V. KLINGLER

Dr. Klingler went to grade and high schools in Hailey. He went to the University of Idaho from 1931–35, and the University of Oregon Medical School 1936–41 (a year out for working). He interned at Emmanuel Hospital, Portland, Oregon from 1941–42.

He served in the 9th Division Infantry from 1942–45. He received the Silver Star, Palm Leaf; Bronze Star; Purple Heart, Palm Leaf, and was a major at the end of the war.

He practiced in Portland, Oregon from 1945–51, then moved to Gooding. He was a member of the staff at Gooding Memorial Hospital.

The Klinglers had two boys and a girl.

DR. KENNETH ALOYSIUS TYLER

Initially Dr. Tyler was from Kalispell, Montana where he was born on April 2, 1912. He then moved to Ithaca, New York when he was eleven. Dr. Tyler's father was a real estate broker. He attended Cornell University and graduated in 1934 with a degree in Animal Biology. He attended the Cornell University Medical College in New York and graduated in 1937. His internship was at the St. Vincent's Hospital in Portland, Oregon.

He began practicing medicine at Boulder, Montana and worked as a part-time physician for the mentally retarded and as the part-time county health officer and county physician until 1941. He then became the staff physician, and surgical assistant for the Montana State Tuberculosis Hospital from 1941–45. In 1945 he became the medical Director for the T.B. Hospital in Cairo, Illinois. In 1946 he moved on to become the medical director of the Idaho State Tuberculosis Hospital. He was a courtesy staff member of Gooding Memorial Hospital and St. Benedicts Hospital. He has been president of the Mt. Powell Medical Society and governor for the Idaho board of Governors American College of Chest Physicians for ten years. He was also president of the Pacific Northwest Chapter of College of Chest Physicians from 1959–60. He married Aileen N. Palmer who was a nurse, and had three children, two girls and one boy.

Early in his practice he delivered babies in miners' cabins and often walked to see his patients especially in the winter when snow drifts prevented passage by car. During a measles epidemic he quarantined a town and prevented the illness from reaching the institution for the retarded. During his work with the retarded institution he removed two beef vertebrae from the upper esophagus of a boy at the school for mentally retarded. He also removed a piece of bed spring from the esophagus of a young man committed to the mental hospital for a thrill slaying of a girl classmate.

DR. B. A. BODMER

Dr. Bodmer delivered five sets of twins in his first three years of private practice after relocating to Gooding, Idaho after his military service was completed. He had been stationed at Perrin Air Force Base in Sherman, Texas as chief of professional services. His father was a school teacher and administrator and two brothers had medical careers. He attended Kansas University from 1947-51 and entered Kansas University Medical school in 1951 and graduated in 1955. His internship was completed at the Sacramento County Hospital in 1955-56. He had three sons.

DR. EDGAR LOCKE SIMONTON

One of the very early physicians in the Wendell area, Dr. Simonton was born in West Virginia on June 24, 1869. His father was a farmer; however, Dr. Simonton's great grandfather was a Revolutionary surgeon. He was an early immigrant to Kansas where his family homesteaded. He attended the University of Kansas Medical School and graduated in 1896 and interned at St. Joseph's Hospital in Kansas City, Missouri. He did extended post graduate work at Bellview Hospital, New York in 1906. His practices were at Wamego, Kansas from 1897-1914 and in Wendell, Idaho from 1914-40. He came out of retirement for the period of 1942-45 because of the shortage of physicians created by the second World War.

During his early practice, surgical cases were sent to Topeka, Kansas City, or Boise. If an emergency surgery was necessary, it was often done on a kitchen table. He traveled a great deal by horse, or horse and buggy to reach his patients. In the 1900s he quarantined 1000 cases of smallpox and vaccinated thousands of others. In 1918 during the flu epidemic, he worked to the point of exhaustion but lost very few patients in the Wendell area. He was the chief medical "man" to the Sisters of St. Benedict at their St. Valentines Hospital in Wendell from 1923 until his retirement in 1940.

He was active in regional medical societies. He enjoyed his genealogy, farming, hunting, camping, wood working, and natural history and reading, especially about Abraham Lincoln. Dr. Simonton married Harriet Vila Dweese on October 19, 1898. They had three daughters, all graduated from college, and two sons that became doctors. Son Richard practiced in Boise until his death and son Kinsey practiced at the Mayo Clinic and was a full professor at Minnesota Medical School.

DR. WALTER EDWARD ANDERSON

Dr. Anderson was born September 13, 1923, Scottsbluff, Nebraska. His father was a salesman. He went through grade school and high school in Scottsbluff, graduating from Chadron High. He attended Doane College, 1941-44 and received his B.A. degree. From 1944-48 he went to Northwestern Medical School, and got both B.M. and M.D. degrees. He had a rotating internship at St. Joseph's Hospital, Chicago, 1948-49, and a general practice residency at St. Joseph's Hospital, Alton, Illinois, 1949-50.

He moved to Gooding in 1950 to start his private practice. From 1955-57 he was on active duty with the U.S. Naval Medical Reserve, and returned to Gooding. For eleven years he was consultant for Idaho State T.B. Hospital, Gooding, and was on the staff at Gooding Memorial Hospital. He belonged to South Central Medical Society, and Idaho State Medical Society.

The Andersons have three sons and two daughters.

LINCOLN COUNTY

In 1882, when the Union Pacific Railroad set up a construction camp at the junction of the main line with the Ketchum branch, it was first called Naples, and later Shoshone. It quickly became a stopping place for miners and others on their way to Bellevue, Hailey, and Ketchum. It grew as a trading post for the settlements along the Snake River.

Sheepmen and farmers began marking off their ranches by planting Lombardy poplars in 1883-84, and it soon became one of the largest sheep areas in Idaho. Lincoln County has a moderate temperature, but occasionally high winds blow across the plains.

DR. CHARLES F. ZELLER

Dr. Charles F. Zeller was a leading physician of Shoshone. Handicapped by the lack of capital with which to pursue his studies, Dr. Zeller worked his way through college, and stood as an example of industry and determination. He was born at Waterville, Kansas, November 17, 1880, one of eleven children of Henry and Julia (Rainbow) Zeller. His father, a native of Germany, came to the United States as a boy, and for many years was engaged in the cattle business. He was a pioneer settler of Kansas.

Charles was the youngest of the children, and his early education was in the public and high schools at Waterville. As a lad he earned his first money working on a transfer wagon, and subsequently secured employment as a farm hand. Eventually he accumulated money enough to enter the medical department of the University of Kansas at Lawrence, where he was graduated in 1903. For one year he served as house surgeon in the University Hospital, then went to Old Mexico as surgeon for the M. C. M. & O. railway. He remained in the employ of that company until 1908, and then moved to Shoshone. Here he opened offices and his practice grew, until he became the leading physician and surgeon in Shoshone.

He was a Republican, and took an active interest in public matters. He became county physician in 1909; belonged to the Lincoln County Board of Health, of which he was secretary. He also was coroner. An outdoorsman, he was fond of hunting and fishing, and took great interest in baseball and football games. Theatricals also claimed a part of his time. He built a beautiful home in Shoshone and invested heavily in real estate.

In October, 1906 Dr. Zeller was married at El Paso, Texas, to Anna T. Bohon, Kansas City, Missouri. They had two children, Winifred G. and Charles W. Dr. Zeller was a member of the Odd Fellows, Knights of Pythias, of which he was chancellor commander, and the Modern Woodmen of America.

DR. WILLIAM H. BAUGH

Dr. Baugh was a well-known physician and druggist at Shoshone, with a wide acquaintance throughout southern Idaho. A native of Missouri, he was born in Booneville, July 28, 1864, and was of German lineage. His grandfather moved from the east to Indiana, and there the doctor's father, Henry Clay Baugh, was born and reared. In 1860 he moved to Missouri and married Elizabeth Steger, of that state. He had previously crossed the plains to California, where he had engaged in mining with fair success. After his return to Missouri he entered stock raising until 1874, when he died of pneumonia. His wife passed away in 1880. They were both members of the Methodist Church.

Dr. Baugh, the eldest of six children, spent his youth in Missouri and acquired his medical education at the Medical College at St. Louis, where he graduated in 1891. He practiced there for two years, then came west to Mountain Home where he formed a partnership with Dr. Smith.

After two years in Shoshone, Dr. Baugh established the first drug store of twenty by ninety feet, which he stocked with drugs, paints, oils, jewelry, stationery, cigars and tobacco. He was also the local physician and surgeon for the Short Line Railroad Company, and was a member of the State Medical Association. In addition to his other business interests, he engaged in sheep-raising, which was then a very important industry in Idaho.

On July 31, 1896, Dr. Baugh married Rose Burke, of Watertown, New York. Dr. Baugh was a prominent Mason, belonging to the Blue Lodge, chapter, commandery and the Mystic Shrine. He was an energetic businessman of marked ability, a progressive citizen and justly popular in his wide circle of acquaintances.

DR. ROYAL GLEN NEHER

Dr. Neher was born April 7, 1920 in Kingsley, Iowa. His father was a farmer and minister. The doctor grew up on a dairy farm, and ran a retail milk route through high school and college. He graduated in 1941 with an A.B. degree from Manchester College, Indiana. In 1944 he received his M.D. degree from Indiana University School of Medicine.

The doctor interned at Lutheran Hospital, Fort Wayne, Indiana 1944–45. He interned in Orthopedic Surgery 1945–46 at Nicholas General Hospital, Louisville, Kentucky, and General Hospital, Manilla, Philippines. In 1946 he was director of Public Health, Chinhae Province, Korea (98th Military Government Group) and was discharged as a captain.

He moved to Shoshone in 1947. In 1949 during a terrible blizzard it became necessary for a bulldozer to tow him five miles to a home delivery. He was snowbound for one month during the blizzard. One morning he left home at five o'clock in the blizzard, and got five miles out of town when he knew he must turn back. He reached home at noon. He also made house calls in a ski-equipped plane.

He was on the staff at St. Benedict's Hospital, Jerome, and was chief of staff in 1953 and 1963. He was also on the staff at Gooding Memorial Hospital. In 1963 he was secretary-treasurer of South Central Idaho Medical Society.

The Nehers had two daughters and two sons.

MINIDOKA COUNTY

In 1810, John Jacob Astor hired Wilson Price Hunt to command an expedition of fifty-six men over much of that part of Idaho which would become the Oregon Trail. Fur trading in the region began with the Northwest Fur Company arrival. A railroad siding built in 1884 became the first permanent settlement. When irrigation water was brought to the land in the early 1900s, thousands of acres were cultivated and crops grew abundantly, making Minidoka one of Idaho's most prosperous counties.

DR. OTTO ALBERT MOELLMER

The son of a Lutheran minister, Dr. Moellmer was born in Hilbert, Wisconsin on July 10, 1905. At the age of twenty-nine, he set up general practice in Rupert. He attended a parochial school in Ludell, Kansas and high school in Brighton, Colorado. A resourceful youth, he worked as a shoeshine boy and a drug store soda jerk in Brighton, as well as a "News Butch" on a narrow gauge railway between Salida and Ouray, Colorado.

By 1930 he had received a B.S. and pharmaceutical chemist degrees from the University of Colorado and later was granted an M.D.

His internship and surgical residence took him to Salt Lake City's L.D.S. Hospital until 1936. Rupert became his home. He rode horseback to see a typhoid patient each day and the roads were blocked by snow, during the winter of 1936–37. Once he rode in a slow plow to a maternity patient who was snowed in, then hung on the back of the plow on the return trip with the patient riding inside the cab. During the winter of 1947–48, the sheriff took the prisoners out of the jail to shovel a path for him into a patient's home after the snow plow had gone as far as it could. One early hospital experience he recalled was an event at the hospital in Rupert, owned and operated by Mrs. Minnie Rasmasson. Every now and then she would get so fed up with the long hours and decide to go to bed. She would discharge all the patients, calling the doctors to say she was sending them home, then she would lock the doors of the hospital. And that was that! No more patients were admitted until she got good and ready.

He was chief of staff at Minidoka County Hospital 1950 and at Minidoka Memorial Hospital 1951, and president of the Idaho Academy of General Practice 1951-52.

DR. WILBERT LOU JAMES

Dr. James was born in Denver, Colorado, July 3, 1918. He was raised in the State Children's Home at Cheyenne, Wyoming. When seven he decided to become a doctor, and worked at anything and everything to accomplish this. The doctor took education along with pre-med, and taught in Lovell, Wyoming prior to entering medical school.

He took pre-med at University of Wyoming, Laramie, Wyoming 1936-40. In 1944 he graduated from the University of Rochester Medical School with M.D. degree.

In July 1945, he finished his internship at the Methodist Hospital, Madison, Wisconsin. He had a surgical residency at Methodist Hospital 1946; an Anatomy & Physiology Fellowship at the University of Rochester 1947-48; a surgical residency in Genesee Hospital 1948-50. He spent twenty-three months in the Army Medical Corps serving at Percy Jones General Hospital, Battle Creek, Michigan, and in Germany.

He started practicing in Midwest, Wyoming, 1950-51; Riverton, Wyoming, 1951-55; Casper, Wyoming, 1955-56. In July 1957 he settled in Rupert, Idaho. He was chief of surgery, Rupert, in 1961. He and his wife have two boys.

DR. THURMAN A. HUNT

Dr. Hunt was born in Stillwater, Oklahoma on June 25, 1919 and lived in Oklahoma until his high school years when the family moved to Texas. He received a B.A. degree from the University of Texas and a medical degree from Southwestern Medical School in Dallas in 1948. He was a member of Phi Beta Pi Fraternity. His internship was at Kansas City General Hospital from 1948-49.

Dr. Hunt then returned to practice medicine for ten years in Memphis, Texas before spending one year in Columbia Falls, Montana and finally settling in Rupert, Idaho. He was a member of the staff at Odom Hospital in Memphis, Texas; Kalispell General Hospital, Kalispell, Montana; and Rupert Memorial Hospital in Rupert, Idaho. He was also a member of the Texas, Montana, and Idaho State Society A.A.G.P.

JEROME COUNTY

First developed as cattle country because of the mild winters for grazing herds, land became the big ticket item after the North Side Irrigation District was completed in 1909. Farming added to the cattle income. The town of Jerome, named for the son of an early-day land developer, became the county seat in 1919. The county was sliced from the old Alturas and the newer Lincoln counties. A point of breath-taking beauty is hidden by the deep walls of Snake River Canyon at Blue Lakes where three small lakes resemble sparkling sapphires. There is no visible inlet nor outlet. Many beautiful waterfalls dot the county.

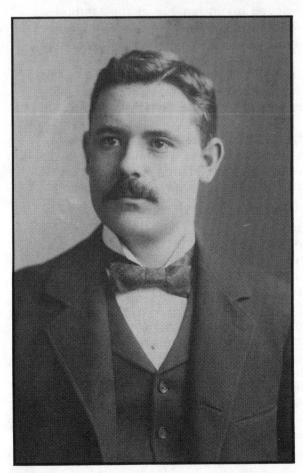

Dr. Edward Douglas Piper practiced medicine in Jerome from 1908 until 1923. As one of the early arrivals in the irrigated area of Idaho, he wisely made land purchases in the area.

DR. MAURICE E. SCHEEL

Delivering a baby at a trading post in the Yukon Territory, along the Alaskan Highway, was probably not what Dr. Scheel anticipated when he entered the medical profession. Born on March 26, 1915, in Hanover, Wisconsin, the family moved to Medford when he was ten years old. He attended Northwest Nazarene College in Nampa from 1934-38 and summer sessions at the University of Washington in 1938, and Oregon State at Corvallis in 1943 and 1945. After graduation, he taught high school for six years before entering medical school.

Dr. Scheel earned his medical degree from Creighton Medical School which he attended from 1945-49. While at Creighton he became a member of Phi Chi Fraternity. Dr. Scheel completed a one year residency at St. Joseph Hospital in Omaha before beginning his general practice in Wendell, Idaho, in 1950.

During his career, Dr. Scheel served in the positions of president and secretary at both St. Benedict Hospital in Jerome and Gooding Memorial Hospital in Gooding. He was medical director at Shadle Sanitarium and Magic Valley Manor both in Wendell. Dr. Scheel was the father of a son and two daughters.

TWIN FALLS COUNTY

Twin Falls County began in 1863, when the first Halliday stage, enroute from Utah to Boise and Walla Walla, made a stop at Rockcreek, the first building in the area, which became a home station. A store was built two years later at the Stricker ranch site. Cattle and sheep raising replaced the flurry of gold mining along the Snake River from 1865–75.

Completely financed and developed by private capital, the Twin Falls Southside Project became the first large irrigation development in the country. Twin Falls city, now a modern and attractive center, was designated county seat in 1904. The county has many attractions including Shoshone, Pillar, upper and lower Salmon and Twin Falls, a 374 feet suspension bridge, Magic Hot Springs and Balanced Rock at Castleford.

DR. CHARLES D. COLLINS

The son of a mechanic, Dr. Collins was born July 16, 1924 and also had one brother who became a doctor. He was raised in South Dakota and received his undergraduate education there. He moved on to the University of Illinois where he received his medical degree. His internship was at the St. Luke's Hospital in Denver, and residency in anesthesiology at the University of Minnesota. He briefly practiced in Sioux Falls, South Dakota before locating to Twin Falls as a staff member at Magic Valley Memorial Hospital. He served as a lieutenant in the Navy and belongs to several professional organizations and societies. He has a son and two daughters.

DR. HARWOOD L. STOWE

Dr. Stowe served as a major in the China-Burma-India area on the hospital staff accompanying Merrill's Marauders in the taking of Myitekina, Burma. He was decorated with the Bronze Star. At one point, he volunteered to perform emergency surgery on the commanding general at the Japanese front in south China. Later, he was decorated by the 47th Chinese Army Commander. Dr. Stowe was also accomplished in the athletic world as the Indoor Big Ten Track Champion of 1926 at the University of Wisconsin where he received his undergraduate and medical degrees. After graduation, he took an active part in professional organizations and served as a member of the Idaho Medical Examining Board and the Idaho State Medical Association.

He was born in Wisconsin in February of 1906. His family came west and he attended high school in Kimberly, Idaho, where he returned for the first six months of his medical career. He moved to Twin Falls in 1935 to practice. His father was a pharmacist and an uncle and a cousin became doctors. He and Mrs. Stowe became parents of two sons and one daughter.

DR. GLENN Q. VOYLES, F.A.C.P.

An active member in a variety of medical associations, Dr. Voyles' career in Twin Falls included serving as the chief of staff at the hospital. He attended Nebraska Medical School from 1937–41. During his residency he was assistant in medicine at the Indiana University School of Medicine, 1945–48. He attended Creighton University, 1934–36 and completed his undergraduate work at the University of Chicago in 1937. He came to Twin Falls in 1948. His wife was active in the Medical Auxiliary and Hospital Guild Music Club while raising a family of three boys and one daughter.

DR. ALFRED A. NEWBERRY

Dr. Alfred A. Newberry, who engaged in the practice of medicine and surgery at Filer, was born near Lockport, Illinois October 22, 1881. He was a son of Stephen and Lucille (Bolin) Newberry. His boyhood days were spent in Cook County, Illinois, where he pursued his education. In 1898, when he was about seventeen, he moved to Denver, Colorado, and there, having determined upon medicine as a life work he became a student at Denver Gross Medical College.

He was graduated in the fall of 1907, and moved to Filer, which was then a tiny hamlet in the midst of a wild country covered with sagebrush. He built one of the first residences in the town, having his office in his home for a time. He was the first physician in that locality, and he saw the town grow from a small village to a thriving place of twelve hundred population. Reading and study kept him in touch with the researches of the medical fraternity.

In 1909, Dr. Newberry was married to Frieda Berger, a native of Washington, and they had one child, Wilmer. Dr. Newberry was a Republican. He belonged to the Independent Order of Odd Fellows and the Masons.

DR. HENRY W. CLOUCHEK

Dr. Henry Walker Clouchek was born in Michigan City, April 7, 1877, and died at Twin Falls, Idaho, February 19, 1934.

He graduated from schools of the medical department of the University of Michigan. He served as intern in the University Hospital one year and as house physician the next. He practiced in Oregon about one year waiting for the opening of the Twin Falls Tracts.

He married Emma Olds June 14, 1904. They moved to Twin Falls that November. He served as physician for Cerey Construction Company, throughout the building period. He was railroad physician for the Union Pacific for several years, during which time he followed private practice, and for a time owned a private hospital on Fourth Avenue East.

He was medical examiner during World War I and served on the State Medical Examining Board as well as being president of South Side Medical Association. Both the Cloucheks were heavily involved in community betterment.

DR. VERN H. ANDERSON

Dr. Anderson was born in Toole, Utah, August 21, 1909. His twin brother was a doctor in Girardville, Pennsylvania. He grew up in Magna, Utah, the second of seven children. In 1931 he received an A.B. degree from the University of Utah, and an M.D. in 1934 from Washington University. He interned at Salt Lake General Hospital, 1934–35.

For two years after his internship he was with the Civilian Conservation Corp, first lieutenant U.S. Army Reserve. He moved to Buhl in 1938 to start private practice. From 1942–46 he was on active duty with the U.S. Navy Transport Service as lieutenant commander.

He belonged to the South Central and Idaho State Medical societies.

The Andersons have one daughter and two sons.

DR. IVAN A. ANDERSON

Dr. Anderson was born in Wenatchee, Washington, May 10, 1903, son of an accountant. Dr. Anderson grew up in Mountain Home, Idaho, and was graduated from high school there. He took agriculture at the University of Idaho, 1922–26, and was instructor of bacteriology at the university, 1926–28, receiving his M.S. in bacteriology in 1928. From 1928–30 he was bacteriologist and serologist at Methodist Hospital.

He took pre-med and two years medicine at University of Utah. From 1934–37 he was with the U.S. Public Health Service, Minneapolis. He received his M.D. from University of Louisville Medical School, and interned at the Emmanuel Hospital, Portland, Oregon.

He moved to Filer in 1940 and started his private practice. He was on the staff of Twin Falls and Magic Valley Memorial hospitals. Dr. Anderson belonged to South Central Medical Society.

He married Marguerite Felthouse of New Plymouth in 1928. They had two sons.

DR. FEN HEBER COVINGTON

On January 13, 1913, in Orderville, Utah, Fen Heber Covington was born. His father was a rancher and carpenter.

He went through high school in Orderville, and went to Dixie Junior College, St. George, Utah, for two years on a scholarship. For pre-med he went to the University of Utah and Utah State University. For his M.D. he attended University of Utah Medical School and New York University. He took graduate work at the university for one year. In 1939–40 he interned at Murray Hospital, Butte, Montana. From 1941–45 he was with the U.S. Army.

He practiced in Utah and California before moving to Twin Falls in 1960, where he specialized in obstetrics and gynecology.

Dr. Covington was on the staff at Magic Valley Memorial Hospital, Twin Falls. He belonged to South Central, Idaho State, and American Medical associations.

The Covingtons have three children, two daughters and a son.

DR. GEORGE WILLIAM WARNER

George Warner was born February 4, 1920, in Gresham, Nebraska. His father was a dentist. The doctor had his early education in Gresham schools, and was active in sports, band, choir, and speech. George attended the first national Scouting Jamboree. He played in dance bands in high school and college.

From 1937–41 he attended Doane College, Crete, Nebraska, and was graduated with a B.S. degree. He attended the University of Nebraska School of Medicine, 1941–44, and received his M.D. degree.

Dr. Warner interned at Colorado General Hospital, Denver, 1944–45. From 1947–51 he had a surgical residency at the University of Colorado Medical Center, Denver. He moved to Twin Falls in 1951.

He was on the consulting staff at Twin Falls Clinic, Magic Valley Memorial Hospital, Cassia Memorial Hospital at Burley, Minidoka County Hospital, Rupert, St. Benedicts Hospital, Jerome, and Gooding Memorial Hospital. He was president of the South Central Idaho Medical Society.

He was a captain in the Marine Corps from 1945–47. The Warners had two girls and three boys.

DR. WILLIAM H. WOODSON

Dr. Woodson was born March 7, 1918 in Virginia. Prior to entering medical school he attended schools in New York, Maryland, and Virginia. He received a B.S. degree in chemistry from Roanoke College, Salem, Virginia in June 1939. From 1939–43 he attended Medical College of Virginia at Richmond. He interned at Virginia Mason Hospital and Clinic, Seattle, Washington, orthopedic residence at Medical College of Virginia, Crippled Children's Hospital, Richmond, and the McGuire V.A. Hospital, Richmond.

He was in the U.S. Army, overseas 1944–46, and was discharged with rank of major. He practiced in Washington, D.C. one and a half years before moving to Twin Falls in 1951.

He and Mrs. Woodson had three boys.

DR. ALBERT F. McCLUSKY

Dr. Albert F. McClusky was born near Oil City, Pennsylvania, July 16, 1876. He began practice in Buhl in 1906.

Dr. McClusky's early education was in the public schools

of his native state, and as a lad of twelve displayed his industry by securing employment at the carpenter trade. He was employed at fifty cents per day at the start, but eventually became a master carpenter, thus earning enough money to carry him through college. He received no outside assistance.

After completing preparatory education and taking a high school course, he took a course in the State Normal School at the age of twenty-four. He went to Michigan for three years during which he attended the University of Michigan at Ann Arbor. Later he moved to Boulder, Colorado. He went to a point known as Santa, in the lumber district, built and conducted a hospital for one year. He returned to Michigan to take a postgraduate course of one year.

In May 1908, he moved to Buhl to open his practice. He belonged to the Idaho State, Twin Falls County, and the American Medical associations. He was a member of the Commercial Club, and president of the first permanent organization. He was a Presbyterian and a Republican. He enjoyed outdoor sports, especially baseball, theatricals, lectures, music, and local lyceum attractions.

On December 23, 1903, Dr. McClusky was married at Ann Arbor, to Louise C. Allmendinger, daughter of Mr. and Mrs. D. F. Allmendinger.

DR. DUNCAN L. ALEXANDER

Dr. Alexander's father, Joseph C. Alexander, was born in Scotland and went to Canada as a young man. There he met and married Isabelle Campbell, who was also a native of Scotland. It was in about 1884 that they crossed to the United States and located in Michigan. He was engaged in the real estate and investment business. He and his wife had five children, Dr. Alexander being the eldest.

He was born in Canada, September 15, 1881, and when three years of age crossed the border into the United States, with his parents who settled in Michigan. His early education was obtained in the public schools of Ontario, Canada, to which he returned for that purpose. He later completed a high school course at Lexington, Michigan. He became a student in the University of Michigan, where he was graduated from the medical department in 1903, with an M.D. degree. After leaving the university he served some time as an intern in the University Hospital at Ann Arbor. He followed that practical experience with two years of independent and active practice in Michigan.

Deciding that the west offered better possibilities in his profession, he located at Tonopah, Nevada and remained there until his move to Twin Falls in 1910. Dr. Alexander was a member and secretary of the Twin Falls Medical Society, the Idaho State Medical Society, and the American Medical Association. He served by appointment as city health officer at Twin Falls.

Fraternally he associated with the Masons, Elks, Odd Fellows, the Knights of Pythias, and the Twin Falls Commercial Club. Dr. Alexander was a Presbyterian. His diversions were found chiefly in hunting and fishing, although in his college days he played baseball and football.

Dr. Alexander saw a bright future for Idaho, not alone as a mining state, but as an agricultural, fruit and lumbering area.

DR. DAN P. ALBEE

Dr. Dan P. Albee, a rancher living on Rock Creek, in Twin Falls County, was born in Accate, California in January, 1856. He was graduated from the medical department of Columbia University, New York in 1888. He started practice in California, but in 1891 moved to Oxford, Idaho, and practiced there until 1894. He then moved to Oakley, Idaho, and followed his profession until 1905. When he moved to Rock Creek, he continued his practice of surgery and medicine in Buhl.

DR. V. ELLIS KNIGHT

Dr. Knight was born February 19, 1916, in Gallatin, Missouri. His mother died when he was fifteen, and he kept house for his father until he entered the university. He made his own way financially through undergraduate school at the University of Missouri from 1935-39.

He enlisted in Army Medical Corps, January 1941, and married Mary (Brown) Knight in June 1942. [She was a graduate Home Economist from Oregon State College. She was president of Idaho State Medical Auxiliary 1961-62, and was actively interested in securing this history on

Idaho medicine.] They had a daughter, Tanis Lee, and a son, Ellis Mc Henry.

He was a lab technician in the United States Army for five years. In 1946 he received his A.B. degree from the University of Missouri Medical School and in 1948 his B.S. in medicine. In 1950 he received his M.D. degree from the University of Maryland Medical School. He was a member of Phi Beta Pi medical fraternity. He interned at Good Samaritan Hospital, Portland, Oregon 1950-51.

He moved to Kimberly, Idaho in 1951. He was chief of the hospital medical division in 1959. In 1960-61 he was a delegate to the Idaho Medical Association from South Central.

DR. MAX WENDELL CARVER

After retiring from the military where he served as a commanding officer, Dr. Carver entered private practice in Filer, Idaho, in 1947. He continued in general practice with an associate, Dr. Anderson, until 1955. He took a surgical residency at U.C.L.A. in Los Angles, 1956-57. He returned to Twin Falls in 1957 to enter his own general practice.

Previously his education was received at Weber College from 1929-31 and continued at the University of Utah from 1931-36. He also attended the two year medical school at the University of Utah and completed his medical education at the University of Louisville School of Medicine from 1937-39. His internship was served at Dee Memorial Hospital in Ogden, Utah.

The son of an attorney, born June 9, 1911, Dr. Carver grew up in Utah and also lived in California and Nevada. In the early years after leaving the military, he did many home deliveries, sometimes trekking across the snow fields to reach a patient's home. He was a pioneer in the use of intravenous solutions of sulfamilanides for pneumonia and had to mix his own solutions. As a result, he was witness to many strange reactions to the new treatment.

Dr. Carver was active in his professional organizations and served two terms as secretary of the South Central Idaho Medical Society as well as a term as chief of staff at Magic Valley Memorial Hospital in 1962. His two daughters entered the medical field, one as his office secretary and the other as a nurse. The Carvers also had two sons.

DR. THOMAS M. BRIDGES

Dr. Thomas M. Bridges was one of the prominent physicians and surgeons in Twin Falls, where he passed away in July 1915, at the age of fifty-seven. He was born in Kentucky in July, 1857, a son of Benjamin and Edna (Miller) Bridges.

Dr. Bridges was reared and educated in Kentucky, pursuing his studies largely under the direction of private tutors. He completed his studies at the University of Louisville, Kentucky, where he was a medical student. He located his practice in Evansville, Indiana, where he remained for a time, after which he entered the U.S. Marine Corps for several years. He then went to Blackburn, Missouri, to practice medicine and surgery until 1894.

He came to the northwest to enter the government Indian service, acting as physician to the Indians of South Dakota, for three years. He was next transferred to the Fort Hall agency, near Pocatello, where he continued for ten years. He then moved to Idaho Falls, where he practiced until his death.

In October, 1885, Dr. Bridges was married to Margaret Green, daughter of Alexander and Elizabeth (Owen) Green.

Dr. Bridges was a member of the Masonic Lodge, the Elks, and his religious faith was Presbyterian. He belonged to the Bonneville County, Idaho State, and the American Medical associations.

DR. GEORGE EMERSON BROWN

The son of a physician, Dr. Brown also had a brother who became a physician. He was born in Miles City, Montana in March of 1913 and lived there until the age of ten, when his father became a member of the Mayo Clinic staff. His began his college education at Carlton College in 1931 but transferred to Michigan to complete his B.A. and on to the Michigan Medical School from 1934–38. His internship was completed at Dansville, Pennsylvania 1938–39. His general practice began in October 1940 and continued until the end of 1943 when he joined the Army as a major in the Army Medical Corps.

He resumed his education in 1946 and received his M.S. degree at Minnesota in 1948. He became an assistant on the Mayo staff in 1947 and completed his training as an internist in 1948. After relocating to Twin Falls, Dr. Brown practiced internal medicine 1948–57. He then became director of medical education at Christ Hospital and an assistant professor of medicine at the University of Cincinnati 1957–60. He returned to Twin Falls in 1960 to practice internal medicine with a major interest in cardiology.

During his early practice, Dr. Brown had to battle the elements as had many in practice before World War II when hospitals were not readily available to all people. He experienced being snowbound when called out to deliver babies for the princely sum of fifteen dollars and was called upon to assist with home surgeries.

An active staff member of the Magic Valley Memorial Hospital, Dr. Brown served on the Executive Committee and as the service chief. He was also the secretary of the South Central Medical Society, president of the Idaho Heart Association, and a charter president of the Idaho Society of Internal Medicine.

Dr. and Mrs. Brown had three sons and two daughters.

DR. GEORGE C. HALLEY

Born in Quincy, Illinois in October 1897, Dr. Halley's father farmed three miles west of Twin Falls. He attended Curry Public Schools and completed his pre-med education at University of Virginia. At the University of Maryland he obtained a M.D. in 1922 and later returned to Johns Hopkins University in 1932 to obtain his M.A. in public health. He also attended the Graduate Medical Field Service School for Regular Army and National Guard Officers in 1928. His student internship was served at the City Hospital in Baltimore, and he did a rotating internship at the University of Maryland, Baltimore in 1922–23 before entering practice in Kimberly, Idaho in 1923.

In 1926 he relocated to Twin Falls where he practiced with the exception of the period he spent as a deputy health officer in Easton, Maryland. Traveling by sled, horse and buggy was not uncommon. He assisted with home surgeries, one of which was on the wife of a doctor in Burley. He delivered babies for about fifteen years. He also did extractions of teeth. He delivered three sets of twins in one month, and two of the mothers were first cousins.

During his service as the health officer of Twin Falls County during the meningitis epidemic, the local physician and nurse died. In the winter of 1935 there were more cases of smallpox reported in the area than in the entire states of Pennsylvania and New York for one year.

Dr. Brown participated in local medical societies and served as the secretary of the South Central Medical Society. He also served as the president of the Idaho State Medical Association and was a member of the Idaho State Board of Medical Examiners for six years from 1941-47. He was president and secretary of staff at the old Twin Falls County General Hospital. For sixteen years he served as a member of the Medical Detachment of Idaho National Guard and reached the rank of major and was the commanding officer. He was in the S.A.T.C. at the University of Maryland in 1918. He had two sons, William and George.

DR. WILLARD H. CLARK

At the age of five, Dr. Clark moved to China from his home in Saskatchewan, Canada, where he was born in November, 1919. In 1938 he returned to the United States to attend the Emmanuel Missionary College until 1940. He then went the Pacific Union College to finish his B.S. His internship and residency were served at the Loma Linda Sanitarium and Hospital 1947-49 when he relocated to Pettsboro, North Carolina for the years 1949-51. He became a staff member of the Riverside Community Hospital in Riverside, California from 1951-54 and in Carona, California from 1951-55.

He served for two years in the military as the Medical Officer in Charge in U.S. Public Health in Claremore, Oklahoma from 1955-57 at a seventy-bed Indian hospital. In 1957 he relocated to Twin Falls to open a practice.

Dr. Clark's father was a minister, but he and his brother, Richard, became doctors. He and his wife, an R.N., had two sons.

DR. HELMUTH FRIEDRICH FISHER

Born in Germany on September 3, 1919, Dr. Fisher's family moved to Italy when he was six. He lived in several Mediterranean and European countries before coming to the United States in 1948 to continue his education, while his family remained in Europe. He attended La Sierra, Pacific Union and San Diego colleges and Loma Linda University. His internship was at the Glendale Sanitarium and Hospital and his rotating residency was at the Contra Costa County Hospital in Martinez, California. He had a fellowship in neurosurgery for one year in Columbus, Ohio.

He was a talented artist and spent one year doing medical art work before entering the School of Medicine at Loma Linda. Many of his drawings appear in medical manuals used today.

Dr. Fisher practiced medicine in Mackay, Idaho, from 1952-53 and in St. Anthony, 1953-56. In Twin Falls he practiced from 1956-62 when he interrupted his practice to complete a residency in anesthesiology. He has now limited his practice to anesthesiology.

He married the former Muriel Spear and they have five sons.

DR. BERNARD L. KREICKAM

Dr. Kreickam was born in Princeton, Wisconsin, March 11, 1916. His father was a teacher and two sisters were nurses.

The doctor was graduated from West High School at Minneapolis in 1932. From 1932-25 he took pre-med at College of St. Thomas, St. Paul, Minnesota. He received an M.S. in anatomy from the University of Minnesota. He was graduated from the University of Minnesota in 1941 with his M.D. degree. In 1948 he received the M.S. degree in internal medicine from the University of Minnesota.

Dr. Kreickam started practicing in Twin Falls January 1949. He was on the consultant staff at Idaho State Tuberculosis, St. Benedict's in Jerome, Magic Valley Memorial, and Cassia Memorial hospitals.

From 1942-46 he was flight surgeon in the 13th Air Force. In 1944-45 he was in the South Pacific. He received the Bronze Star, and was a captain.

The Kreickams have six daughters and two sons.

DR. BEN E. KATZ

Dr. Katz was born in Osage, Iowa, September 11, 1921. He went through high school in Osage. In 1943 he got his B.A. from the University of Iowa and received his M.D.

degree from the University of Iowa College of Medicine in 1946. He took a postgraduate course at the New York University Medical School, 1949–50.

From 1946–47 he interned at Salt Lake County General Hospital; pediatric intern at University of Minnesota, 1950; pediatric fellowship at Minnesota, 1951–52.

He moved to Twin Falls in 1952. He was on the staffs at Magic Valley Memorial in Twin Falls, St. Benedict's, Jerome, and Cottage Hospital, Burley. He belonged to the American, Intermountain, and Idaho Pediatric societies, Idaho Heart Association, American Board of Pediatrics, South Central Medical Society, and American Medical Association. He was a consultant to the Idaho State Tuberculosis Hospital and Idaho Crippled Childrens Service, and director of Twin Falls Cerebral Palsy School.

The doctor was a medical officer with Des. Division 92, San Diego, and Mare Island Naval Hospital.

The Katzes had two daughters and three sons.

DR. CHARLES W. CULLINGS

Charles Cullings was born December 27, 1918, Derry, Pennsylvania. His uncle and a cousin were physicians.

For four and a half years he was an engineering officer as lieutenant commander. From 1941–46 he was on active duty in U. S. Navy, and spent three and a half years in the South Pacific. In 1938–40 he attended the U.S. Naval Academy, Annapolis; West Virginia Wesleyan College, Buckhannen, West Virginia, 1936–38; University of Pittsburgh, 1946–50, where he received his M.D. He interned at Uniontown Hospital, Pennsylvania, 1950–51.

From 1951–59 and again in 1960–61 he practiced in Waynesburg, Pennsylvania. In 1959–60 he practiced in Filer, Idaho, and moved to Buhl in 1961. He was on the staff at Magic Valley Memorial Hospital, Twin Falls.

Dr. Cullings and his wife, Muriel, have two daughters and a son.

DR. DEAN H. AFFLECK

Dr. Affleck was born in Grand Rapids, Michigan, August 15, 1905. His father was in the logging business, and he spent his early life and schooling in Grand Rapids.

He attended the University of Minnesota and received a bachelor of architectural engineering in 1928, bachelor of medicine in 1932, and doctor of medicine in 1933. Dr. Affleck interned at the University of Minnesota, and Alameda County Hospital, California. At Tulane Medical School he had a fellowship in OB/GYN, and at Johns Hopkins in surgical pathology.

Dr. Affleck moved to Twin Falls in 1937. He belonged to American College of Surgeons. He was a major in the Medical Corps, for four years during WWII, and was chief of general surgery at the 307th General Hospital.

The Afflecks had one daughter and one son.

DR. GEORGE T. DAVIS

George Davis was born September 15, 1913, Roanoke, Virginia. Before entering medical school he was a chemist for the Eastman Corporation in Tennessee.

He received an A.B. degree from Asbury College, in 1936, and an M.D. in 1943 from University of Tennessee Medical School. He interned at Baptist Hospital and for three years had a residency at John Gactin Hospital, both in Memphis.

Dr. Davis moved to Twin Falls in 1950. He was on the executive staff at Magic Valley Memorial Hospital, and belonged to American Board of Urology; had a fellowship in American College of Surgeons. From 1943–46 he was a captain in the U.S. Army.

The Davis family have three daughters and two sons.

DR. F. WAYNE SCHOW

Dr. Schow was born in Lehi, Utah, May 4, 1911. His father was a field man for Amalgamated Sugar Company. His brother, Douglas Schow, was a doctor in Twin Falls.

Wayne was raised in Rupert and worked as janitor in the local hospital while attending high school. He attended Idaho State College 1930–32; University of Idaho 1932–33; University of Nebraska, 1933–37, where he received his medical degree. He interned at L.D.S. Hospital where he also took his residency. Dr. Schow first practiced in Hailey and spent five years in the Army as major and wing surgeon. In 1946 he moved to Twin Falls.

He was president and secretary of the Magic Valley Memorial Hospital staff, and a member of the executive staff. He was a councilor of Idaho State Medical Association.

The Schows had two children, a son and a daughter.

DR. PAUL B. HEUSTON

From his birth on January 29, 1921, Dr. Heuston's life was spent in the Tacoma area until he began attending Jefferson Medical College in Philadelphia in 1943 after graduating from the College of Puget Sound. As a young man, he was an active Boy Scout and attained the rank of Eagle Scout and received the Bronze Palm. While attending Jefferson Medical College (1943–46), he served as vice-president of his class. He participated in the medical fraternity and was on the Dean's Committee.

Dr. Heuston served his internship at Lenox Hill Hospital from 1946–47 until he began his active duty in the Navy. The majority of his active duty was spent aboard the USS Consolation Hospital Ship as a radiologist with the rank of lieutenant j.g. until 1949. After the Navy, he returned to Lenox Hill Hospital to complete his residency in radiology from 1949–51 and received an appointment as adjunct radiologist to the staff of Lenox Hill until March 1952.

He moved to Twin Falls, Idaho, to serve on the staff at Magic Valley Memorial Hospital from 1952 to 1953. He began his private practice in therapeutic and diagnostic X-ray, and became radiologist for the Twin Falls Clinic, St. Benedict's, Cassia Memorial, Gooding County Memorial, Sun Valley, Minidoka County hospitals and consultant radiologist for the Idaho State Tuberculosis Hospital.

He served as secretary-treasurer and president for the South Central Idaho Medical Society, councilor for the Idaho State Medical Association, and chairman of the Public Health Advisory Committee.

Dr. Heuston, his wife Ann, a former school teacher, and their three daughters enjoy spending time at the family's Sun Valley cabin and frequent outings to explore old mines and surrounding primitive areas.

DR. HARVARD C. LUKE

A Twin Falls physician since 1951, Dr. Luke was a native of Utah, born December 26, 1912. His father was a science professor. Dr. Luke received his bachelor of science degree in 1939 from the University of Idaho but had also attended the University of Utah (1937) and Idaho State (1935). He completed his first year master program at Johns Hopkins University in 1940 and received his M.D. degree from the University of Southern California.

His internship and residency were completed in Los Angeles County from 1950-51 and he then located in Twin Falls. He served as chief of South Center District Laboratories and was an epidemiologist and parseitrologist for the State of Idaho.

He was in the Army and served as a major in the Sanitary Corps four years. He later became a professor of bacteriology at the University of North Carolina.

He and his wife had two daughters.

DR. VICTOR VIRGIL TELFORD

The son of a refrigeration worker, Dr. Telford of Twin Falls also had working experience with frigid weather. Called out on a frozen November morning to see a sick child, Dr. Telford was met at the door by a distraught mother who announced her child was a stutterer. After the surprised doctor recovered his own speech, he asked to see the child but was informed the child was sleeping and could not be disturbed. The mother paid for the doctor's visit with cold cash retrieved from the frost chest of an ice box.

DR. LYLE E. WONDERLICH

Breeding and raising registered Welsh ponies carried on the tradition of farming in Dr. Wonderlich's family. He was the father of a large family of two girls and five boys. The doctor was born on February 24, 1923 in Bloomington, Kansas. He obtained his undergraduate education at the University of Kansas. He began his medical education at Yale but finished at the University of Kansas Medical School. In addition, he was a Fellow of the American College of Anesthesia and a Diplomate of the American Board of Anesthesia. His internship was at the Salt Lake County Hospital and his residency in anesthesiology at the V.A. Hospital and University of Colorado. He spent one year in general practice in Osborne, Kansas in 1948 and then specialized in anesthesia beginning in 1949 in Concordia, Kansas. As a member of the U.S.A.F., he served as a captain in the medical corp in Biloxi, Mississippi from 1950-51 and then relocated to Twin Falls in 1954 to practice.

CASSIA COUNTY

It was the excellent grazing land that attracted cattlemen and sheepherders to Cassia County and resulted in the cattle owners establishing "Deadline Ridge" through the entire county. No sheep could pass over the line for grazing. Notorious Diamond Field Jack convinced some sheepmen they could cross the line and a man was killed. Jack was in and out of court for a long time before being convicted of murder. He was saved by reprieves and finally pardoned.

Indian fighting also took place in Cassia. The City of Rocks was the site of a massacre by Chief Pocatello, and Connor Creek is named for General Connor who won an 1864 battle with the Bannock and Shoshoni. Irrigation water made Cassia an important agricultural county.

DR. C. I. SATER

C.I. Sater went by the name of "Doc" from the time he worked in a drugstore at Weiser and became interested in acquiring the nickname officially. He was the third child born to John Henry and Emeline Norehead Sater on Mann's Creek, near Weiser, on September 13, 1882. He had five brothers and four sisters. After completing high school, he went to Barnes Medical School (now Washington University) at St. Louis, Missouri, graduating in 1909. He married Stella Landwehr on May 3, 1909, and came to Malta, Idaho. She joined him in 1910. They had five children.

As far as money was rated, he was a "poor" person, but insofar as helping others he was rich, indeed. When someone was struggling to pay what they owed him and he knew they just could not afford it, he would say, "Don't worry, I'll catch you next time." There was not a "next time" unless the former patient walked into his office and paid him. One man in Burley said, "Doc charged six dollars for delivering my brother, and when I was born several years later, his price had only risen to seven dollars." In his later years of practice the fee was twenty-five dollars no matter how far he had to travel to deliver the baby. Many couples had large families, some not paying for the delivery of any of their children. Dr. Sater never refused to go to the aid of anyone, nor did he harbor any resentment against those who had not paid.

In the early years he traveled by horse and buggy, and later was able to buy a Model T. He had a difficult time learning to drive it, and received a few kicks from the crank. He was highly intelligent and could recite many of Shakespeare's work verbatim. Mathematics came quickly to mind, while someone else was struggling to come up with the correct answer. His family said his motto was: "Burn the midnight oil."

He was interested in many things. He liked farming and raised alfalfa, had sheep, cows, pigs, turkeys and chickens. At one time he kept bees. His love of roses was well known and he did so well with them that in the early 1940s, an Idaho Falls florist beseeched him to go there and graft roses. Instead, he went to Dubois, Idaho, where he felt he could do more good as a doctor for the Civilian Conservation Corps. He wanted to share his professional knowledge and skills with anyone interested. His wife of many years was a strong support and helped him through the lean, tough years. In 1936 they moved to Albion where he was doctor for Albion State Normal and surrounding communities.

His wife died in 1940 and he in 1946. One woman said, "I was twelve years old before I could be convinced that Dr. Sater wasn't God!"

DR. JAMES RAYMOND KIRCHER

A native of Highland, Illinois, Dr. Kircher was born January 2, 1919. He moved from Illinois to Wisconsin during infancy, and from Wisconsin to Idaho in 1933. He worked two years after high school before studying at the University of Idaho from 1938 to 1941. Graduating with a bachelor of science degree, he continued on to the University of Northwestern Medical School and graduated in 1944. He interned in Cook County Hospital, Chicago, 1944-45.

He served as a medic in the U.S. Army from 1945 to 1947, attaining the rank of captain. Dr. Kircher practiced in Albion in 1947 and 1948. Burley, Idaho became his home after 1948. In 1945, he married and they had two children before she died in 1955. He married again in 1956.

Doctor Kircher was on the staff of Cottage Hospital in Burley, 1947-60; practiced at Cassia Memorial in Burley and was chief of staff 1960-61.

DR. JAMES FRANK KURFEES

Born in Louisville, Kentucky on January 22, 1931, Doctor Kurfees attended the Kentucky Military Institute for four years and Vanderbilt University for two years 1948-50. After two years at the University of Louisville, he worked as an industrial paint chemist and lab technician. His medical degree was from the University of Louisville School of Medicine in 1956. He interned at Macon Hospital, Georgia for one year followed with a general practice residency.

In July 1960 Doctor Kurfees opened practice in Albion, but closed up in October 1961 to teach full time. He spent two years in the Navy as a lieutenant, senior grade, and was a destroyer squadron doctor. He was also an active staff member of Cassia Memorial Hospital. He had three children, including twin girls.

DR. DEAN MAHONEY

Born on July 28, 1929 in Albion, Doctor Mahoney set up practice in Burley after three years in the U.S. Air Force. Before entering medical school, he taught chemistry. Southern Idaho College was his choice to get a B.S. degree in 1949. Two years later he started medical school at the University of Utah, 1951-55, and joined Phi Beta Pi fraternity. His internship was at Ancker Hospital in St. Paul, Minnesota. He continued training when in service as captain and flight surgeon in the Air Force from 1956-59.

DR. AXEL O. NIELSON

Doctor Nielson was born in Copenhagen, Denmark, October 25, 1868 and after graduating from high school there at sixteen years of age, came to the United States with his brother, Doctor Alexander Nielson who practiced at Emphraim, Utah.

He knew but a few words of the English language when he entered Brigham Young Academy at Provo, Utah, and graduated before he was twenty. He taught at Ogden, before accepting the position of principal of the Cassia State Academy. Soon, he was elected superintendent of public schools of Cassia County. The doctor carefully saved his earnings, and two years after his own arrival sent for his parents and two sisters.

In 1900 Doctor Nielson began the study of medicine at Illinois Medical College of Chicago, graduating in 1905 with an M.D. degree. He was truly a country doctor. The people in the Oakley and Burley area called him by his initials A.F.O. and he knew everyone, as he had delivered 1,358 babies.

In 1908, to further advance his surgical skills, he went to Europe for postgraduate work and spent several months in London and Vienna. He also studied in the medical centers of New York, Chicago, California, and other places. For more than two weeks each year, throughout his career, he attended clinics or medical schools in the larger centers. He practiced in Oakley until a year before his death when he moved his office to Burley.

Like all the pioneer doctors, he was like a light upon a hill. In addition to caring for the physical ills, he was the spiritual and educational advisor. He fought against the prejudices of people, and many times was called in at the last moment, when everything else had failed, and his reputation had to suffer from the superstitious dread of patients. Once he was beaten by a father because he could not cure his daughter of her illness. At any and all hours of the day or night, he was called to brave winter storms and travel roads which were difficult and dangerous. His matched team of white horses was well-known for not letting other horses pass them on the road. He had several narrow escapes, being thrown from the buggy or sleigh in which he was riding. Medical practice often meant days away from home and family in order to care for other families. Surgeries were performed in his own office or at the Fremstead Hospital in Burley.

In some cases, Doctor Nielson was forced to operate in private homes, using the dining table as operating table and cooking utensils to sterilize instruments and dressings. As many people as possible would pack into the room and even the windows were darkened by the heads of spectators. Sometimes a number of these people would fall in a faint while the operation was in progress. With no trained nurses at hand it was not unusual for one farmer to give the anesthetic and another, scrubbed up and dressed with a mother-hubbard apron, to hand him his instruments and hold retractors.

While a horse and buggy had served him well, he was the first to bring a car, a "horseless carriage," into the community and it provided merriment on the part of the townspeople. It would get stuck in the heavy mud of spring and a farmer would have to come and pull him out.

His early life as a teacher caused him to serve as chairman of the Oakley School Board. He married Ettie Hunter, who died in 1899, the mother of one son, Elmo, whose death occurred one year prior. In October 1900, the doctor married Louisa Haight and together they had six sons, all of whom became attorneys.

DR. SAMUEL PATTERSON

Doctor Patterson was born May 4, 1875 in Morengo, Iowa, and had two physician brothers, Charles and James, in Iowa. Doctor Samuel Patterson practiced in Mackay, Idaho and in Victor and Breda, Iowa.

He attended high school in Morengo, and later received his medical degree from Creighton University in Omaha, Nebraska. The Holy Cross Hospital in Salt Lake City, Utah was where he did his residency.

DR. CHARLES A. TERHUNE

After several moves during his early years, Dr. Terhune settled in Burley and operated the Cottage Hospital for twenty-five years with Drs. H.D. Dean and L. M. Kelly. He served as chief of staff and of surgery at Cottage Hospital and chief of surgery at Cassia Memorial Hospital in 1961-62. He was president of South Central and the Idaho State Medical associations.

Dr. Terhune was an Army lieutenant colonel from 1941-45 and was awarded the Bronze Star.

Dr. Terhune was born in Savannah, Missouri, and the family soon moved to Kansas City, then on to Twin Falls in 1911 where he began first grade. During the year the family again moved, this time to Burley where he graduated from high school in 1924. He attended the University of Idaho from 1925-29 and received a B.S in pre-med. He graduated from Northwestern University in Chicago with an M.D. in 1933, and did his residency at

Harborview Hospital, Seattle, 1934. He was a member of Signa Chi and Phi Chi medical fraternities. Dr. Terhune and his wife, Ruth, whom he describes as "a swell gal," had two sons and a daughter.

DR. WALTER RAY PETERSEN

When Dr. Walter Petersen started practice in Burley in 1966 there were six physicians. There are now twenty. He knew for a long time that he would like to go into medicine, but was "afraid I wasn't smart enough to make it, and scared to death of shots." He knew that his mother also wanted him to become a doctor, and he couldn't get it out of his mind.

This is how he describes what became D-day (Decision day) for him. "It was a day of decision that autumn afternoon in 1957 when I walked into the office of Dr. Irvin Jolley, pre-med advisor in chemistry at the University of Idaho. I had been majoring in civil engineering in my two years of college before my Latter Day Saints mission, and also that quarter at Brigham Young University after my return from Uruguay in March. Because it would have taken me longer to get my degree in B.Y.U.'s five-year engineering program, I was back at the University of Idaho, where I had started as a freshman in 1952.

"I had been thinking a lot about medicine versus engineering, and decided it would be helpful to talk it over with the pre-med advisor. Dr. Jolley had helped so many young men and women choose a successful and rewarding career in medicine. He was so well thought of by medical schools for sending such good pre-med students, that he was able to get Idaho grads into top-ranked medical schools throughout the nation. Within two hours after our talk, I was transferred out of my engineering into pre-med courses."

With the change to pre-med, he remembered his happy thought after the college freshman chemistry class, "That's the last chem class I will ever have to take!" Now, there was quantitative and qualitative chemical analysis, organic and physiologic chemistry. With these difficult studies he didn't stop to think that on June 10, 1963, when he received his M.D. degree, he would say, "Now I know I could never be happy in anything but medicine. I would have been happy as an engineer, never having known medicine—but now I couldn't."

Walter was born April 17, 1934 to Raymond Orlinzo and Jane Maria Prescott Petersen, and had two sisters. He and his wife, Eileen, live with their family in Burley.

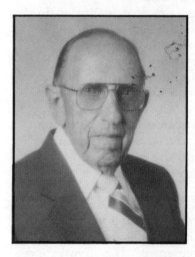

Dr. Richard P. Sutton practiced at Burley, in the heartland of a great agricultural area.

DR. RICHARD POMEROY SUTTON

When Dr. Richard P. Sutton, Burley physician, began practice there were three doctors in town, all in general practice. He thinks that they all practiced from seventy-five to one hundred hours a week many times. He delivered more than 4,000 babies and was on call day and night, seven days a week.

He remembers well a five-year-old girl, struck by a car and bleeding profusely from her head. He shaved and cleaned her head, put in stitches, during which he felt an irregularity in the skull bone. He sent her to Cottage Hospital for X-rays and enroute she went into a coma with seizures. The doctor called a neurosurgeon in Salt Lake, who told him the emergency was such that he had no time to send her anywhere, that Dr. Sutton would have to operate immediately. He and another doctor lifted the depressed piece of bone, suctioned the clot and relieved the pressure on the brain. The little girl relaxed and started to cry. Dr. Sutton sent her to the neurosurgeon for follow-up care and she recovered with no ill effects. He had other emergencies, but none so dramatic.

Dr. Sutton was born February 7, 1912 at Chicago, son of a pioneer physician, Dr. Richard J. and Mrs. Sutton. He attended the University of Utah from 1930 to 1931 and from 1937 to 1941. Medical school was at Northwestern University, 1941–43. His internship and residency were served at the L.D.S. Hospital in Salt Lake City.

Following a year at Magda, Utah, as an employee of Utah Copper Company, he entered military service, and became a captain in the Army Medical Corps. After the war, he moved to Burley to practice with his father, who had suffered three heart attacks and was overworked with offices in both Burley and Oakley.

He was in practice from 1947 until retirement in 1980. Dr. Sutton and his wife Gwen became parents of four children, Dorene, Norma Jean, Robert and Steven.

DR. CONSTANTINE ANNEST

Dr. Annest was born in Pocatello, April 18, 1919. His brother was a doctor in Tacoma, Washington. He was raised near Declo and went through high school. He took pre-med at the University of Utah, and received his M.D. from the University of Louisville School of Medicine in 1943. He had an externship at Kentucky Baptist Hospital, where he met his future wife. He interned in Texas hospitals before moving to Burley in 1948.

He was on the staff at Cottage and Cassia Memorial hospitals and belonged to the South Central and Idaho Medical associations. In the U.S. Naval Reserve, he spent two years at the Navy Hospital, Corpus Christi, Texas.

He owned his own plane, and spent lots of time with his three sons.

DR. J. B. KENAGY

John Brough Kenagy, born February 13, 1863, at Bellefontaine, Ohio, educated in Missouri and Kansas, and was teacher, principal and superintendent in Nebraska and Colorado. He married Harriet Sliffe in 1890, and they had a son, Fayre, and daughter, Louise. He had always wanted to study medicine and knew if he didn't do it soon he would never be able to. So he gave up working in education, moved his family to Boulder and entered the School of Medicine.

Graduating in 1906, as a physician and surgeon, he

moved his family to Boulder, prepared for practice. He soon heard of the opening up of the Minidoka Irrigation Project in Cassia County and he was intrigued with the prospect of pioneering in such a new area. That September when the family got off the train at Rupert, they found a general store, butcher shop, hotel, and three saloons around a square in the center of the new town for a future park. Tents and shacks were scattered in the outlying area and the Kenagys lived at the Martin Hotel until there was a house for them.

In the early years, he was a true horse and buggy doctor, driving across the sandy country roads to his patients. In the winter he bundled up in six coyote skins that Fayre had trapped, tanned and made into the robe for his dad. When drifting snow made buggy travel impossible, he saddled up his horse, "Ned," and always reached his destination. When the Downard, Montgomery or Howell ferries were frozen into the ice, he would tie his horse and make his way on foot, with lantern and medicine bag, to see a patient or deliver a baby.

Medical fees were small, one dollar for an office call and twenty-five dollars to deliver a baby, which included six months prepartem care and several weeks after. Half the patients had no money and some never paid. One touching instance was of a good patient bringing the doctor one-hundred pounds of wool to pay her bill. She had laboriously plucked the wool from fences where sheep had left wool on the barbed wire. He sent the lot to Utah Woolen Mills and received several beautiful blankets in return.

DR. FAYRE KENAGY

In 1919, Dr. Fayre Kenagy joined his dad in the Rupert office. He also graduated from Colorado School of Medicine, and the younger doctor was able to assume more and more of the load the senior doctor had carried for years. Dr. Fayre enjoyed those years with his father, who was a devout Methodist and was on the board of trustees and sang in the choir at the church. During his entire practice he was surgeon for the Union Pacific Railroad, and there, too, his son was able to assist. The father died November 17, 1934, at the age of seventy-one.

CHAPTER
13

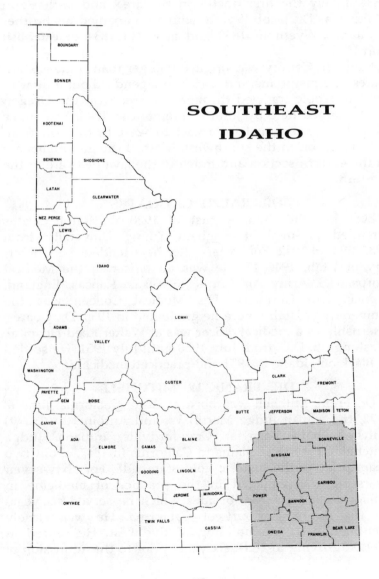

SOUTHEAST
IDAHO

BINGHAM COUNTY

Major Andrew Henry and what he referred to as his "first Americans" wintered in what was to become Bingham County in 1810, followed by several exploring and trapping parties. Wilson Price Hunt's expedition came in 1911; Captain Bonneville's party in 1832, and again in 1834. Likely the first doctor in the area, and perhaps in Idaho, was Dr. Jacob Wyeth, who accompanied his brother Nathaniel Wyeth in 1832 and again in 1834 to establish Fort Hall.

Bingham County was originally larger than some eastern states and historians find it rich in legend. About a quarter million people traveled through the area over the Oregon Trail mapped here by John C. Fremont in 1843. The Snake River cuts a diagonal from east to west to the American Falls reservoir in the southwest. Most of the mountains are in the eastern section and much of the lava beds are in the western.

DR. RALPH G. GOATES

Born in Lehi, Utah, August 10, 1920, Dr. Ralph Goates attended pre-med at Brigham Young University from 1937–39 and 1942. Four years later he attended the University of Utah, 1946–47. He was an officer in the Medical Corps, U.S. Army Air Corps, in Texas, Kansas, England, France, and Germany. His Medical College was the University of Utah where he graduated in 1950. Dr. Goates' internship as a medical officer was at Walter Reed Hospital, Washington, D.C. from July 1950 until July 1951. He settled in Blackfoot, Idaho in 1951 and practiced medicine.

DR. FRANK W. MITCHELL

Dr. Frank Mitchell was born at Adin, California, June 6, 1872, the son of Judge Martin W. and Antoinette (Curry) Mitchell, both born at Crawfordville, Indiana. Judge Mitchell crossed the plains to California in 1847, about two years prior to the historic gold stampede. For sixty-seven years he was engaged in the practice of medicine in California and Oregon, besides which he served six years on the Supreme Court of California. He was closely identified with the building of the west. He retired at Weiser, arriving in 1884, six years prior to the admission of

Idaho Territory to the Union. His wife died in Weiser, November 9, 1911.

Dr. Mitchell was the youngest of five children and a lad of twelve years when they came to Idaho. He completed high school at Weiser, attended business college in Portland and in 1892 received a degree in pharmacy from Willamette University. He entered Rush Medical College, Chicago, and graduated in 1894 with an M.D. degree. He practiced in the St. Louis, Missouri hospital, until entering Barnes Medical College there, where he received a supplemental degree in 1903. He interned in the St. Louis City Hospital. Later he served a second internship in the general hospital at Rock Springs, Wyoming. In 1907 he took post-graduate work at Chicago Polytechnic, and in 1910 studied at Chicago medical schools and hospitals.

October 10, 1903, Dr. Mitchell established his home and office at Blackfoot. His cash capital when he started practice at Blackfoot was eighty dollars. He was vice president of the Idaho State Medical Society and was a member of the American Medical Association. He was medical examiner for fifty-two life insurance companies with business in Idaho. He was a Mason, Odd Fellow, and Modern Woodman of America, a Democrat, and he and his wife were members of the Protestant Episcopal church. He was president of the Parker Mountain Mining Company.

December 2, 1897, he married Winifred Hopkins, daughter of Andrew J. Hopkins, who moved to Idaho when she was a girl. Dr. and Mrs. Mitchell had no children.

DR. CLAYTON AUGUSTUS HOOVER

Dr. Hoover was born in Washington, D.C. in 1853 and was a boyhood friend of Tad Lincoln, son of the president. They went to school together, shared the same bench and lunch pail. Clayton enjoyed playing at the White House after school and remembered playing marbles on the floor of the Blue Room. He remembered the lanky president, hearing their shouts of joy, joining them, kneeling down to best them in a game of marbles.

As a graduate of George Washington Medical School, he was sent west as a government doctor and was at Montpelier, Idaho, in 1882. He was the only physician within a radius from Evanston, Wyoming to Boise and from McCammon to Butte, Montana. He was also surgeon for the Union Pacific until 1905.

He practiced continuously for fifty-seven years and was the first president of both the Idaho Medical Society and the State Board of Medical Examiners. In 1905, he moved to Blackfoot after being appointed superintendent of the State Mental Institution for sixteen years. He visited every patient every day.

Dr. Hoover married in Washington, D.C. and they had a son, Alfred, who became a druggist at Shelley. After the death of his first wife, he married Bessie Brown of Liberty, Idaho, and they had five children. In 1928, one year after he had spent six months in the east studying and being honored as the oldest living graduate at George Washington Medical School, he was stricken with a stroke and died.

DR. WALTER GRIMMETT HOGE

The son of a dentist, Dr. Hoge was born March 13, 1914 in Paris, Idaho. He had two cousins who were physicians, Alfred and Bruce Budge of Boise. He was educated at Idaho State College, 1938-37 and went to the University of Utah from 1937-38. He graduated from Brigham Young University in 1936 with a B.A. degree. He did graduate study in bacteriology at the University of Idaho in 1937-38 and graduated in 1939 from the University of Hawaii with an M.D. in bacteriology. He was an instructor in bacteriology at the University of Idaho from 1939-41.

His medical education was at Northeastern University, receiving his B.M. and M.D. degrees in 1944-45. His rotating internship was at the Cook County Hospital in Chicago, 1944-45. He practiced at Preston, 1947-48 and Shelley, 1948-52; and started at Blackfoot in 1921. He was a captain with the U.S. Army, 1945-47 in Germany as regimental surgeon. Hospital staff appointments were at Bingham Memorial Hospital in Blackfoot; two terms as chief of staff at Idaho Falls Hospital; chairman of the Record Committee, and staff member of Sacred Heart Hospital in Idaho Falls. Memberships were in Idaho State Medical Society, Necrologist during 1961-62. He was secretary of the Idaho Academy of General Practice for two consecutive years. He and his wife had four children.

DR. A. E. MILLER

In 1986, Dr. Miller wrote a feature story, "When did the joy leave the practice of medicine?" which was distributed nationally by the Associated Press, being published in hundred of papers across the country. AP editor Jack Capon liked the story so well that he sent a photographer from Los Angeles to Blackfoot to illustrate the feature. A small part of it is included here.

Dr. Miller was attending a medical conference and overheard a group of doctors saying what he had heard many times before, of bureaucratic hassles, senseless regulations, endless raises in insurance premiums. Four of them had recently been sued and two of them devastated by the experience. Three of them wanted out. The eldest asked the question that haunts America's doctors, "When did the joy go out of medicine?"

"I know what it's like to be a family doctor in Blackfoot, and I've known it for a long time. There has been a Dr. Miller in Blackfoot for the past fifty-four years. My father came here in 1933, at the height of the Great Depression. I was born in November," Dr. Miller wrote. He went on to describe the wondrous things in a doctor's office, types of infections and illnesses, and of the healing drugs that have helped cure diseases of the past.

With heart-rending sentences he told of elderly patients he and his father had tended, and the rising costs of medicine, equipment that will do things never dreamed of in earlier days, and he said that his nurse for twenty-three years, Florence Jex, had been replaced by a physician assistant, two nurses, receptionist, bookkeeper, cleaning lady and occasionally, a medical manager. "Florence would hate the telephone today," he wrote. "She would not believe sixty to seventy calls a day. Bills were posted once or twice a year, usually after the crops were in. Dad had strong feelings about overcharging. He once told a young surgeon, 'You're going to make a lot of money. Stop trying to make it all at once.'

"The blind shall see, and the lame shall walk. Cataracts and hips are no longer miracles, even in a small town like ours. How can it be that this same medical technology has created a hell on earth? We are told, 'Keep good records to defend yourself in a lawsuit.' The medical record is no longer there for patient care. It is a legal document. The physician has been blamed for outrageous medical expenses beyond his control. On the other hand, people are paying an outrageous price for their medical care.

"It's time folks got together."

DR. LYNN H. ANDERSON

Dr. Anderson was born in Idaho Falls, August 16, 1923. His father was an accountant and cabinet maker. In 1944 he received a degree in pharmacy from the University of Idaho, Southern Branch. He went to Northwestern University Medical School from 1944-48 and got his M.D. degree. He got his master degree in pharmacology in 1948. From 1948-49 he interned at St. Luke's Hospital in Chicago. He had a residency at the same hospital, 1949-51, in internal medicine. For six months he was with the Army Medical Corps at San Antonio, Texas.

After army training in psychiatry, he was assigned to Field Hospital in Wurzburg, Germany, as a psychiatrist, from 1951-53. His last year of residency was internal medicine at Veteran's Hospital, Chicago, 1953-54.

He started practice in Blackfoot, September 1954, as specialist in internal medicine. He was on the staff at Bingham Memorial Hospital; Bannock Memorial Hospital, Pocatello; St. Anthony Hospital, Pocatello. He belonged to the Idaho Society of Internal Medicine.

The Andersons had one son.

DR. GERALD J. CONLIN

Dr. Gerald J. Conlin, Blackfoot, died October 1, 1965, in Denver Colorado. Born August 9, 1918 in Blackfoot, he received his M.D. degree from the Washington University School of Medicine in 1943. He interned at Barnes Hospital, Children's Hospital, and the Maternity Hospital, St. Louis, followed by pediatrics residency at St. Louis Children's Hospital.

Dr. Conlin entered the Army in 1945, and retired as a lieutenant colonel in 1954. He was licensed to practice in Idaho, January 13, 1959, and was employed at State Hospital South.

BONNEVILLE COUNTY

The Snake River cuts through the county flowing across a quiet, green valley that is between the Caribou Range and the Big Hole Mountains. It is a scenic county with many creeks flowing into the Snake. The county is named for the renowned captain who passed through in the early nineteenth century. Heavy traffic beat a path through the county from Salt Lake to the Montana gold mines. The first settlers built their cabins at the Eagle Rock ferry in 1864. Eagle Rock was later named Idaho Falls, and by 1880 farms were doing well. The Latter Day Saints (Mormons) came in from Utah and built irrigation systems which further enriched the farming areas.

DR. THOMAS C. WILLSON

The urge to "go west" was strong within young Dr. Thomas C. Willson of Virginia. In the spring of 1890, he, his wife, and infant son gave way to the urge and left the Old Dominion and moved to Montpelier, Idaho and opened an office. Soon he had established a satisfactory practice.

Thomas C. Willson was born in Richmond, Virginia in 1863. He spent his boyhood in that immediate vicinity. He first became a pharmacist and later studied medicine. For several years he was associated with Dr. Leigh in Clarksville, Virginia. On January 17, 1899, he was married to Adeline Shangle, the daughter of a Methodist Minister. On October 25 of the same year their first child and only son, Harry Leigh, was born.

In the summer of 1890, after his arrival in Idaho, he had occasion to make a trip through Star Valley, Swan Valley, and on down the Snake River Valley, returning to Montpelier via Soda Springs. The doctor was so impressed with the vast undeveloped Snake River Valley and its future possibilities that he closed his affairs in Montpelier and moved to the little town of Eagle Rock. Later that year the name "Eagle Rock" was changed to Idaho Falls.

In Eagle Rock, Dr. Willson opened an office and developed a large practice. At that time there were no telephones, and travel was by horse and buggy or sleigh when roads were passable, otherwise by horseback. There were no hospitals, no trained nurses, or other trained help except another over-worked doctor. In consequence of these circumstances, the patients' relatives or friends had to assist the doctor as best they could and the doctor's responsibilities were heavy. Despite the handicaps, these pioneer doctors did some remarkable work.

On October 23, 1893, a daughter and last child, Mary Wrenn, was born to Dr. and Mrs. Willson. The daughter, Mrs. Harold Holman, resided in Silver Spring, Maryland and the son, Dr. Harry L. Willson, practiced medicine in Idaho Falls until his death in 1959 from a cerebral hemorrhage.

Dr. Thomas C. Willson practiced medicine for fifty years in Idaho Falls. In addition to his practice, he was active in civic affairs and in the development of the resources of Snake River Valley. He was a Past Master of the Masonic Lodge, a member of the Elks and Odd Fellows Lodges. He was a Baptist but usually attended the Methodist Church to which his wife and children belonged.

Dr. Willson died from coronary thrombosis, December 14, 1940, after a few hours illness. His wife died in October 1943 from a cerebral hemorrhage.

DR. MARK BAUM

Concern for sun exposure is not a recent concern of the medical society. In the late 1940s Dr. Baum, a dermatologist, was concerned because as he said, "As the sun increases in its intensity each year, I see more and more sun dermatoses." This Idaho native, son of a Justice of the Peace and seed potato dealer, was born and raised in Ashton. He graduated from College of Idaho with a B.S. in chemistry in 1940 and secured a three month job with the Pure Food and Drug Administration testing apples for lead content. He then entered the George Washington University Medical School and received his M.D. in 1944. While attending George Washington University he was a member of Phi Chi Phi.

Dr. Baum interned at the U.S. Naval Hospital in Long Beach from 1944–45 and completed a residency in dermatology at Indianapolis General Hospital in 1947–49. Dr. Baum held a staff appointment at both L.D.S. and Sacred Heart hospitals in Idaho Falls and was vice president of Rocky Mountain Dermatological Society.

Dr. Baum served twenty-two years as a Naval reservist and saw active duty in World War II and the Korean War. He achieved the rank of commander and held the positions of commanding officer of Naval Reserve Research Co. 13-6, and president of Idaho Falls Chapter of Naval Reserve Association. He married the former Charleine Chenoweth of Glendale, California.

DR. FRED E. WALLBER

Dr. Wallber was born June 5, 1919 at Milwaukee, Wisconsin. His father was a banker. Dr. Wallber got his grade and high school educations in Milwaukee. From 1937-40 he took pre-med courses at the University of Wisconsin, receiving his BS degree in 1941. In 1942 he received his medical degree from the Medical School at the University of Wisconsin.

He interned at St. Joseph's Hospital, Phoenix, Arizona and completed a rotating residency in ophthalmology (1944), John Gaston Hospital, University of Tennessee, Memphis, Tennessee, 1949-50. He started his practice in Idaho Falls in 1951.

Dr. Wallber was on the general staff of the Idaho Falls Hospital and Sacred Heart Hospital, also was a past president of the general staff of the Sacred Heart Hospital. He was a past president of the Idaho Falls Medical Society; program chairman of the Idaho State Medical Association, 1958; Councilor for District 4, Idaho State Medical Association, 1958-61. From 1944-46 he was a captain in the U.S. Army Medical Corps, 94th Field Hospital.

The Wallbers have three daughters and one son.

DR. ARTHUR R. SODERQUIST

When Dr. A.R. Soderquist died in 1964 at Idaho Falls, age eighty, he was the oldest practicing physician there. When he arrived in Idaho at age twenty-four, in 1908, the town was known as Eagle Rock, and he helped establish the first hospital there.

He was born June 4, 1884, at Lafayette, Minnesota to a farming family. Dr. Soderquist worked on the farm, and attended grade school and high school in Lafayette. In 1902-03 he took a pre med. course at Gustavus Adolphus College. He received his Doctor of Medicine from Hamline University Medical School, where he went from 1904-08.

He went to Idaho Falls, Idaho November 1, 1908, and practiced until 1963. He was chief of staff at the Latter Day Saints Hospital, secretary of the Idaho Falls Medical Society, and a captain in the State National Guard.

A rose garden, fishing, and hunting were his hobbies. He had one son.

DR. GUY CURTIS WAID

Medicine skipped a generation in Dr. Waid's family. His father was a railroad agent and telegrapher, but his grandfather practiced medicine in Kansas starting in the 1890s. Dr. Waid was born in Downey, Idaho on May 16, 1921. He was educated at the University of Idaho from 1938-42 and received his medical degree from Stanford University in 1945. He was a member of the Alpha Kappa Kappa Medical Fraternity and also the Alpha Omega Alpha Honor Medical Society. His internship was served at San Francisco Hospital from 1945-46. He became an assistant resident in the same facility from 1948-50.

In 1950 he moved on to become an assistant resident in internal medicine in Salt Lake City until 1951 when he became chief resident at the same hospital. In 1952 he moved to Idaho Falls to become a member of the medical staff at Idaho Falls L.D.S. and Sacred Heart hospitals. During his career he was president of the Idaho Falls Medical Society and served as president of staff of the Sacred Heart Hospital in 1963-64. His military career was served in the Navy as a lieutenant junior grade from 1946-48. He married in 1948 and had three children.

DR. CLIFFORD M. CLINE

The son of a druggist, Dr. Cline was born in Iowa on August 11, 1884. He attended the University of Iowa before entering medical school at Northwestern University at the age of twenty. His residency and internship were served at the Chicago Pli Clinic Hospital from 1905-07.

He went to Idaho Falls from 1907-08 and then practiced for a year in Boise before returning permanently to Idaho Falls in 1909. He performed tonsillectomies and deliveries in the homes of his patients and also experienced scarlet fever, small pox and influenza epidemics. His methods of transportation ranged from horse and buggy, sleds and later automobiles. He was a pioneer in certain types of surgeries (i.e. thyroids) in the Idaho Falls area. His early hospital experiences were in Village Improvement and Idaho Falls General. He later served as chief of staff of L.D.S. and Sacred Heart hospitals. He spent five years in the Selective Service. He had one daughter and two grandchildren.

DR. GEORGE L. VOELZ

As chief of medicine for the Atomic Energy Commission in Idaho Falls, Dr. Voelz was one of those to treat the victims of an early atomic accident that exposed victims to high levels of radioactivity never encountered before.

This Wisconsin native, born October 13, 1926, started his education at the University of Wisconsin only to have it interrupted by eighteen months in the U.S. Navy as an electronics technician. He return to the University of Wisconsin and received his B.S. in 1948 and continued on to the University Medical School and received his M.D. degree in 1950. He relocated to the University of Oregon Medical School and Hospital in Portland, Oregon to complete his internship in 1951.

Dr. Voelz received a fellowship in Industrial Medicine from the Atomic Energy Commission at the University of Cincinnati, Kettering Lab from 1951–52 and did further in-plant training at Los Alamos Scientific Lab in New Mexico from 1952–53. He remained at Los Alamos as a staff physician in the Industrial Medicine Group from 1953–57 and then moved on to become the chief of the Medical Services Branch of the Idaho Operations Office for the Atomic Energy Commission in Idaho Falls in 1957.

Dr. Voelz is married with three children.

DR. DAVID HARLIN SMITH

Born in Fillmore, Utah on February 7, 1915, Dr. Smith went through school in Idaho Falls. He returned to Utah and the University of Utah from 1937–39 and continued his education at the University of Tennessee until he graduated in 1943. His nine month internship was served at the San Bernadino County Hospital.

He worked for Hanford Engineer Atomic Installation until 1945 and then moved to Shelley, Idaho and practiced from 1945–48. In 1948 he relocated to Idaho Falls. He served as chief of staff for the L.D.S. Hospital in Idaho Falls and also the president of the Idaho Falls Medical Society. Six of his ten children were adopted. He enjoys fishing, hunting and raising quarter horses and purebred German Shorthair bird dogs.

DR. L. JOHN BINGHAM

Dr. Bingham's medical practice got off to a rather unusual start. His first two patients were of the canine variety—the first required treatment for a broken leg and the next needed an amputation of the tail. As he put it, "It caused me to check my shingle."

The report of a man thrown from his horse during a hunting trip with a possible back injury came during a Sunday afternoon church meeting. Dr. Bingham went on the call driving his jeep up the side of a very steep mountain. The mountain was so steep the jeep rolled over a cliff. Vehicles were without seat belts in those days, and the doctor was thrown from the jeep. Fortunately, he received only minor contusions, abrasions, and cracked glasses. The hunting party righted the jeep and the doctor and party continued on to find and treat the patient without further incident.

Because of the twenty-five miles between the doctor and hospital, a wild race with time and the stork was common. Not only was distance a problem; obstacles in the form of livestock on the road could create hazards. Luckily only in one case did the doctor and patient not quite make it to the hospital on time. Just about to the hospital the doctor had a flat tire. After a hasty change, just as he and the patient entered the hospital, his last daughter was born.

The doctor was born on December 15, 1918 in Ogden, Utah and had the usual growing up experiences with few calamities and various jobs as a teenager. He did spend two years as a missionary in Germany and the United States just before entering medical school. He attended the University of Utah from 1935–41 and went to the University of Pennsylvania from 1941–43 to receive his M.D. His nine month internship was at the L.D.S. Hospital in Salt Lake City and in addition he did a nine month residency in OB/GYN at General Hospital in Salt Lake City, Utah. He practiced in Kamas, Utah in 1947 and also in Salt Lake City. He also practiced in Blackfoot, Idaho from 1954–55 before coming to Idaho Falls in 1955. His military career was in the U.S. Army where he served as a captain.

Dr. Bingham had staff apointments at Sacred Heart, and was president of staff at the Idaho Falls L.D.S. Hospital in 1961. He also served on various committees. He married Helen William on December 10, 1943 and had three sons and two daughters.

DR. DAVID S. BURNET

A former major in the Army, Dr. Burnet served in the Medical Corps from 1947-52 in Germany and Korea as well as in the United States. He received his education at the University of Virginia and received his B.A. in 1943 and continued on to graduate from the Department of Medicine in 1946 with his M.D. His internship was served at the Orange Memorial Hospital in Orange, New Jersey from 1946-47. After his military service, he began his residency in neurology and psychiatry in 1962 at the University of Virginia Hospital and completed his training in 1955.

Dr. Burnet was born in Charlotte, North Carolina on February 26, 1921 and his father was a commissioner of the Internal Revenue Service. He was a staff psychiatrist at State Hospital South, Blackfoot and also on the staff of Sacred Heart and L.D.S. hospitals in Idaho Falls. He was a delegate to the Idaho State Medical Society for two years and also a member of the American Psychiatric Association, Intermountain Psychiatric Association, and the American Association of Mental Deficiency. He had three children, two daughters and one son.

DR. JACK RODERICK CAREY

A native of Wenatchee, Washington where his father was a barber, Dr. Carey was born on February 26, 1920. He attended the University of Washington and then Northwestern University Medical School and graduated in 1944. His internship was at St. Luke's Hospital in Chicago, Illinois from 1944-46 and he then moved on to King County Hospital in Seattle, Washington from 1948-51.

In 1951 he moved to Idaho Falls, Idaho where he practiced at Sacred Heart Hospital and L.D.S. Hospital. His military service was served in the Army as a captain from 1946-48. He has three daughters and one son.

DR. GEORGE H. COULTHARD

Dr. Coulthard was born on a farm near Missouri Valley, Harrison County, Iowa on March 9, 1878. He was the son of William and Jane (Eddee) Coulthard, who were numbered among the early settlers of that section of the Hawkeye state, and became prominently identified with its pioneer development and upbuilding. The father secured a tract of government land in Harrison County, and developed it into a valuable and productive farm.

Dr. Coulthard, who was the third of nine children, gained his early experience in connection with the work and management of the farm. He attended the public schools and the Woodbine Normal School at Woodbine, Harrison County, from which he was graduated in 1900. He attended the medical department of the University of Iowa, Iowa City, and was graduated with the class of 1904, with his M.D. degree. That same year he moved to Idaho Falls and established his practice.

In 1907 Dr. Coulthard was elected to the city council. During the administration of Governor Brady, he served as a member of the State Board of Health. He was one of the organizers of the Idaho Falls Club of Commerce, and was its first president. The doctor was a Mason and passed various official chairs in the Masonic bodies; was a past master of the Eagles Lodge, and the Elks. He enjoyed hunting and fishing, and was president of the Idaho Falls gun club. He was also a member of the American Medical Association and Idaho State Medical Association.

DR. GLENN W. CORBETT

Glenn Corbett was born February 1, 1915, in Grace, Idaho. His father was a farmer. He attended grade and high school in Grace, and took pharmacy at Idaho State. In 1936 he received a B.S. degree from the University of Idaho, southern branch. He attended the University of Utah for two years, and then Temple University School of Medicine, where he received his M.D. in 1942.

From 1942–43 he interned at Good Samaritan Hospital, Los Angeles, and Childrens Hospital, Hollywood. He was in the Air Force from 1943–46, in Santa Ana, California and Yuma, Arizona. In 1950–51 he took graduate training in surgery at the Evangelist School of Medicine in Los Angeles.

He started practicing in Preston, and then moved to Idaho Falls. In 1944-45 he was chief of staff at Sacred Heart Hospital in Idaho Falls. The doctor was also chief of surgery at Sacred Heart Hospital and L.D.S. Hospital.

The Corbetts had two daughters and one son, all golf enthusiasts.

DR. ERVINE STEPHENSON BILLS

After an eleven year career as a commander in the U.S. Navy, Dr. Bills came to Idaho Falls to practice in 1954. He was a staff member of the Idaho Falls L.D.S. Hospital and Sacred Heart Hospital. His education was obtained at the University of Utah from 1934-38 and the University of Utah Medical School from 1938-40. His internship was at the hospital of the University of Pennsylvania in Philadelphia. He was born in Salt Lake City on October 8, 1926 but grew up in Blackfoot, Idaho. His father was an automobile salesman but his brother, named Jack W. Bills, is also a doctor in Van Nuys, California. He has three children, one girl and two boys.

DR. ELLSWORTH P. BLAIR

Awarded the Purple Heart and Bronze Star during a three year period (1942-45) in the military during World War II, Dr. Blair returned to his practice in Idaho Falls in 1945. Previously he had briefly practiced medicine in Arcola, Illinois from March of 1941 until January 1942. He established his Idaho Falls practice in January of 1942 and began serving his time in the military in August.

The son of a farmer, born July 7, 1912, Dr. Blair received his education at the University of Idaho, University of Utah, University of Chicago, and Rush Medical School. He did a one year rotating internship at the Illinois Center in Chicago and spent three months at the Contagious Disease Hospital also in Chicago. Prior to medical school he spent two and one-half years as a missionary at an L.D.S. Church in Germany.

He was a member of the L.D.S. Hospital and Sacred Heart Hospital staff in Idaho Falls, Idaho and was also the chief of staff at the L.D.S. Hospital. He was the president of the Idaho Falls Medical Association and also president-elect of the Idaho Chapter of the AAGP.

DR. J. DOUGLAS DAVIS

Dr. Davis was born February 13, 1918, in Delta, Utah; the family home was in Provo, Utah. His father died when he was one year old, and his mother worked, supported, and educated five children. The doctor worked his way through college and medical school.

In 1943 he received his A.B. degree from Brigham Young University, and his M.D. from University of Utah in 1946. From 1945–49 he was on active duty with the U.S.N.R. He interned at the U. S. Naval Hospital, in Seattle, and the U.S. Naval Hospital in Bremerton, Washington.

He started practicing in Idaho Falls in 1949. Dr. Davis was on the staffs at L.D.S. Hospital and Sacred Heart Hospital in Idaho Falls. He belonged to the Idaho Falls Medical Society.

The Davises had two boys and two girls.

DR. JOHN HARPER CULLEY

Son of a pharmacist, John Culley was born January 23, 1909, in Ogden, Utah. He attended the Ogden public schools. He went to the University of Utah, and received his B.A. degree in 1930 from the University of Southern California. In 1933, he received his M.D. degree from the University of Pennsylvania. From 1934–35 he interned at Alameda County Hospital, Oakland, California, and at Polyclinic Hospital, New York City from 1940–41. He moved to Idaho Falls in 1941.

The doctor was on the staffs of L.D.S. Hospital and Sacred Heart in Idaho Falls. He belonged to the Upper Valley Medical Society and Idaho Falls Medical Society.

He was a captain in WWII from 1942–46, and a major in Korea from 1950–52. He was awarded an air medal; WWII Victory medal; American Campaign medal; Asiatic-Pacific campaign medal with three battle stars; Korean campaign medal; United Nations medal; Army Reserve medal with x device; National Guard medal with x device; rated A.A.F. flight surgeon. He was ready army reserve officer with rank of colonel; on staff of Idaho Adjutant General; and, state medical officer for Army National Guard.

The doctor owned his plane, and was active in the Army National Guard. He and his wife, Margaret, had two sons.

DR. MAURICE KING HENINGER

A native of Canada born on December 16, 1917, Dr. Heninger grew up on a farm in Canada. He came to the U.S. to study at Brigham Young University where he studied for his bachelor of arts degree. After his graduation he married and returned to Canada to study at the McGill University in Montreal in 1941 and graduated in 1945 with his M.D. degree. His internship was served in Montreal hospitals and then he completed three years of training in radiology at St. Paul's Hospital in Vancouver, B.C.

During his training, he joined the Royal Canadian Army Medical Corps and served as a captain for three years. He spent one of those years at the Prisoner of War Camp in Northern Alberta. After he completed his military service, he established a practice at Lethridge, Alberta for one year.

He then relocated to Idaho Falls as a radiologist at the L.D.S. Hospital. He was also a consulting radiologist at the Sacred Heart Hospital in Idaho Falls and at the Bingham Memorial Hospital and the State Hospital in Blackfoot. He was active in the Idaho Falls Medical Society and has served as the chief of staff for the L.D.S. Hospital. He and his wife have six children, four daughters and one son.

DR. HARVEY EARL GUYETT

Born at the turn of the century on April 22, 1900, in Woodbine, Iowa, Dr. Guyett did not stray from the state of Iowa until he began his internship. He grew up and was educated in Woodbine and continued on to Iowa University and also the College of Medicine. Before becoming a doctor, he worked as a high school teacher and athletic director in Oklahoma schools. After graduating from the medical school in 1929, he began his internship in Salt Lake City at St. Marks Hospital. After completing his internship in 1930, he established a practice in Shelley, Idaho and practiced until 1932 when he relocated permanently in Idaho Falls. In his early practice he traveled by horse and sleigh to make winter calls. Home surgeries and deliveries were also very common.

While in college Dr. Guyett was a member of the R.O.T.C. from 1926-29. He then entered the Medical Reserves as a first lieutenant. He served active duty during World War II from 1940-46 as a major and continued on in the Medical Reserves as a major until he retired in 1960 from the reserves. He was also active in professional societies and was a staff member at L.D.S. Hospital and Sacred Heart Hospital in Idaho Falls. His only daughter became a teacher.

DR. SILVIES S. FULLER

Originally from Harrisburg, Idaho where he was born on February 27, 1875, Dr. Fuller and his mother moved to Kansas after the death of his father in 1892. He taught high school for five years in the Kansas public school system and then entered the Kansas City Medical College and graduated in 1903. While he was in medical school, he taught a chemistry class to help pay for his own schooling. After graduation in 1903, he returned to Hutchinson, Kansas to practice for two years.

Dr. Fuller relocated to the Idaho Falls area and established Fuller Hospital in 1909. He was an active member of several fraternal organizations and was also a firm believer in the opportunities present in Idaho for anyone willing to work hard.

DR. RONALD K. LECHELT

Another Iowa native, Dr. Lechelt grew up in Cedar Rapids, Iowa and attended Britt Junior College from 1947–49. In 1949 he served in the U.S. Navy as an airman. From 1950–52 he attended the State University of Iowa and in 1952 entered the College of Medicine. He earned his M.D. in 1956 and began his internship at Broadlawns General Hospital in Des Moines, Iowa. In 1957–59 he also trained at Raymond Blank Memorial Hospital for Children in Des Moines. In 1959 he moved to Idaho Falls and established his practice. He is a staff member of Sacred Heart and Idaho Falls hospitals and a member of the Idaho State Medical Society. He is married and has two children.

DR. DAUCHY MIGEL

The son of a silk manufacturer, Dr. Migel came to Idaho Falls after serving in the Army Medical Corp in the U.S and South Pacific. He was born in Brooklyn, New York on November 5, 1913 and was raised in Pelham Manor, New York. He attended college at Hotchkiss and Colgate universities and also attended the Harvard Medical School from 1934–38. His internship was served in Springfield, Massachusetts and he completed a surgical residency from 1940–43 at the New York Postgraduate Medical School and Hospital.

He was affiliated with Idaho Falls L.D.S. Hospital and Sacred Heart Hospital. Courtesy staff positions were at Madison Memorial Hospital in Rexburg, Ashton Hospital, and Steele Memorial Hospital in Salmon. He was active in the local medical society and was a former governor of the Idaho Chapter of the American College of Surgeons. He and his wife, Frances, had one daughter and three sons.

DR. C. RICHARD NIXON

Dr. Nixon was a practicing pharmacist, as was his father, before becoming a medical doctor. He earned his pharmacy degree in 1950 from the Idaho State College. In 1957 he earned his M.D. from George Washington University and began his internship at L.D.S. Hospital in Salt Lake City, Utah. In 1958 he began his practice in Blackfoot, Idaho where he was a staff member of the Bingham Memorial Hospital. Dr. Nixon and his wife, the late Phyllis Barle, became the parents of three boys and one girl.

DR. ALBERT W. KROLL

A Washington state native, Dr. Kroll attended Walla Walla College from 1934–39 earning his B.A. and Loma Linda University from 1943–47 to earn his M.D. He established general practices in Los Angeles, California and Rosalia, Washington. He also studied pathology and completed a pathology residency in the Veterans hospitals in Denver from 1954–56 and in Milwaukee from 1958–60. He then served as pathologist at the Milwaukee Veterans Hospital from 1960–61 and then became the pathologist at the L.D.S. Hospital in Idaho Falls. He was an active member of the U.S. Army Reserves from 1950–62 holding the ranks of captain and major. He is the father of three sons.

DR. RHEIM MAGLEBY JONES

The son of a doctor, Dr. Rheim was born on July 29, 1919 in Monroe, Utah. He and his brother, Nyles, both became doctors. After studying at the University of Utah, he attended the University of Pennsylvania Medical School and graduated in 1943. He completed his internship and residency in U.S. Public Health Service hospitals in Baltimore. In 1952 he practiced in Galveston, Texas also in the U.S. Public Health Service with the rank of lieutenant colonel. In 1953 he relocated to Idaho Falls to establish a practice. Two of his four daughters and his son attended Brigham Young University.

DR. THOMAS T. McCOMB

Thomas McComb was born in Pittsburgh, Pennsylvania on November 19, 1878. When he was two, his family moved to Iowa where he lived until he went to an academy in Minneapolis, Minnesota. He returned to Iowa to attend the State College at Ames. He continued his education at the University of Iowa Medical School and graduated in 1905. After completing his internship at Onawa, Iowa, Dr. McComb worked as a physician and surgeon for the Lost River Irrigation Company until 1911. He then relocated to Idaho Falls and went into practice with Dr. G. H. Coulthard. After a year, he began his private practice. He also became one of the owners of Idaho Falls General Hospital and took an active part in its management. He is a member of the Bonneville County Medical Society and the Idaho State Medical Society as well as several fraternal organizations. He married Massie Thomas of Iowa.

DR. FRANKLIN LaRUE

Dr. LaRue was born January 10, 1854, in Zanesville, Ohio, and died November 1, 1928, in Phoenix, Arizona. Early in his life, he was riding range for thirty-five dollars a month, and was thrown from a horse, breaking his ankle. During his convalescence he decided to become a doctor.

The doctor went to Jefferson Medical College. He started practicing in Zanesville, and then moved to Idaho Falls. He made his calls with a horse and buggy, and when the weather got thirty degrees below, it was hard on both him and the horse. In January 1906, he performed an emergency appendectomy, with the patient on the kitchen table. He had only a small kit of knives with a sheepherder to help him. The patient was up and around in a few days, and Dr. LaRue gained statewide fame for the case.

The LaRues had five sons.

CARIBOU COUNTY

The nickname of an early settler prospector, "Caribou" Fairchild, was given to Idaho's newest county. The county was traversed by the earliest expeditions west and the Oregon Trail here made a triple fork, leading to Fort Hall, Salt Lake City, and California. At the peak of the westward movement more than a thousand people daily passed by Soda Springs. The bubbling waters of the numerous natural springs remain an attraction to the travelers of today. Both Captain Bonneville and John C. Fremont wrote of the "beer springs" in their reports. Cattlemen brought in herds to take advantage of the large grazing ranges. Latter day discoveries of phosphate rock has brought much wealth to the area. Anaconda Mining Corporation filed more than twenty patented claims and built the first modern plant for the production of phosphate rock in 1920. Others followed. Nine separate ranges and ridges make up the Peale Mountains in the eastern section of the county.

DR. ELLIS KACKLEY

This tribute to Dr. Ellis Kackley was given by Nadine Jenkins at a Speech Festival held in Bancroft, Idaho May 30, 1954. The information she gathered from life-time residents in the valley and from the *Soda Springs Sun* published at the time of his death.

Dr. Ellis Kackley was born in the Smokey Mountains in east Tennessee, July 15, 1871. He spent the first twenty-seven years of his life there. Then it is said he came out west to die. Afflicted with a lung infection and spitting blood, he was attracted to Soda Springs by an advertisement in a medical publication. This ad told of the serious need for a doctor in this area. Young Kackley sent an inquiry to Mr. Eastman, a druggist in Soda Springs. He replied that Soda Springs had an ideal climate for a man with lung trouble, and that any doctor who settled here, tended to business, and did not drink or gamble would make a lot of money.

So the day after his graduation from the University of Tennessee he left for Soda Springs. Arriving there April 2, 1898, he was a total stranger. He was slight in stature, pale, and weak. He occupied a room in the back of Eastman's

Drug Store for about a year. As he walked through the drug store one day, one of the men said, "We'll be burying that fellow in a couple of weeks."

The doctor didn't die according to plan. Living a good life, breathing the cool mountain air, and using his own determination to get well he began to recover and to build up a following and a professional practice which in those days could hardly have been dreamed.

One of his early cases was a man from Chesterfield, Idaho. He had broken his leg and two men started by team to take him to Montpelier to Dr. Hoover. It was night when they arrived at Soda Springs, so they spent the night there, intending to continue the remaining thirty miles the next morning. Dr. Kackley heard of the case and called on the man. He examined the broken leg; then took off his coat and vest and went to work saying, "I want you men to know that you don't have to go to Montpelier to get a doctor."

During the years that followed, the young doctor, who came out west to die, was kept busy answering calls over a fifty mile radius. In those days he used horses with buggies in the summer and sleigh in the winter, and often rode horseback. If the snow was too deep he used skis; but whatever mode of travel, he never let his patients down. It is said that one time he had to swim across the Bear River in order to answer a call in a hurry. Another time during the winter he was traveling on a hand car on the railroad when he hit a freight-train. His bag snapped open and instruments flew in all directions. He found some of the instruments the next morning, some he didn't find until spring, and some he never found.

At that time he had no hospital, so most of the patients were cared for in their homes, where many times surgery was done by the light of a flickering kerosene lamp. Dr. Kackley is said to have performed operations on a bunk in a lonely sheep camp and on a pool table in a saloon.

One time he was called to the home of a very sick woman, and he could see immediate surgery was necessary. The only one with her was a fourteen-year-old daughter. Dr. Kackley had the daughter turn her chair so that she couldn't see him operate and she gave anaesthetic to her mother as he directed her. The mother was on an old fashioned bed, the springs were made by lacing rope together. He successfully operated and removed one of the woman's kidneys. Years later as the doctor was telling his one son, Evan M. Kackley, M.D., of the operation, the son just laughed and said, "Dad you're the biggest liar ever, that kind of an operation would be hard even now with modern hospitals." As they were talking, a young lady came into the office and said, "Dr. Kackley I don't suppose you know me, but I am the girl who gave the anaesthetic to my mother while you operated on her."

He liked animals and had horses, sheep, cattle, chickens, and geese in the yard. There were always cats around and one or more dogs, all friends and pals of the doctor. Usually when you saw the doctor, you saw at least one of his dogs. His flock of geese numbered close to a hundred, probably the most favored and pampered flock of geese in the world.

A part of each evening he would spend reading. He had a remarkable memory and a forceful vocabulary, supplemented with a long list of explosive words (sometimes called swearing but seemingly natural when used by him).

In later years, his office patient-load became so great, he could not continue making calls and he remained in his office most of the time. He had his own private hospital until Caribou County built a hospital and made him superintendent.

He practiced for forty-five years. He was seventy-two when he passed away in 1943. A high school gymnasium was not large enough to hold all the grateful people who came to his passing ceremony. All came to pay tribute to one who gave so freely and asked so little in return.

DR. EVAN M. KACKLEY

Following in his father's footsteps, Dr. Evan Kackley practiced eleven years in Soda Springs from 1931 until 1942. He was born in 1906. By the time he was seventeen, he was attending Stanford University's medical school. Seven years later, in 1930, he finished at Harvard with his medical degree. He remembers a good many home surgeries during the early 1930s when the roads were closed for months by snow in the eastern end of Idaho. The usual means of transportation in the winter was a sled and many miles of walking year-round. Doctor Kackley never sent a bill to a private patient or kept records of charges.

During WWII, with the U.S. Navy he was a commander, taking in the Solomon Island campaigns. Later, he became chief of urology at Bremerton Naval Hospital. Back in Soda Springs, he was superintendent of the Caribou County Hospital and became a member of the State Board of Medical Examiners under Governor Bottolfsen. He and his wife raised two sons, Ellis N. and Alvin E. Kackley.

DR. RUSSELL TIGERT

Dr. Tigert was born July 24, 1915, Soda Springs, Idaho. His father and his brother were also physicians in Soda Springs. He attended elementary and high school in Soda Springs and received a B.S. degree in pre-med from the University of Idaho. From 1937–39 he was assistant chemist and engineer for Anaconda Copper Co., Conda, Idaho.

In 1943 he was graduated from Washington University, St. Louis, Missouri with his M.D. degree. He had a rotating internship at St. Louis City Hospital, St. Louis for nine months, followed by nine months as an assistant residency in surgery. He practiced in Montpelier, Idaho from 1947–42. From 1945–47 he was with the U.S. Army medical corps, rank of captain. He was in Soda Springs, Idaho from 1952–64.

In 1949 and 1950 it was a very severe winter, which required state snow equipment and state police patrol cars for escort, radio contact. etc. He went horseback once into a rough mountain area.

He was president, Bear River Medical Society of Idaho. Dr. Tigert was a member of board of directors of South Idaho Medical Service Bureau; Industrial Accident Committee of Idaho; and Idaho State and American Medical Societies.

He and his wife had two daughters.

BANNOCK COUNTY

The Portneuf River flows south to the center of Bannock County and enters the American Falls Reservoir. During Idaho's early history, there were more trails along the Portneuf than any other in the region. Fort Hall Trading Post on the Oregon Trail was located here, pathfinder John C. Fremont explored the area, early stages and Wells Fargo were routed through the area. Trappers were among the first settlers, followed by colonizers of the Latter Day Saints Church. The largest city, Pocatello, became a principal division point on the Union Pacific Railroad.

DR. RICHARD KENNETH GORTON

A Soda Springs native born June 17, 1918, Doctor Gorton practiced in Pocatello other than time away for service. He was chief of surgery in a mobile hospital (U.S. Army, 1951–52) and later chief at an evacuation hospital.

His undergraduate work was at the University of Idaho, graduating in June 1941. Four years later he graduated from Temple Medical School in Philadelphia. His fraternity was Phi Beta Pi. His internship, 1945–46, was at Jersey City Medical Center. He did his surgical residency from 1946–50, and thoracic residency from 1950–52 at New York State Hospital.

He became chief of staff at the Bannock Memorial Hospital in Pocatello during 1960 and 1961.

DR. NEAL MALLISON

Doctor Mallison graduated from Boise High School in 1905 and attended Creighton University at Omaha in the medical department. He graduated with the class of 1912 with an M.D. He came to Pocatello in May 1913 and opened his practice. He married Dorothy Heaston June 10, 1908 and they had one daughter, born in 1912.

DR. FRED M. RAY

Dr. Fred Ray was born February 11, 1882 on a farm near Bedford, Indiana, the tenth of twelve children and the eighth successive son. He attended grades and one year of Normal School at Beaver Dam, Kentucky, and taught five grade schools, taking spring and summer courses at the end of the terms. In this way he earned enough money to enter college and received his certificate in 1908.

He graduated from Northwestern Medical School June 9, 1909, having been excused a month earlier to accept an obstetrics internship in Chicago. He went into practice in Malad for six months and then on to Leadore for fifteen months, after which he moved to Pocatello in 1911. In 1914, he took a general course in Wesley Hospital, Chicago. From 1912 to 1921, he delivered about two-hundred babies a year.

Other physicians in his family were Dr. Charles Ray, Salt Lake City; Dr. Dailey Cooper Ray of Pocatello. He and his wife, Rachel, had a son, Ralph M., who became a doctor in Portland. The Rays had five grandchildren.

DR. FRANCIS SAMUEL MILLER

Dr. Francis Miller was a physician, surgeon and a veteran of two wars. He was born January 7, 1879 at Jonesboro, Tennessee and died at the age of eighty-four in Pocatello. He spent his early life in Tennessee where he attended local schools. In 1898 he enlisted in the U.S. Army during the Spanish-American War and served in the Philippines. He then attended Grant University Medical School at Chattanooga. After graduation he opened his practice at Oaksdale, Washington in 1908.

On June 3, 1908 he married Grace Gray at Oaksdale and they came to Pocatello in 1913 where he practiced with a brother, Dr. James Miller. He served as a medical officer with the U.S. Army in France during World War I. He retired in 1948.

Interested in outdoor activities, he won awards for his rifle marksmanship. He was an honorary member of the medical staff of St. Anthony Hospital.

DR. MELVIN MacPIKE GRAVES

Dr. Graves was born at Niagara Falls on May 20, 1912 and after the age of twelve, lived in Cleveland, Ohio. He had an uncle, Hubert, who was a doctor in Ohio.

His B.A. degree from Western Reserve University in 1934, where he was Phi Beta Kappa was followed by study at Harvard Medical School, graduating in 1937. He was an intern at St. Luke's Hospital in Cleveland and was a resident in surgery at Cleveland City Hospital from 1938 to 1942. The next four years were spent in Warsaw, New York, at the Wyoming County Community Hospital where he was an assistant in surgery. After 1946, he moved to Pocatello for private practice as a surgeon. He was named a Fellow of the American College of Surgeons in 1945 and a Diplomate of the American Board of Surgery and National Board of Medical Examiners in 1946.

In 1955 and 1956 Doctor Graves was president of staff of Bannock Memorial Hospital. In 1960 and 1961 he was president of staff of St. Anthony Mercy Hospital. From 1962–63 he was vice-president of the Board of Trustees of Northwest Medicine Medicine. He joined the American and Idaho Medical Associations. In 1956 he was the president of Southeast Idaho Medical Association. In addition, he became a 32nd degree Mason, Shriner and belonged to the Elks Club.

Doctor Graves married Dorothy Fisher in 1939 and they had two boys and two girls.

DR. JAMES H. BEAN

Dr. James H. Bean was one of Pocatello's earliest doctors, and was well-known in southern Idaho. He also ran a drug store. A native of Boston, he was born October 23, 1856, of Scotch-Irish ancestry. His father, James, was born in London, and there married Harriet Harvey. In 1856 they came to the United States, locating in Boston, where the father was a florist. He was also in the coal trade for twenty-five years. His mother died in 1876, at the age of fifty-seven.

The doctor was educated in Medford, Massachusetts. He began the study of medicine with an army physician, after which he entered the medical department of Dartmouth College and was graduated in 1873. He entered Jefferson Medical College in Philadelphia and graduated in 1877. For a year he practiced in a hospital in that city, and then moved to Denver where he remained until 1882.

In that year he came to Idaho as assistant surgeon for the Union Pacific Railroad Company. He carried on a general practice at Eagle Rock, now Idaho Falls, going to Pocatello in 1888. In 1884 he married Della Priestley of Lawrence, Kansas. They attended the Episcopal Church. The doctor was a master Mason in the Eagle Rock Lodge No. 19, A.F.&A.M; charter member of the Idaho State Medical Society and an organizer of the Rocky Mountain Interstate Medical Society.

DR. EMMETT GOODE WARD

Dr. Ward was born September 9, 1905 in Nashville, Tennessee. His father was a Methodist Bishop. The family moved to Houston, Texas, when he was one year old. He lived in Houston and Dallas until he went to Webb Prep School at Bell Buckle, Tennessee, 1920–24. He returned to Dallas, and got his premedical training and degree at Southern Methodist University. He joined SAE fraternity. From 1927–31 Dr. Ward attended the University of Texas Medical College, Galveston, and received his M.D. degree.

He interned in Southern Pacific Hospital at Houston, 1931–32. From 1947–50 he had a residency in psychiatry, Hastings State Hospital, Nebraska. He had a general practice in Dallas, 1932–36. From 1936–41 he was with the Texas State Hospital system, and was assistant super-intendent at State School, Austin. He had a general practice in Beaumont from 1941–47. From 1950–52 he was staff psychiatrist with the Texas State Hospital system. He was staff psychiatrist at the Veterans' Administration, Houston; and at Perry Point, Maryland, and Salisbury, North Carolina 1952–55. From 1955–57 Dr. Ward was staff psychiatrist at State Hospital South, Blackfoot. In 1957 he went into private practice at Pocatello.

He was a member of the American, Idaho and Southeast Idaho Medical Societies, and Intermountain Psychiatric Association. The Wards had one son, an engineer.

DR. WILLIAM H. ANDERSON

Dr. William H. Anderson came to Soda Springs, Idaho in 1897. His profession had honored him, first electing him to the office of second vice-president of the Idaho State Pharmaceutical Association, and later first vice-president. The doctor established a drugstore as soon as he located.

Dr. Anderson was born at Florence, Pennsylvania, February 14, 1835, the son of Robert S. and Dorcas Hopkins Anderson. He received his early education in Pennsylvania and Ohio, and the Kolectic College of Medicine and Surgery at Cincinnati. He graduated in 1855, at twenty, and began the practice of medicine in Newark, Iowa. Four years later he moved west, settling in Utah, and practiced in Cache and Malad counties, as well as in Oneida County, Idaho. In 1897 Dr. Anderson began his full-time practice in Idaho.

Public service was a big part of Dr. Anderson's activity, and for twenty-five years he was justice of the peace in Utah. At one time he was regimental surgeon in the Nauvoo Legion of Cache County, Utah, and postmaster of Portage, Utah for thirty years. He was a member of the Church of Latter Day Saints and served as counselor to the bishop.

The children of Dr. and Mrs. Anderson are William, Dorcas, and Mary.

DR. DEAN ELMO CALL

Dr. Call was born July 27, 1918, in Philadelphia. His father and a brother were also doctors. He went to Idaho State College, and received a B.S. degree from B.Y.U. He received his medical degree from Jefferson Medical College in 1951. The doctor interned at Salt Lake City Hospital, and had a residency at University of Utah Medical School for over four years. He was in China with the U.S. Army four years.

He moved to Pocatello in 1957 and was on the surgical staff at Bannock Memorial and St. Anthony hospitals. He belonged to the Southeastern Idaho and Idaho State Medical associations. He and his wife had six children.

DR. E. V. SIMISON

Following the tradition of his father, Dr. Simison and his brother became doctors. He was born July 11, 1912 in Hawley, Minnesota where his father practiced. He left Hawley to attend North Dakota State in Fargo 1929–32. He went to the University of Missouri School of Medicine 1932–34 when he earned his B.S. In 1936 he was graduated from Rush Medical University of Chicago with his M.D. He was a member of social and honor fraternities. His internship was at St. Lukes Hospital in Chicago for two years and a one year residency at University Hospital in Missouri.

He practiced in Pocatello, 1939–61, with staff appointments at St. Anthony's Mercy Hospital as chief of staff and on the executive committee. At Bannock Memorial Hospital he was president of staff and member of the executive committee. He was active in the local and state medical societies. He married Dixie Wood in 1938, and they have a son Philip and daughter, Karen.

DR. CALVIN BUHLER

The son of a farmer in Bern, Idaho, Calvin Buhler became a doctor after farming. He was born October 11, 1925. To earn money while in medical school, he drilled water wells during his vacations. He attended the University of Utah and earned his B.S. in 1950 and his M.D. from the University's Medical School in 1954. His rotating internship was at the L.D.S. Hospital in Salt Lake City in 1954–55 as well as a fifteen month surgical residency from 1955–56. He began practice in Pocatello in August 1956 and remained there throughout his practice. He and his wife, Elizabeth, have three sons and two daughters.

DR. DENNIS L. WIGHT

As a youngster, Dennis Wight worked on his father's dairy farm helping deliver milk to customers in and around Brigham City, Utah. He was born in Thatcher, Utah, January 12, 1919. His B.S. degree in pharmacy was earned at the Idaho State College from 1937–39, and he also attended the Utah State University for one year from 1943–44. He obtained his M.D. from Western Reserve Medical School from 1944–48 and was a member of Alpha Kappa Kappa.

His internship was at Emmanuel Hospital in Portland, Oregon and residency at the University of Utah Medical School Hospitals in Salt Lake City. He had a three year OB/GYN residency. He practiced in Fort Riley, Kansas, 1952–54 and Pocatello from 1954 on. He served as head of OB/GYN at Bannock Memorial Hospital. In 1959 he was the secretary for the Southeast Idaho Medical Society and was also president. While in the Army at Fort Riley, Kansas as a captain, he was the head of the OB/GYN department. He and his wife had one son and one daughter.

DR. JOHN EMERSON COMSTOCK

The son of a banker, Dr. Comstock was born March 31, 1925 in Rexburg, Idaho. His family relocated to Pocatello when he was seven and he attended grade school and high school there. He began his education at the University of Idaho but graduated from the University of California in 1945 with his A.B. and his M.D. in 1948. He trained at the San Francisco City and County hospitals from 1948-55 when he completed a year of senior residency in medicine.

He returned to Pocatello in 1955 to remain. He was a staff member of St. Anthony and Bannock Memorial hospitals. His served in the U.S. Navy as part of the V-12 program from 1942-46 and then in the U.S. Army as a captain. He was active as the secretary and later as the president of the Southeastern Idaho Medical Society and was appointed to the State Board of Medicine in 1962. He and his wife had four children.

DR. M. J. SHARP

Before Dr. Sharp began his medical career, he spent fifteen years as an industrial chemical engineer for the government and in private industry. He was the son of a farmer in Lewisville, Idaho and born on March 12, 1915. He attended Idaho State College, 1932-36 and again in 1947-48. He earned his A.B. in Chemistry at B.Y.U. in Provo in 1941, graduating Magna Cum Laude, and attended the University of Utah College of Medicine, graduating with an M.D. in 1951. He interned as an assistant surgeon at the U.S.P.H.S. Hospital in Seattle from 1951-52.

He returned to Pocatello in 1952. His staff positions were at the Bannock Memorial and St. Anthony's Mercy hospitals. He was secretary of medical staff in 1958-59 at B.M.H. and A.A.G.P. representative to the executive staff in 1960. His military service was in the Coast Guard form 1951-52, as an assistant surgeon. He enjoys working for his church and the Boy Scouts. He has lectured to youth groups throughout the state on communism, morality, freedom. He is married with two sons and three daughters.

DR. ROBERT J. EMERSON

A native of Eugene, Oregon, Dr. Emerson was born on June 28, 1929 where his father was the Deputy Superintendent of the Oregon Department of Education. Before entering medicine, Robert worked at the Atomic Energy installation, now the National Reactor Testing Station as a research biochemist at the Hanford facility. He obtained a B.A. degree from Linfield College in McMinnville, Oregon, 1947-51 in deputation and public relations. He was also a biology research and lab instructor at Linfield. He had a strong interest in drama and was in four productions; he was listed in *Who's Who in American Colleges*, and a member of Theta Chi Fraternity.

After a summer at the University of California, he attended the University of Oregon Medical School from 1952–57 and earned his M.S. and M.D. degrees. His masters degree was in biochemistry and he published five related publications. Dr. Emerson's general internship was served at the Good Samaritan Hospital in Portland and he also finished internal medicine residency, 1958–59. He did a one year residency at the Holcomb Diabetic Clinic in Portland.

Dr. Emerson opened practice in Pocatello in 1959 and served on the surgery committee at the St. Anthony Hospital. The doctor and Mrs. Emerson are the parents of two sons.

DR. LOUIS N. DIANA

Dr. Diana received his B.A. in 1938 from New York University; his M.D. in 1942 from New York Medical School. In 1943 he interned at Newark City Hospital; his later studies included New York Post Graduate Medical School, Basic Science Ophthalmology, 1955–56, and Brooklyn Eye and Ear Hospital, 1956–58.

He moved to Pocatello in 1955 and was on the staff at Bannock Memorial and St. Anthony Mercy Hospitals. He belonged to the Southeast Idaho, Idaho, and American Medical associations, and Diplomate of the American Board of Ophthalmology.

Dr. Diana and his wife have a daughter and two sons.

DR. JAY PETERSON MERKLEY

Dr. Merkley was born September 25, 1920, Wapella, Idaho. He attended the University of Idaho Southern Branch, 1938–40. From 1944–47 he went to Centenary College, Shreveport, Louisiana, and University of Utah Medical School 1947 through 1950, earning his M.D. and B.S. degrees. He was in the Air Force from 1943–46; an aviation physiologist, he operated the attitude chamber unit. While he was stationed at Barksdale Field, Louisiana, he took his undergraduate work at Centenary College.

In 1950–51 he interned at the U.S. Marine Hospital, Staten Island, New York, and had a residency at Welborn Clinic, Evansville, Indiana, 1951–52.

He started his Pocatello practice in 1952 and belonged to

the Southeastern Idaho Medical Society, and was active with the cancer society.

Dr. Merkley is active in breeding and showing Arabian and other horses. The Merkleys have two sons and three daughters.

DR. JOSEPH BENTON KOEHLER

Dr. Benton Koehler was born in Denver, Colorado, August 25, 1907. He was graduated from West Denver High School in 1925. In 1930 he received a B.S. degree in chemical engineering from University of Colorado and his M. D. in 1937. He did graduate work at the University of Pennsylvania, 1948-49, and at Western Reserve, Cleveland, Ohio, 1949-51. He interned at the University of Colorado Medical School 1937-38, and had a residency in Optholmology, St. Luke's Hospital, Cleveland, 1949-51.

From 1938-42 Dr. Koehler had a general practice in Grace, Idaho, and in Soda Springs from 1942-48. He moved to Pocatello in 1951, and was an eye, ear, nose, and throat specialist.

Dr. Koehler was on the executive staff at St. Anthony Mercy Hospital, and Bannock Memorial Hospital. He belonged to the Southeast Idaho Medical Society.

The Koehlers had a daughter and a son.

DR. EDWARD A. ROBERTS

Dr. Roberts was born in Ottawa, Illinois, July 20, 1885. His brother, son, and uncle were doctors. He attended grade and high schools in Ottawa. In 1910 he was graduated from Northwestern University. He interned at L.D.S. and Judge Mercy hospitals, Salt Lake City. From 1912-58 he practiced in Pocatello. He was division surgeon for the Union Pacific Railroad from 1912 to 1948.

He was on the staffs at Bannock Memorial Hospital and St. Anthony Hospital. From 1933-45 he represented Idaho in the House of Delegates of American Medical Association. He was a charter member of American Association for Trauma Treatment, and belonged to the American College of Surgeons. He served as first lieutenant in the Army Medical Corps from 1918 to 1919.

He enjoyed oil painting. On May 27, 1915 he married Florence Bloom in West Burlington, Iowa, and they had three daughters and two sons.

DR. CLARK PARKER

Clark Parker was born in Emporia, Kansas, May 22, 1915. His father was a lawyer. In 1938 he received an A.B. degree from Kansas State Teachers College, and his M.D. degree in 1946 from University of Kansas School of Medicine. He had a rotating internship at St. Margaret's Hospital, Kansas City, and a three year residency in general surgery at St. Margarets.

He practiced in Pocatello from 1950-54. From 1954-57 he was in the Army at the Medical Center in Landstuhl, Germany. After his discharge, he returned to Pocatello to private practice. He was director of Student Health Service, Idaho State College, and surgeon for the Union Pacific Railroad.

He was on the staff at Bannock Memorial and St. Anthony hospitals, and belonged to the Southeast Idaho Medical Society.

Dr. and Mrs. Parker have three sons.

DR. CORWIN ELLIOT GROOM

Corwin Elliott Groom was born July 5, 1913, at Afton, Wyoming. He went to school in Pocatello and the New Mexico Military High School. Corwin attended the University of Idaho Southern branch in Pocatello, Northwestern University and the University of Pennsylvania. He pledged Alpha Kappa Kappa fraternity.

His internship was at Minneapolis General and residency at the Atlantic City Hospital, New Jersey. With a specialty in urology, he practiced at Pocatello. Dr. Groom was chief of staff at both St. Anthony and Bannock Memorial hospitals and president of the Southeastern Idaho Medical Society and councilor for the Idaho State Society. Dr. Groom was a major in the Air Force during World War II.

Two brothers-in-law, Dr. W.R. Hearne of Pocatello and Dr. L.J. Bear of Dearborn, Michigan, were in practice. He and Marjorie P. Collins were married July 7, 1936, and had five children.

DR. DAN C. McDOUGALL

Dr. McDougall was born in Malad in 1899 and died on March 9, 1951. After graduating from George Washington Medical School in Washington, D.C. in pediatrics in 1927, he was licensed in Idaho in 1931 and practiced in Pocatello.

DR. THOMAS J. McDEVITT

A member of the well-known McDevitt family of Pocatello, Thomas was born March 27, 1933, and attended Idaho State College from 1951–52, where he was a finalist in the Rhodes Scholar competition. He then went to the University of Idaho from 1954–57, and Marquette University, 1957–61. He interned at St. Benedict's Hospital in Ogden, Utah, and began Pocatello practice in 1962.

Dr. McDevitt was with the 5th Regimental Combat team 1952–53 and was awarded the Korean Presidential Citation and the Combat Infantryman badge.

DR. EUGENE W. EARL

After growing up on the Burley farm where he was born May 26, 1924, Dr. Earl went to the University of Washington but graduated from the University of Oregon. He also attended the University of Oregon Medical School and graduated in 1948. His internship was at the San Bernadino County Hospital, from July, 1948 until July, 1949. His pediatric internship was at the St. Thomas Hospital in Nashville, Tennessee from 1949–50. His pediatric residency was at the Childrens Hospital of Michigan in Detroit from 1950–51. He was certified by the American Board of Pediatrics in 1961.

He began practicing in Pocatello in 1952 to the present except for a two year period as a Navy lieutenant from 1952–54. He is a member of the St. Anthony Mercy Hospital staff. The Earls have three daughters and two sons.

DR. E. LEON MYERS

Dr. Myers was born June 7, 1920, Newtonia, Missouri. His father was a physician in Joplin, Missouri. Leon attended Tulane and American College of Radiology, and interned at Baptist Hospital, New Orleans. In New Orleans he had a residency at Charity Hospital, and in St. Louis at Barnes Hospital. He was a U.S. Air Force major in 1952, and after service moved to Pocatello in 1953. From 1963–64 he was chief of staff at St. Anthony Hospital.

Astronomy and carpentry were his hobbies. He and his wife, Ruth Ann, had two sons.

DR. FRANK M. SPRAGUE

Before doctors were listed as child specialists, Dr. Frank Marion Sprague of Pocatello and Boise was one. From 1912 until 1947 when he retired, he devoted most of his career to the caring for children. He was born in Morrill, Kansas, October 11, 1875, and moved to Pocatello in 1898, where he operated a drugstore with his brother, Charles H Sprague.

Within a few years, he decided to study medicine and was graduated from the Jefferson Medical School in 1907. He also took advanced study at Harvard, and was a graduate of the University of Kansas in Lawrence. Upon his return to Idaho, he practiced in Pocatello from 1912 until 1945, when he moved to Boise to continue his practice. He also practiced briefly in San Francisco.

During World War I, Dr. Sprague served in the Army, and in World War II was associated with the Boise Induction Board. He was a member of Pocatello's Portneuf Lodge No. 18, AF and AM, York Rite, and in Boise was a member of the El Korah Shrine and the Rotary Club.

When he died on November 8, 1949, in Boise, he was survived by his wife, Ethel Linda; brother, Charles of Pocatello; and two sisters, Sadie Harris of Boise, and Nettie Nance, Uniontown, Kansas.

DR. DAVID CAROLLO MILLER

David Miller decided at age six that he would become a doctor and lived the dream. He practiced internal medicine in Pocatello forty years after opening an office in the Yellowstone Hotel in 1950. In 1953, he and other doctors built the Medical Arts Building. He died March 6, 1993, after an illness of about a year. He was a community and state, as well as medical, builder serving as chairman of the Idaho Board of Medicine, Union Pacific staff physician, three times St. Anthony Hospital staff chief, medical director of Geriatric and Hillcrest Haven convalescent centers; and many committees. He organized the first emergency call system of physicians and assisted in organizing the first intensive care unit and nursing program at St. Anthony Hospital.

Dr. Miller was born March 28, 1919 in Kemmerer, Wyoming, and moved with his family to a ranch near Lava Hot Springs when he was a year old. He earned a bachelor of science degree from Idaho State University's College of

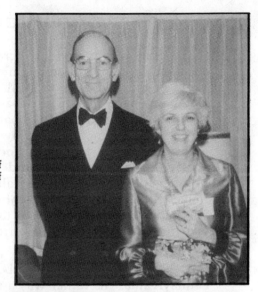

Dr. David and Phyllis Ann Miller of Pocatello attend an Idaho Board of Medicine dinner in Boise, 1974.

Pharmacy in 1941; attended Case Western Reserve University Medical School in Cleveland and received his M.D. in 1944, specializing in internal medicine. That year he married Phyllis Ann Boyce in Cleveland, Ohio, and they had four daughters, Joanne, Louise, Amy, and Coletta, who is now a doctor in Chicago; and one son, Robert.

In 1946-47 he was with the Army of Occupation in Wiesbaden, Germany.

DR. RICHARD HOWARD

Dr. Howard was born to pioneer physicians W.F. and Minne Howard, who moved to Pocatello in 1901, and had three brothers who also became doctors. He began his Pocatello practice with Dr. Dan McDougall, with whom he attended Johns Hopkins School of Medicine. Both young doctors did lab work for other doctors to augment their income during the depression years.

Dr. Richard was greatly influenced by traveling with his father to care for patients in outlying areas when he was a child. They would travel as far as the train could take them and then hire a horse and buggy to reach the patients. In those years doctors could ride trains at reduced fares to reach patients in the hinterlands.

Dr. Richard lived to be the senior practicing physician in Pocatello.

POWER COUNTY

The Snake River stretches across the county which holds so much of Idaho's dramatic history and lies on the direct route of the Old Oregon Trail. An American Fur Trading Company party met with disaster in the first attempt to navigate American Falls by boat and because of that event the falls have since been known as American. A point of great interest is Massacre Rocks, where an Indian war party attacked a westbound wagon train in 1862. A number of travelers were killed, wagons burned, and horses stolen. In 1925, the entire town of American Falls was moved a half-mile when the dam was finished and a lake formed. Rich farmlands surround the town.

DR. THOMAS E. DILLON

Dr. Dillon was born December 16, 1931, McKees Rocks, Pennsylvania. His father was a fireman for the railroad. In 1954 he received a B.S. degree from the University of Pittsburgh, and M.D. from Jefferson Medical School, 1958. He interned at Madigan Army Hospital, 1958–59, Tacoma, Washington.

For four months he practiced in Grangeville, and moved to American Falls, October 1961. He was on the staff of Power County Hospital, and belonged to the American Medical Association and South East Medical Society.

Dr. Dillon and his late wife, Ellen, have two sons and a daughter. He now resides in Caldwell and has remarried.

DR. FRANK LOUIS HARMS

One of his interesting experiences, during his practice of medicine, was wheeling a patient from home to the highway in a wheelbarrow because of lack of other transportation. He also used skis, snowmobile, and airplane to make calls, home deliveries, and surgery during the bad winter of 1949.

Dr. Harms was born March 8, 1914 at Cordell, Oklahoma. His father was a physician with a practice in Cordell. Two brothers were doctors: Dr. Edwin Harms, Wichita, Kansas, and Dr. Harold Harms, Ruston, Louisiana. He also had a doctor brother-in-law, Dr. David Pankratz, Memphis, Tennessee.

Dr. Frank Harms lived in Cordell until time of internship. He attended schools there, and was valedictorian of his high school class. He became a member of the General Conference Mennonite Church when he was fourteen.

He was graduated from the Medical School, University of Oklahoma, Oklahoma City, with a B.S.M degree in 1937, and an M.D. degree in 1939. In 1939 he received an honorary A.B. degree from Bethel College, Newton, Kansas. For one year the doctor interned at Good Samaritan Hospital, Portland, Oregon. Starting in 1940, he practiced in Aberdeen, Idaho for thirteen years, and then moved to American Falls. At American Falls he was chief of staff at American Falls Hospital; president of the Southeast Idaho Medical Society, and education chairman for A.A.G.P. in Idaho.

His wife, Lois Kliewer Harms, was graduated from Bethel College, with majors in English and Economics. She was elected to Who's Who Among College Graduates in 1938. The Harms had one daughter and two sons.

ONEIDA COUNTY

In 1854, a family of Mormons from England arrived as the first settlers of a county that then stretched from the Montana border on the north to Utah on the south, and included a part of what is now Wyoming. The family was forced out by a series of Indian raids and it was ten years later that a family by the name of Peck became the first permanent settlers. Despite the blight of several years of crickets eating the seed crops, the farmers remained to work in mining and other endeavors. The crickets disappeared in 1879, farming resumed, and has been profitable. Dairying and cattle-raising are the primary sources of income.

DR. ORSON H. MABEY, SR.

Before studying to become a professional doctor, Orson Mabey taught school for two years after receiving his teacher's certificate in 1911 from the University of Utah. Eight years later, in 1919, he graduated from Jefferson Medical College. He performed many home surgeries the first years of practice and remembered especially the flu and small pox epidemics.

He was born in Malad, Idaho in 1890 to parents who enjoyed the farming profession. After he received his medical degree, he did residency in 1919 at St. Francis Hospital in Hartford, Connecticut and moved on the next year to complete his training at the general hospital in Salt Lake City, Utah. He made his home in Garland, Utah for two years and then Lehi, Utah until 1924.

Finally, he returned home and practiced in Malad, Idaho until his retirement.

FRANKLIN COUNTY

Thirteen Latter Day Saints families arrived in covered wagons to settle on the present site of Franklin in 1860. They thought they were in Utah, but soon learned they had established a town and a county, both named Franklin, in Idaho. As other families arrived, Pack Ferry was established to cross the Bear River. At the toll bridge, which came about nine years later, an overland stage and mail station called Bridgeport was built at the crossing.

The U.S. government answered an appeal to protect the people from marauding Indians by sending General Patrick E. Connor and two hundred troops, who helped pave the way for expanded settlement. Farming communities of Clifton, Weston and Dayton were set up in 1864, '65, and '67.

The first railroad in Idaho Territory was the Utah & Northern Railroad, built from Brigham City, Utah, to Franklin in 1873. The Mormon Church advised its members in the area to help build the road, and the professional railroad builders were amazed at the numbers of men who turned out and sped up the process.

DR. GEORGE T. PARKINSON

Doctor George Parkinson practiced in Preston from 1910 and was a county physician of Franklin County at one time. Dr. Parkinson represents one of the pioneer families and is the son of a physician from Utah where his family had been located since pioneer days.

George Parkinson was born at Coalville, Utah, December 27, 1883. His parents were Dr. W. B. and Clarissa Parkinson. His father, a native of England, came to America when four years old, and with his parents, rode behind an ox team over the plains until they came to the vicinity of Caldwell, Utah where they were among the first settlers. His father spent his early years attending school there and later graduated from the medical department of Utah University.

The second in a family of five children, George, while attending the public schools of Utah and partly through the example of his father, was determined to make medicine his profession. He graduated from the Medico-

Chirurgical College of Philadelphia. After obtaining his degree in medicine, he first located his practice at St. Anthony, but after a short time he moved to McCammon and finally came to Preston, where he built up a very large practice. At Salt Lake City on August 19, 1902, he married Florence Wilson and together they raised four children.

In politics, Doctor Parkinson was an independent and his religious relations were with the Church of the Latter Day Saints.

DR. LEO ROGERS HAWKES

No matter how far he traveled, Preston, Idaho called Dr. Hawkes to return to his home. Born on November 19, 1911 in Preston, he attended elementary and high school in the area before being called to Germany for two and one-half years as an L.D.S. Missionary. Upon returning to the U.S., he received a B.S. degree from Utah State University and completed two years of medical studies at the University of Utah where he was a member of Phi Kappa Phi and Delta Phi. He was also a Rhodes Scholar candidate while at Utah State University which he attended from 1930-37, before graduating from the University of Chicago, Rush Medical College in 1939. He was a member of Alpha Omega Alpha honorary medical fraternity.

Dr. Hawkes interned at L.D.S. Hospital in Salt Lake City from 1939-40 before beginning practice in Preston in 1940. He served on the medical and surgical staff at both Franklin County General Hospital and Logan L.D.S. Hospital. He served as president and later as secretary of the Bear River Medical Society and secretary of Cache Valley Medical Society. Dr. Hawkes was the father of three sons and one daughter.

BEAR LAKE COUNTY

A mountainous county on the east and west, the Bear River runs right through the center from north to south. Thirty-mile long Bear Lake rises a mile above sea level, creating an area rich in farming, cattle and sheep raising, and recreation. The area's original name of "Miller," given by the Wilson Price Hunt expedition of 1811–12, was changed six years later when the Donald McKenzie party found so many black bears they renamed the river and lake. Paris was the first permanent settlement by Mormon families from Utah. In 1883 Union Pacific constructed its main line through Bear Lake County in crossing Idaho.

DR. LEON PAUL GAERTNER

Dr. Leon Paul Gaertner received his Idaho license to practice medicine and surgery on October 9, 1919. He devoted his career to the citizens of Montpelier, Idaho. He served in organized medicine in a number of capacities and was president of the Bear Lake-Caribou Medical Society in 1951. Born in Wayne, Nebraska on October 21, 1889, he died at age seventy-three in Phoenix, Arizona.

DR. JOHN WEBSTER LANGFORD

Dr. Langford was born in Illinois in 1841, and at age twenty-two he enlisted in the First Regiment, Wisconsin Heavy Artillery, to serve in the Civil War. He was in Washington, D.C. when President Lincoln was assassinated. He had a ticket for the play at Ford's theater that night, but stayed on guard duty to replace a sick buddy. He heard shots fired in the darkness and learned that they were fired by the pursuers of John Wilkes Booth.

He married Martha Gott of Wisconsin. They had five children. They moved first to Wyoming and later to Wardboro in Bear Lake County, Idaho. They became members of the Latter Day Saints Church and John took a second wife, Rhoda Ann Dimick. They had seven children. Many of their direct descendants still live in the area.

The Langford family was the first white family to spend a winter in Wardboro and "Doc" pulled teeth, delivered babies and tended the ill. Dr. Langford died at Wardboro in April 1916. His first wife, Martha, died in 1919 and Rhoda Ann died in 1928.

DR. J. H. MOON

Dr. J. H. Moon located in Montpelier, Idaho in 1887. He was prominent in business circles, having a drug store in Afton, Wyoming and Montpelier. At the time of his death, he was opening a third in Idaho Falls.

Born in New York he received his education in the east. He served in the Army through the entire Civil War. Later, he was several times commander of the Grand Army of the Republic. At one time he was professor of anatomy in the Medical College of Chicago. He also served as representative in the Michigan legislature. Dr. Moon was an active member of W.H.L. Warren Post 17, G.A.R. He died suddenly in February, 1891 from a heart attack.

DR. ARTHUR D. COOLEY

Dr. Cooley was a young physician when he arrived in Bear Lake County, Idaho, in 1911, and located in Paris. He had excellent educational training. In Paris he became associated with Dr. G. F. Ashley and built a hospital at Montpelier with Dr. Ashley practicing there.

He was born at Salt Lake City, Utah, March 2, 1885. His father was Andrew Wood Cooley, a native of Michigan who came to Salt Lake City at an early period, and became a school teacher. His mother was Ann Hazen, born in England, who at the age of three years accompanied her parents to America and across the plains to Utah in the early '60s. Dr. Cooley was the sixth of seven children. He attended the high school at Logan, Utah; the University of Utah, Salt Lake City and Northwestern University, Chicago, completing his medical course in 1911.

During the summer months, he took a special language course at Boyd College, Chicago. He was an intern in the Latter Day Saints Hospital, Salt Lake City before coming to Paris, Idaho. He selected this location believing it had very bright prospects, especially if more attention was given to dairying. Dr. Cooley learned early the valuable lesson of industry and secured his collegiate education by means of his own work. He was a Democrat, and was affiliated with the Latter Day Saints.

On September 4, 1912, at Paris, Idaho, Dr. Cooley was united in marriage to Miss Louise Price, daughter of William and Lottie (Ennis) Price, pioneers of the region.

CHAPTER
14

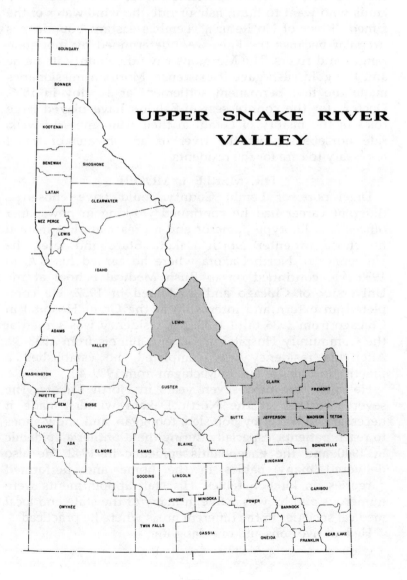

UPPER SNAKE RIVER
VALLEY

LEMHI COUNTY

A monument celebrates the birthplace of Sacajawea, "the bird woman," who accompanied the Lewis and Clark expedition and found her brother near the spot when the party arrived. One of the most ruggedly beautiful of any of the counties, it draws sportsmen from many states and lands who want to hunt, fish, or ride the whitewater of the famed "River of No Return." Lemhi's eastern boundary is irregular because the lines were determined by mountain ranges and rivers. The Mormons gave the county its name and the gold rush gave it existence. Mormon missionaries made the first permanent settlement at Tendoy in 1855. Doctors for the county seat of Salmon have played large roles in the history of Lemhi in their willingness to walk, ride horseback, float the river or any means of travel necessary to care for the residents.

DR. MERLE J. MOORE

Dr. Moore of Lemhi County could have chosen a different career had he continued working in newspaper offices as a linotype operator and a pressman, but instead he chose to enter North Dakota State and later the University of North Dakota where he earned his B.A. in 1935. He continued on to Rush Medical School at the University of Chicago and graduated in 1937. He completed an extern and internship at the Grant Hospital in Chicago from 1936 until 1938. His residency was served at the Community Hospital in Geneva, Illinois from 1938-39. After his residency was completed, he established a practice in Chicago and in Michigan from 1939-40.

He spent the next seven years in North Dakota. The severe weather of the North Dakota winters made it necessary to travel by bob sled, toboggan, and snow shoes to reach patients, especially during the diphtheria epidemic in 1940 and the encephalitis epidemic in 1942. He also delivered many babies in the home and performed surgeries on kitchen tables. His staff appointments were numerous and he was active in many of the state and local medical societies in the different areas where he practiced.

He had two sons and one daughter.

DR. JOHN L. MULDER

Born in Chicago, Illinois on October 7, 1891, Dr. Mulder was the first of several doctors in the family. His son and a brother-in-law also became doctors. He received payment for his services in meat, wood, and vegetables and a variety of other ways for the many deliveries and surgeries sometimes performed on the "kitchen table." When weather conditions had been extremely bad, he even drove his car up and down the railroad tracks because they were the only clear path available to reach his patients. He dealt with epidemics, severe weather, and travel conditions that many of today's doctors would not dream of enduring to reach his patients.

Dr. Mulder served in the U.S. Army during World War II during his internship. He attended the Hope College in Holland, Michigan from 1911 to 1914 and the University of Minnesota Medical School from 1914-18. He practiced in Chaska, Minnesota (1919-21), Cavalier, North Dakota (1921-37), and Twin Falls, Idaho (1937-38) before coming to Salmon, Idaho in 1938 until he retired in 1962. He was active in professional societies as well as community groups. His son became a doctor and practiced in Seattle and his daughter became a teacher.

DR. ZACH A. JOHNSON

A former high school teacher, Dr. Johnson served five years in the military before entering the University of North Dakota to earn his B.S. degree in 1948. He was drafted with the North Dakota National Guard in 1951 as a private but soon transferred to the Air Corps and completed his service as a major. After the earning his B.S., he went on to the University of Colorado and completed his M.D. degree in 1950 and then did an internship at the Marine Hospital in Seattle, Washington in 1950-51.

Dr. Johnson practiced briefly in Glendive, Montana before establishing his practice in in Salmon, Idaho in 1952. He served for five years as the chief of staff for the State Memorial Hospital in Salmon.

He is the father of two sons and two daughters.

FREMONT COUNTY

Captain Andrew Henry had left Montana due to Blackfoot Indian ferocity and came into Idaho in 1810 and built Fort Henry on the North Fork of the Snake River. The next spring he abandoned the fort and it was used that same year by the Wilson Price Hunt expedition. Many years later, in 1879, the first settlement was made at Egin Bench, and named St. Anthony Falls for the similarity to falls seen on the Missouri River. A bridge was built over the river and the town of St. Anthony came to be.

One of the oldest post offices of the area, Rea, became the center of a cattle and sheep raising industry. Mormon settlers came and transformed the rugged country into farms and ranches. Fremont is a beautiful county, with most of it above 4,600 feet. A semi-circular mountain section projects into Montana with Henry's Lake as its center. It is the access county to Yellowstone Park and has many tourists.

DR. KARL R. MALOTTE

The youngest of four children, Karl Malotte, born April 1, 1887, obtained his early education in the public schools of Graham, Missouri. He credited much influence from his father, Reverend James Malotte who, during the Civil War, enlisted in the Southern army as a private and fought gallantly at the Battle of New Orleans. After marrying Mary Eddy, born in Missouri, and entering the ministry, his father moved to Kansas where he had charge of a Baptist Church. His last pastorate was in Maryville, Missouri where he died October 16, 1900.

Karl graduated from Northwestern University at Evanston, Illinois with a Bachelor of Arts degree. In 1910 he became a Doctor of Medicine and interned at Chicago Hospital for a year.

Starting westward on a vacation the spring of 1911, Dr. Malotte was so favorably impressed with the future and beauty of Idaho that he opened an office at St. Anthony in 1911, and built up a good practice. Doctor Malotte married Isora Graham on September 6, 1906 and they had two children, Karl and Mary Donna.

The doctor was a member of the Idaho and the American Medical Associations.

DR. WILLIS ARTHUR MELCHER

Born April 9, 1909 in Omaha, this was where Willis Melcher was to attend pre-med school at the University of Nebraska and Creighton University. Willis graduated from the University of Nebraska Medical School in 1939. He traveled to Charleston, South Carolina for his internship at Roper Hospital and to Woodard Hering Hospital in Wilson, North Carolina for his residency, finishing in 1940.

Called to the service in 1940, Dr. Melcher had an eventful military career before returning to private practice and eventually moving to Ashton, Idaho, in July of 1955. He was on active Army duty in September 1940 and served at Camp Jackson, South Carolina and Blanding, Florida until March 1941, when he went to Panama until 1943. He was a regimental surgeon at Fort Davis with the 15th Infantry Division (Panama Canal) in 1941, post surgeon at Fort DeLesseps through 1943 and post surgeon of the Atlantic Sector. In Cristobol and Colon, Panama, he was a consulting surgeon with the American forces in revolution against Dr. Arias, President, Republic of Panama. In the fall of 1943 he was stationed in Ogden, Utah at the Italian Prisoner of War Camp. Later, he was sent to England and France. He received a Bronze Star and Certificate of Merit for his work in caring for 17,600 enlisted men with the assistance of only nine enlisted men and one dental officer. He was honorably discharged from the Army in 1945.

By then, he and his wife Ivy Lois Melcher were moving to a new home in South Carolina where he had interned and received his medical license. Mrs. Melcher writes, "He immediately began training me to assist him. I found it hard to understand these southern people and they found it just as hard to keep up with these western folks. We had hardly unpacked when we were called to go out in the country to deliver a baby. We loaded the car with sterile supplies and the home delivery table and followed the expectant father out into the country.

"When we arrived, we found a two room house that had surely been there since before the Civil War. It had real air conditioning, holes in every wall. The only means of heating the house was a fireplace and we asked the expectant father to get some wood. We moved the bed close to the fireplace and hoped the mother would keep from freezing. The grandfather and the children were in another bed across the room, trying not to look in our direction. The only chair I could find had only three legs, but as things progressed, I propped it by the patient's head and sat on it to give the anesthetic. Just then the wee one decided to be born and the fire got hot as the dickens. Doctor Melcher was frying on the fanny end, and soon invented 'the twist' to keep from burning. The baby arrived, hale and hardy and in a puff of steam. Just then the chair broke, and I fell on the floor. But the doctor kept things under control and never again complained about being cold behind.

"Our bill was thirty-five dollars and he could not pay, but we gave him a package of cigarettes to celebrate the new baby, and they were grateful. It was a good beginning. We delivered 1,500 babies while we lived in the deep south."

Seven years later they moved to Ogden, Utah for a three-year stay where he was a Weber County physician and had a private practice. In 1955 they moved to Ashton and practiced there for many years.

DR. MILLER M. HARSHBARGER

Dr. Miller M. Harshbarger, physician and surgeon in St. Anthony, was born in Woodbine, Iowa, June 1, 1875. His parents were Henry Clay and Nettie (Edgerton) Harshbarger. His father went to Iowa in early life, settling at Woodbine, where he engaged in the real estate business. He became mayor and served for one term as a member of the State Legislature. He enlisted at Omaha in the First Nebraska Infantry at the time of the Civil War, and served throughout. He then went to the western frontier and fought the Indians for six months. He was wounded in the battle of Shiloh, and on many a battlefield gave proof of his valor.

Later he farmed in Woodbine, and in 1901 moved to Fremont County, Idaho, where he purchased land near St. Anthony. This he improved and cultivated throughout his remaining days. He died March, 1912, and his wife died April 9, 1891.

The youthful days of Dr. Harshbarger were spent in

Woodbine where he attended public school. He afterward entered Hamline University at St. Paul, Minnesota. He joined 21st Kansas Infantry for service in the Spanish-American, and was with the Hospital Corps until the end of the war and returned to Hamline University. He completed a course in medicine with the class of 1902.

Dr. Harshbarger moved to St. Anthony and opened an office. He practiced there with the exception of a period of two years in Brownsville, Texas, and three years at Mount Vernon, Illinois. He took post graduate work in New York. He also homesteaded in Madison County, and proved up on the property. In October 1911, Dr. Harshbarger married Grace Campbell. They had two children, Raquel G., born July 1915, and William M., March 1917.

Dr. Harshbarger was a Republican; belonged to the Masons and the Mystic Shrine, Elks and Knights of Pythias, Modern Woodmen of America, and Woodmen of the World. He was a member of the Idaho State and American Medical Associations.

DR. ROBERT RUDOLPH KLAMT

The son of a building contractor and native of Ashton, Robert was born March 6, 1920 and lived there until entering Idaho State College from 1938 until 1942. Following graduation with a B.S. degree in pharmacy, he served in the U.S. Navy until entering medical school. From 1944 to 1948 he attended Creighton Medical School in Omaha. His internship was at the U.S. Naval Hospital in Long Beach, California until 1949. He practiced in Basin and Greybull, Wyoming, where the hospital was a converted old home, from 1949–50 and came to St. Anthony.

He recounts that a jeep was needed to get to a patient, but especially recalls going thirty miles by snowplane to treat an elderly man with a cervical vertebrae fracture. While practicing in St. Anthony, he was on the Fremont General Hospital staff and was instrumental in getting this hospital constructed and completed in 1959. Over the years, he held offices of president, vice president, secretary, and treasurer of the Upper Snake River Valley Medical Society and was a District Medical Director for the Cancer Society.

JEFFERSON COUNTY

Jefferson County is a uniformly level bit of Idaho geography and encompasses a part of the Snake River Plain. About sixteen miles of the eastern boundary line is formed by the Snake River before it makes a semi-circle and flows back out of the county south. Jefferson never experienced an early-day mining boom, but had its share of visiting colorful characters, including Annie Oakley and Mrs. Emma Ott, the 450-pound troubleshooter for the Pony Express Stage Line. Rigby is the county seat and a number of Idahoans have held that name, including medical practitioners.

DR. RAY HOMER FISHER

Patients said, "Like father, like son," of Dr. Ray Homer Fisher of Rigby in Jefferson County (formerly Fremont), because he was courageous, would put in long hours at his practice, and was eager for knowledge. His father, William F. Fisher, was a rider for the famous Pony Express, riding from April, 1860 to July, 1861 from Salt Lake to Ruby Valley, Nevada, and to California. He was one of the hardiest and speediest riders in the service and his record of thirty-four hours and twenty minutes continuously in the saddle, during which he made three hundred miles, still stands.

Many of these courageous men were killed by hostile Indians or by hardships faced during their travels. Mr. Fisher managed to come through unscathed, partly because of his knowledge of the Bannock and Shoshone Indian languages, both of which he spoke fluently. He became the first assessor of Oneida County, when it embraced the territory from Utah to Montana. They had eleven children, of whom Dr. Fisher was the next to the youngest.

The professional career of Dr. Ray Homer Fisher made him known as one of the most capable young physicians in Fremont County. A native of Idaho, with the true westerner's love for his own country, he added to its prestige in the field of medical science and in his official capacity as county physician. Dr. Fisher's family was long connected with Idaho's history. His brother, State Senator

George Fisher, was prominent in Democratic politics, and his father could have claimed being one of those who blazed the trails for the pioneers to this state.

Ray Homer was born March 9, 1883, at Oxford, Bannock County, Idaho and was the son of William and Millenium (Andrus) Fisher. He attended public schools in Utah and the Utah Agricultural College, from which he received a Bachelor of Science degree in 1904. He then entered the University of Colorado, graduating in 1909 with the degree of Doctor of Medicine. He entered practice at Helper, where he was substitute division surgeon for the Denver & Rio Grande Railroad. Later, Dr. Fisher spent one year in practice at Oxford, but July 1, 1910 went to Rigby, and on opening his office was appointed assistant surgeon for the Short Line Railroad.

He built up an excellent practice, and his success in a number of complicated cases made his name well-known in Idaho medical circles. He was appointed county physician in 1911, and served for several years. Dr. Fisher was a member of the American, Cache Valley, and the Idaho State Medical and the Southern Idaho District, and Pocatello Medical Societies. He was a member of the National Medical Fraternity, and Omega Upsilon Phi. He invested in several enterprises, and had an interest in the State Bank and the City Pharmacy. He belonged to the Church of the Latter Day Saints.

On June 8, 1909, Dr. Fisher was married at Louisville, Colorado, to Blanch Dierden, daughter of Jabez and Mary Dierden. They had one child, Fred Dierden Fisher, on May 25, 1910, at Lewisville, Idaho.

DR. ALFRED M. PALMER

Prominent among Idaho's medical men of southeastern Idaho was Dr. Alfred M. Palmer of Rigby. In these modern days, when the course of medical training is long and strict, the practitioner newly-graduated is often better prepared than the physician of half a century ago was after years of practice. Dr. Palmer enjoyed the benefits of a thorough preparatory training, and subsequently kept fully abreast of the advances and discoveries in his profession. He built a large and representative professional business.

Alfred M. Palmer was born March 31, 1885 at Logan,

Cache County, Utah, and is a son of William and Linnie May (Fisher) Palmer, natives of Utah. His father, a well-known civil engineer and bridge constructor, met an accidental death on the Short Line Railroad at old Kansas Station, Idaho, during the same year that Dr. Palmer was born. His mother was married ten years later to J.H. Carlson, of Oxford.

Alfred was the only child born to his parents, and his early education was secured in the public schools of Oxford. He later became a student in the Utah Agricultural School, where he took a five-year course, then entered the University of Colorado to start his medical studies. Following this, he attended the Denver-Gross College of Colorado. At that time, Dr. Palmer became house surgeon at the Latter Day Saints Hospital at Salt Lake City, where he spent one year, then choosing for his field of practice the town of Rigby. He settled in Rigby for the fact that it was the location of his uncle, Dr. Ray Homer Fisher, with whom he formed a partnership on his arrival. Dr. Palmer belonged to the American Medical Association and the Idaho State Medical Society, and was also a member of the Omega Upsilon Phi medical fraternity.

Politically a Democrat, he served as city physician of Rigby. His religious belief was that of the Church of the Latter Day Saints, in which his family was always prominent.

On June 12, 1912, he was married in Salt Lake City, Utah to Miss Bertha Wells. On May 25, 1913, at Rigby, a son, William Wells, was born to Dr. and Mrs. Palmer.

DR. EARL EAMES

Dr. Earl Eames was born in Menan, in what was then Fremont County, now Jefferson, in 1890. He was reared in Menan and attended school in Idaho Falls. He attended the University of Valparaiso, Indiana and graduated from Rush Medical College in 1917. He spent a year in hospital work in San Francisco and later joined the Army and served in France. Upon his return to the states, he opened an office in Newdale and later moved to Teton, although he kept his practice in Newdale. He died in 1953.

MADISON COUNTY

Latter Day Saints farmers from Utah traveled north to Madison County to take advantage of the farming resources in the area. They were the first permanent settlers and established Sugar City in 1878 and Rexburg in 1883, with other villages to follow. Rexburg is the county seat and the site of Ricks College, which was founded in 1888 as Bannock State Academy. The only mountain range in the county is the Big Hole in the southeastern section. Many good fishing streams come from the mountains and attract sportsmen from all parts of the country.

DR. M. F. RIGBY

Dr. Rigby, a member of a family of thirteen children, was born a twin on June 7, 1905 in Newton, Utah. His twin brother became a dentist. His father was a professional man, a bank president and also manager of a grain company. As a young boy, Dr. Rigby worked on cattle ranches and farms before attending Utah State University and later the Universities of Utah and Louisiana. In New Orleans, Dr. Rigby received his residency training at the Louisiana State Charity Hospital.

He married Miriam Young of New Orleans. He practiced in Rexburg, Idaho from 1937 until he retired.

DR. O. D. HOFFMAN

Opening and operating the first hospital in Teton Valley at Driggs, Idaho, in May of 1939 was just the beginning of many hospital and medical society associations for Dr. Hoffman. He was later chief of staff for three years at Madison Memorial Hospital in Rexburg and a member of the courtesy staff of L.D.S. and Sacred Heart hospitals in Idaho Falls. He was a member of the American Medical Association; Idaho State Medical Association; Upper Snake River Valley Medical Society—president for two different terms; a member of numerous committees in Idaho State Medical Association and counselor for district four in Idaho State Medical Association. He was also a consulting and examining physician for Selective Service for twenty-four years.

Dr. Hoffman was born May 24, 1910 in Logan, Utah where he attended public school. He graduated from Utah

State University in 1932 with a B.S. degree then attended the University of Utah Medical School for two years before graduating from the University of Louisville in 1937 with an M.D. degree. His internship was at Thomas D. Dee Hospital in Ogden from 1937–38. Dr. Hoffman began practice in Driggs in 1938 and moved to Rexburg in 1946. Dr. Hoffman and his wife, the former Lois Choules, had one son and three daughters.

DR. LESTER J. PETERSEN

His father was a school teacher when Dr. Lester Petersen was born on May 31, 1932 in Rexburg, Idaho. He states there were no other family members who were physicians. During his high school days, he was student body president. While attending the University of Utah, he obtained a B.S. degree in 1954 and his M.D. degree in 1957. He belonged to the Phi Rho Sigma fraternity. His internship was at Owyhee, Nevada from 1958 to 1960 and he worked for the U.S. Public Health Service as an assistant surgeon in his early professional years.

Dr. Petersen was president of the Upper Snake River Valley Medical Society in 1964. From 1963 to 1965 he served as chief of staff of the Madison Memorial Hospital. With his wife, Lola, they had four children, Mark, David, Suzanne, and Michelle.

DR. HARLOW B. RIGBY

Harlow B. Rigby went back to the town in which he was born on New Year's Day 1893, to begin his practice as physician and surgeon. Rexburg was where he was born and educated through two years at Ricks College. His parents were Joseph E. and Mary (Beck) Rigby. He received his Bachelor of Science degree from the University of Utah in 1918.

His M.D. from Harvard came in 1920, and he spent three months in continental Europe with an interstate medical group before returning to Idaho. His was the 1,223d license to practice in Idaho and he built and owned the Rexburg General Hospital. Dr. Rigby belonged to Rotary and was a delegate to the International Convention in Dallas, 1929. He was a Phi Beta Pi and a Republican. His church was the Latter Day Saints (Mormon). He was married to Elsie Graham in Oklahoma, May 13, 1922.

CHAPTER
15

THE "PLUS" PEOPLE

William T. Wood, recently retired M.D., and a friend were discussing his career from the time of medical study through his practice in his hometown of Coeur d'Alene. They talked of the heartaches, sorrows, joys, and wonders of the practice of medicine. "If you had it all to do over again, Bill, would you become a doctor?" His wife, Dolores, interjected with, "Oh, yes!" Bill, taking a few seconds of thinking, replied, "The answer would be 'Yes' if I could start over at that same time in medical history when I began, and continue to practice as it was up until about ten years ago. As it now is, the answer would be 'No'."

Dr. Bill, who had delivered hundreds of babies and cared for hundreds more during his career, told of how M.D.s who finished training when he did and up until the decade ending in 1980, look at the broad field of medicine today and cannot recognize the scene. An overwhelming federal government interference, multitudinous and complicated paperwork required by the government and by the insurance companies, prestige eroded, and ability challenged by litigious patients, startling increases for malpractice insurance, and other continuously annoying problems, have brought about a great degree of dissatisfaction among a large number of doctors.

"So," Dr. Bill went on, "I would not recommend to any of my children or grandchildren that they study medicine. It just isn't worth it."

The years have passed, picking up an awesome speed as they rolled by. The frontier changes from the days of the trapper and explorer to those of the pioneer settler, still with a gun at his side as he turned and broke up the soil to plant his crops. He then moved to build a more solid home for his family and a new era began.

And yet, in Idaho there remain those communities that keep close to the frontier spirit and, certainly, to rugged individualism. This is a good thing. Many of the hard-working and weary medical men and women seek out just those spots—the back country, the lakes, the hills and the treeclad mountains—for renewal, for recreation, and for recovery of strength and perspective.

The signs are hopeful that some of the young men and women who are studying, or plan to study, medicine are doing so with the desire to practice in rural and, in some cases, remote areas. They like the idea of being able to serve those who are quite a distance from the cities and all the facilities of modern hospitals and clinics.

Katie James Reynolds of Grangeville, daughter of Darcy and the late Mr. James, did her pre-medical study at the College of Idaho in Caldwell, and is now at the University of Washington Medical School. On an Albertson's grant, Katie not only studied, but has had two summer rotations of actual practice as an aide to a nurse practitioner in Idaho's heartland, Stanley Basin. In an area guarded by the jagged peaks of the Sawtooth Range, it would be difficult to find a spot that better fit the word "rural." This Presidential Award student has already had experience in giving emergency aid to those injured in accidents, wrecks, and mountain activities.

The two sons of Jim and Judy Eisses of Hayden Lake, Michael, twenty-three, and John, twenty-four, are both thinking of practicing rural medicine because they feel there is a great need for doctors in the hinterland. John has already received his Master's degree in New Testament study and Michael, after one year of pre-med at the University of Idaho, is entering the University of Washington for three years to receive the all-important letters "M.D." after his name. Both will be studying under the WAMI program, as is Katie James Reynolds.

From the medicine practiced by the Indians, the trapper, the horse-and-buggy doctors, to the medical experiments continuing in space, discoveries have been made that boggle the mind. Still much of what is called "granny medicine" is found to soothe, heal and effect cures. And we know that none of this could have come about without those sturdy medical men and women who went before. What of them?

What would you say is the outstanding mark of the pioneer doctors? Bible reading, churchgoing and prayer? These are indispensable, but external, signs of their spirits. What was inside? And in what order? Optimism? Charity? Patience? Not distinctive enough. "What *do* they *more than others?*"

In that question, asked nearly 2,000 years ago from a mountain above the Sea of Galilee, there is the clue to the outstanding mark of the early doctors. What did the pioneer doctor *more* than others? These men and a few women, striding across the great panorama of the west with a daring and adventure that was their life, what did they? The emphasis should be put on the word "more," for this is what they did. They did more. They were the plus people.

They were more compassionate. They were more generous. They were more loving. They were more steadfast. They were the plus people: the plus Americans, the plus Idahoans. They were both Dr. Boecks, Drs. Taylor, Braxtan, Ustick and Calloway of Boise, the Drs. Platt and McGahan of St. Maries, the Drs. Whitwell of Salmon and Finney of Harrison, and many others of whom you have read in this book.

It took a special brand of moral courage and tenacity of purpose. You will have read of those who willingly participated in every war in which America has been involved: the Revolutionary, the Civil, the Spanish American, World Wars I and II, the Korean and Vietnam. They gave *more* to relieve distress; *more* to heal the sick; *more* to bind up the wounds of battle; they preserved life and they helped to build strong communities. What a heritage have the medical people of today. And not the medical people only. This is our heritage. The question is, "What *do* we *more* with it?"

CHAPTER
16

PHYSICIANS UNITED

IDAHO MEDICAL ASSOCIATION

On June 21, 1893, a call for a meeting to plan a state medical society was sent from Boise by Dr. Carroll Lincoln Sweet to all physicians in the state, urging a September meeting to organize to protect themselves in professional matters. They met September 12, 1893, in Boise City Hall. They were told of strong support by the Pacific Medical Record of Portland, and its offer to be the official organ for the group. A listing of "doctor eagles" from Moscow south to Silver City, Hailey, Pocatello, and Boise signed the request for the meeting.

From Boise, signers were C.L. Sweet, George P. Haley, E.L. Perrault, F. Thompson, William Stephenson, and L.C. Bowers; from Caldwell: W.C. Maxey, Ed E. Maxey, Charles E. Lee, and A.F. Isham; Payette: C.M. Scott, I.E. Burr, and G.W. Stephenson; from Weiser: C.B. Shirley; from Silver City: John W. Weston and A.C. Lippencottt; from DeLamar: J.J. Plummer; Mountain Home: W.F. Smith; Shoshone: W.H. Baugh; Hailey: D.W. Figgins and N.J. Brown; Pocatello: I.H. Moore, J.H. Bean, F.B. Toms, and O.B. Steely; Moscow: W.W. Watkins, C.E. Worthington, and R.C. Coffey; and Lewiston: C.W. Shaff.

Dr. W.W. Watkins of Moscow was elected chairman and Dr. Carroll Sweet of Boise, secretary. The credentials committee reported that twenty-five doctors had applied for membership. Doctors C.B. Brierly, J.A. Hansel, and J.H. Finfrock of Boise; J.W. Givens, Blackfoot; O.W. Hall, Star; J.B. Morris, Lewiston; and G.W. Pendleton, Idaho Falls, also attended.

Later in the session, applications were received from R.M. Fairchild and W.D. Springer, Boise, and J.H. Murray, Nampa.

To effect a permanent organization other officers were named: I.H. Moore, vice president; Carroll Sweet became treasurer as well as secretary; and Doctors Perrault, Brown, W.C. Maxey, and Shaff as a Board of Censors.

The first legislation proposed on higher standards for doctors failed to pass. It is said it was defeated by "two or three well-known men, who could not meet professional requirements recommended." They were better organized at the 1896 Legislature, and had "bought" a diploma from a diploma mill in Chicago in the name of a "Dr. Rogers," who was actually an Idaho senator, to show how weak the law was under which physicians in Idaho registered. When Senator Rogers found himself a registered M.D., he and others were convinced and the legislation passed.

In the 1897 Legislature, an amended form of the bill was passed and signed by Governor Frank Steuenberg. The Supreme Court declared the law unconstitutional. The committee felt that its labors had been in vain, but the

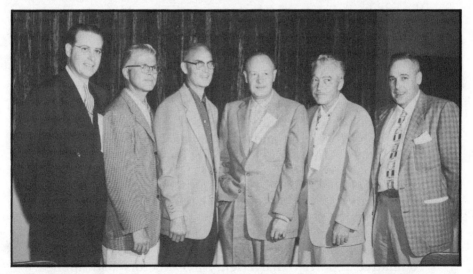

Idaho Medical Association officers at the 1954 convention in Sun Valley are, *left to right:* Doctors Vic Simison, Pocatello, retiring president; Alexander Barclay Jr., Coeur d'Alene, incoming president; Robert McKean, member; Asael Tall, Rigby, president-elect; Donald Worden, Lewiston, delegate; Quentin Mack, Boise, secretary-treasurer.

(Courtesy Alma Barclay)

1898 session decided to try again with a similar act. It did pass, but not until the 1899 session, and with amendments over the years, remains on the statutes.

The ninth annual meeting established district societies, with each to elect one Fellow for every five members, with the Council and the Fellows to make up the governing board, and modifications have taken place over the years.

Praise was often heaped on *Northwest Medicine*, "one of the very few best State Journals published."

PAST PRESIDENTS
IDAHO MEDICAL ASSOCIATION

*W.W. Watkins, Moscow	1893	*W.R. Howard, Pocatello	1912
*W.W. Watkins, Moscow	1894	*J.W. Gue, Caldwell	1913
*L.H. Moore, Pocatello	1895	*F.W. Mitchell, Blackfoot	1914
*C.L. Street, Boise	1896	*J.M. Alley, Lewiston	1915
*M.H Wood, Boise	1897	*T.O. Boyd, Twin Falls	1916
*C.A. Hoover, Montpelier	1898	*C.S. Moody, Hope	1917
*C.W. Staff, Lewiston	1899	*W.F. Smith, Boise	1918
*E.E. Maxey, Caldwell	1900	*W.F. Smith, Boise	1919
*J.R. Numbers, Weiser	1901	*C.P. Stackhouse, Sandpoint	1920
*H.A. Castle, Pocatello	1902	*H.W. Wilson, Twin Falls	1921
*Geo. Collister, Boise	1903	*M.T. Smith, Wallace	1922
*J.L. Conant, Genesee	1904	*J.R. Gray, St. Anthony	1923
*R.L. Nourse, Hailey	1905	*Fred A. Pittenger, Boise	1924
*J.B. Morris, Lewiston	1906	*C.W. Pond, Pocatello	1925
*L.P. McCalla, Boise	1907	*N.R. Wallentine, Sandpoint	1926
*E.W. Kleinman, Hailey	1908	*D.L. Alexander, Twin Falls	1927
*J.L. Stewart. Boise	1909	*Alex. Barclay, Sr., Coeur d'Alene	1928
*J.M. Taylor, Boise	1910	*H.P. Ross, Nampa	1929
*J.W. Givens, Orofino	1911	*H.D. Spencer, Idaho Falls	1930

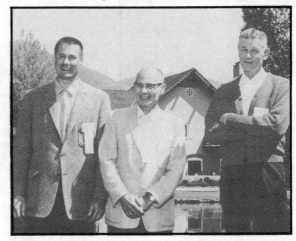

In 1963, the Idaho Medical Association named, *left to right*: Dr. Paul Heuston of Twin Falls, president-elect; Dr. Manley Shaw of Boise, president; and Dr. Robert Staley of Kellogg, past president. The photo was taken at the annual meeting at Sun Valley.
(Courtesy Marie Whitesell)

*D.S. Cornwall, St. Maries	1931	*Manley B. Shaw, Boise	1963
*J.N. Davis, Kimberly	1932	Paul B. Heuston, Twin Falls	1964
*E.N. Roberts, Pocatello	1933	*Corwin E. Groom, Pocatello	1965
*J.S. Springer, Boise	1934	*Wallace H. Pierce, Lewiston	1966
*C.R. Scott, Twin Falls	1935	*A.Curtis Jones, Jr. Boise	1967
*J.R. Crampton	1936	James R. Kircher, Burley	1968
*D.C. Ray, Pocatello	1937	*O.D. Hoffman, Rexburg	1969
*A.C. Jones, Sr., Boise	1938	John M. Ayers, Moscow	1970
*F.C. Gibson, Potlatch	1939	Wm. R. Tregoning, Boise	1971
*F.M. Cole, Caldwell	1940	Geo. W. Warner, Twin Falls	1972
*A.M. Newton, Pocatello	1941	J.E. Comstock, Pocatello	1973
*Paul M. Ellis, Wallace	1942	E.R.W. Fox, Coeur d'Alene	1974
*Geo. O.A. Kellogg, Nampa	1943	R. Geo. Wolff, Caldwell	1975
*Parley Nelson, Rexburg	1944	Ben L. Kreilkamp, Ketchum	1976
*W.O. Clark, Lewiston	1945	D. R. Bjornson, Idaho Falls	1977
*O.F. Swindell, Boise	1946	R. J. Ellsworth, Boise	1978
*Geo. C. Halley, Twin Falls	1947	H. Kent Staheli, Pocatello	1979
*A.B. Papenhagen, Orofino	1948	Don. D. Price, Caldwell	1980
*F.B. Jeppesen, Boise	1949	W.Dyce Thurston, St. Maries	1981
*W.R. West, Idaho Falls	1950	Clayton C. Morgan, Boise	1982
*R. T. Scott, Lewiston	1951	R. W. Newcomb, Twin Falls	1983
Alfred M. Popma, Boise	1952	Wilfred E. Watkins, Nampa	1984
*Wallace Bond, Twin Falls	1953	John W. Gerwels, Lewiston	1985
*E. V. Simison, Pocatello	1954	Howard E. Adkins, Boise	1986
*Alexander Barclay, Jr., CdA	1955	J.O. Nicholson, Twin Falls	1987
Robert S.McKean, Boise	1956	T.J. Setter, Idaho Falls	1988
*Chas. A. Terhune, Burley	1957	A.W. McRoberts, Pocatello	1989
*Hoyt B. Woolley, Id. Falls	1958	Robert S. West, Coeur d'Alene	1990
*Don. K. Worden, Lewiston	1959	David M. Barton, Boise	1991
*Quentin W. Mack, Boise	1960	J. E. Scheel, Twin Falls	1992
Asael Tall, Rigby	1961		
*Robt. S. Staley, Kellogg	1962		*Deceased

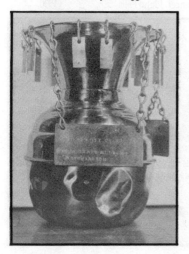

THE ROYAL GABON: Working daily in matters of life and death, medical people take every opportunity to lighten their lives with laughter and joking. For years, this battered old spittoon was awarded to a doctor at the annual IMA meeting. His name was imprinted on a metal card and another notch added to hang it on the rim. The presentation speech pointed out the ridiculous situations in the life of the "winner," who had the honor of displaying it for a year. Dr. Paul Ellis of Wallace missed having the award in his office, so had a picture taken to hang on the wall.

(Courtesy Paula Stephenson)

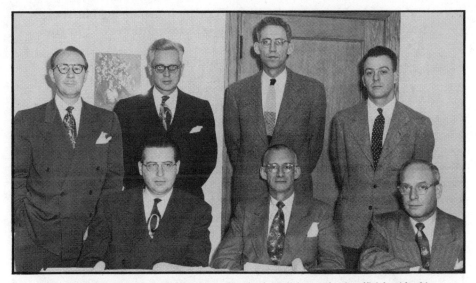

The original board of the Idaho State Board of Medicine make it official with this photograph after their first meeting. *Left to right,* seated Doctors Vic Simison, Pocatello; Paul Ellis, Wallace, and Sam Poindexter, Boise. *Standing left to right:* Armand Bird, executive director; Doctors Harlan Stowe, Twin Falls; William Ross, Nampa; and Gedney Barclay, Coeur d'Alene.

(Courtesy Paula Stephenson)

IDAHO STATE BOARD OF MEDICINE

Confused in some minds, the Idaho State Board of Medicine is separate from the Idaho Medical Association. The Board of Medicine was set up by statute to represent the public in dealing with the profession and to it come the complaints and requests for help. The Medical Association was set up by the members for group action. The confusion likely comes from the days during which both were housed in the same office with the late Armand Bird, former Associated Press representative in Boise and later a writer for the Idaho Department of Public Health, in charge. Bird served for about fifteen years until he retired in 1975. Donald Deleski, who had been administrative assistant to the board, was named executive director to the board and Donald Sower hired by the associaion. Sower has since been succeeded by Robert Seehausen. Deleski received his education in Burley and was graduated from

Idaho State University with a B.A. in journalism. He took graduate study at the University of Utah and served in the U.S. Air Force.

In 1976, legislation was enacted to set up a Board of Medical Discipline to police the medical profession and enforce professional standards. Membership is composed of five physicians appointed by the Board of Medicine and one public member. Current (1993) members are Doctors Michael Estess, Wayne Allen, Brent Payne, Donald Bjornson, and Louise Shadduck. The Disciplinary Board "investigates or inquires into misconduct or unprofessional behavior, whether real, apparent or merely suspected, and take action . . . deems best in interest of the public and justice."

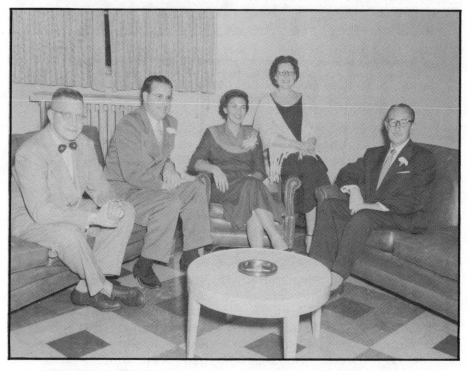

Shoshone County Medical Association and Auxiliary entertained for visiting state officers in 1953. *Left to right:* Dr. Glen Whitesell of Kellogg, County president; Dr. Vic Simison, Pocatello, IMA president; Helen (Mrs. Robert) Smith, Boise, Auxiliary State president; Margaret (Mrs. Pete) Peterson, Wallace, Shoshone County Auxiliary president; the late Armand Bird, executive Director, Idaho Medical Association.

(Courtesy Marie Whitesell)

THE AUXILIARY
LOOKING TO THE FUTURE

Fourteen wives of Idaho doctors accompanied their husbands to the Tri-State meeting of Medical Associations in Yellowstone Park on August 28, 1928. It was a propitious gathering for both. The Idaho Medical Association asked the women to organize an auxiliary, which they were happy to do and began to plan events for future conventions. As the years passed, they did many things to help the communities and state. The American Medical Association Auxiliary had organized six years previous and urged all states to do so.

Until 1941 the wife of the I.M.A. president served as auxiliary president. First president of the new organization was Mrs. Alexander Barclay Sr., Coeur d'Alene. Other officers: Mrs. H.P. Ross, Nampa, vice-president; Mrs. D.E. Cornwall, St. Maries, corresponding secretary; Mrs. J.N. Davis, Kimberly, recording secretary; Mrs. D.L. Alexander,

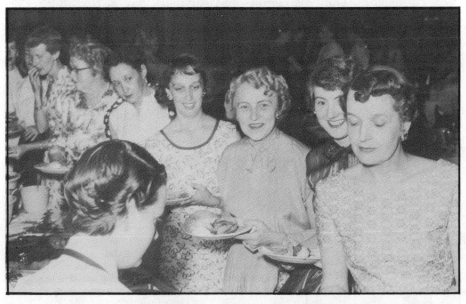

The ladies line up for an Auxiliary buffet at the 1953 meeting of both the IMA and auxiliary in Sun Valley. *Left to right:* Mrs. Clarence (Jean) Gibbon, who appears perplexed by the multiple choices; Mrs. Paul (Elizabeth) Ellis, past president, Wallace; Mrs. Vic Simison, Pocatello; Mrs. Glen (Marie) Whitesell of Kellogg; Mrs. Wallace Bond and daughter, Twin Falls; and Mrs. Robert (Dorothy) Staley, Kellogg.

(Courtesy Marie Whitesell)

Twin Falls, treasurer. In 1941 the custom of electing the auxiliary president was changed. Mrs. Harmon Tremaine of Boise was elected on her own and members pledged support. This was also the first year that Idaho had a representative on the national board, with Mrs. Arthur C. Jones of Boise named fourth vice president. She was assigned to organizing auxiliaries in the west.

Projects upon which the Auxiliary worked included: visiting the retarded at Nampa School and Colony, financing summer camp for underpriviledged youngsters, funding infantile paralysis treatment, teaching first aid and home nursing, recruiting nurses and funding student nurse loans and scholarships, donating to Red Cross for flood relief in Idaho, and sponsoring Doctor's Day with medical exhibits. In addition, they produced slides on "Poisons in the Home," for use in grade schools, films on medicine and nursing for school and college libraries, a booklet on health careers in Idaho which was given to high school guidance counselors. They also sponsored Auxiliary day at the Idaho Legislature and a home centered health care program.

Kootenai County was the first to organize an auxiliary, shortly after the Yellowstone session. By 1942 the membership had reached thirty-seven and ten years later, 1952, had reached 292 and has grown to nearly 450. However, as the early doctors learned, Idaho's populated districts are widely separated and it is difficult to meet often.

In 1963, Mrs. E.R.W. Fox of Coeur d'Alene was elected as a director to the national board and named national reports chairman. She had served as Idaho Auxiliary

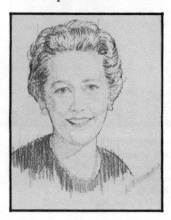

Ellen (Mrs. E.R.W.) Fox of Coeur d'Alene served for a number of years on the national board of the Auxiliary to the American Medical Association. She also served on the Idaho Auxiliary Board and compiled a fifty-year history of the Idaho Auxiliary.

(Courtesy Dr. E.R.W. Fox)

president in 1959 and on numerous state committees. In 1966, she was elected national secretary and re-elected for a second term. In 1968, Mrs. Fox was named national finance secretary, a position she held for seven years. At the Atlantic City convention in 1975, the Auxiliary to the A.M.A. presented her with an honorary membership. She was the twenty-fifth woman to be so honored during the fifty-three years of the Auxiliary existence.

At that convention, Mrs. Ben Katz of Twin Falls, Idaho Auxiliary president in 1971, was elected to serve two years as national director.

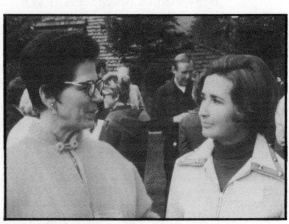

Idaho Medical Auxiliary president Kathy (Mrs. H. Don) Moseley of Coeur d'Alene chats with Boise member Alice (Mrs. Gustav) Rosenheim at 1972 convention in Sun Valley.

PAST PRESIDENTS
IDAHO MEDICAL AUXILIARY

1928	*Agnes Barclay (Mrs. Alex., Sr.)	Coeur d'Alene
1929	*Margaret Ross (Mrs. H.P.)	Nampa
1930	*Anna E. Spencer (Mrs. H.D.)	Idaho Falls
1931	*Mrs. D. E. Cornwall	St. Maries
1932	*Mrs. J. N. Davis	Kimberley
1933	*Mrs. E.N. Roberts	Pocatello
1934	*Mrs. J. S. Springer	Boise
1935	*Grace Scott (Mrs. C.R.)	Twin Falls
1936	*Mrs. J. H. Crampton	Lewiston
1937	*Mattie Ray (Mrs. D.C.)	Pocatello
1938	*Lois Jones (Mrs. A.C.)	Boise
1939	*Mrs. F. C. Gibson	Potlatch
1940	*Leila Cole (Mrs. F. M.)	Caldwell
1941	*Mrs. Harmon Tremaine	Boise
1942	*Emma Beck (Mrs. W. W. Sr.)	Blackfoot
1943	*Mrs. R. T. Hopkins	Orofino
1944	*Mrs. George O. A. Kellogg	Nampa
1945	*Mrs. J. H. Murphy	Twin Falls

1946	*Elizabeth Ellis, (Mrs. Paul M.) .... Wallace
1947	*Beulah Freeman (Mrs. Roy) .... Boise
1948	*Dixie Simison (Mrs. E. V.) .... Pocatello
1949	*Margaret Wood (Mrs. John T.) .... Coeur d'Alene
1950	Mary Lesser (Mrs. L. F.) .... Boise
1951	*Addie West (Mrs. Walter R.) .... Idaho Falls
1952	Mildred Bonebrake (Mrs. H. E.) .... Wallace
1953	Noma Creed (Mrs. J. Woodson) .... Twin Falls
1954	Helen Smith (Mrs. Robert S.) .... Boise
1955	*Miriam Rigby (Mrs. Murland F.) .... Rexburg
1956	Hazel J. Carver (Mrs. Max. W.) .... Filer
1957	Marguerite Burton (Mrs. Jerome K.) .... Boise
1958	*Harriett Woolley (Mrs. Hoyt B.) .... Idaho Falls
1959	*Ellen Fox (Mrs. E.R.W.) .... Coeur d'Alene
1960	Ione Bell (Mrs. Max. F.) .... Boise
1961	Laurene Gorton, Mrs. Richard K.) .... Pocatello
1962	*Mary Knight (Mrs. V. Ellis) .... Kimberly
1963	Marie Whitesel (Mrs. Glen M.) .... Kellogg
1964	Judy Carlsson (Mrs. E. R.) .... Nampa
1965	Phyllis Ann Miller (Mrs. David C.) .... Pocatello
1966	Enid Husted (Mrs. Otto M.) .... Coeur d'Alene
1967	*Virginia Tregoning (Mrs. Wm. R.) .... Boise
1968	Fran Migel (Mrs. Dauchy) .... Idaho Falls
1969	Myrtle Peterson (Mrs. Willard M.) .... Twin Falls
1970	Ida Smithson (Mrs. Carl B.) .... Boise
1971	Gloria Katz (Mrs. Ben E.) .... Twin Falls
1972	Kathy Moseley (Mrs. H. Don) .... Coeur d'Alene
1973	Lois Harms (Mrs. Frank L.) .... American Falls
1974	Zoe Ann Shaub (Mrs. Roy O.) .... Twin Falls
1975	Barbara Quickstad (Mrs. Quentin L.) .... Boise
1976	Barbara Hoge (Mrs. Walter G.) .... Blackfoot
1977	Mary Lou Truxal (Mrs. A. C.) .... Rupert
1978	Lola Peterson (Mrs. Lester J.) .... Rexburg
1979	Carol Newcomb (Mrs. Russell W.) .... Twin Falls
1980	Cathy Thompson (Mrs. C. E.) .... Coeur d'Alene
1981	Lois Hatten (Mrs. Harold W. Jr.) .... Boise
1982	Dee Palrang (Mrs. A. M.) .... Caldwell
1983	Eileen Petersen (Mrs. Walter R.) .... Burley
1984	Kaye Knight (Mrs. Lawrence) .... Boise
1985	Yolande Waid (Mrs. G. Curtis) .... Idaho Falls
1986	Karen McLandress (Mrs. Richard) .... Coeur d'Alene
1987	Pat Fulwyler (Mrs. Robert) .... Boise
1988	Ione Horrocks (Mrs. Sydney A. Bert) ...... Pocatello
1989	Jackie McRoberts (Mrs. Andrew) .... Pocatello
1990	Elaine Kimball (Mrs. Frank) .... Coeur d'Alene
1991	Kay Merrick (Mrs. David) .... Boise
1992	Tommie Holm (Mrs. Eugene) .... Burley
1993	Carol Skellenger (Mrs. William) .... Coeur d'Alene

*Deceased

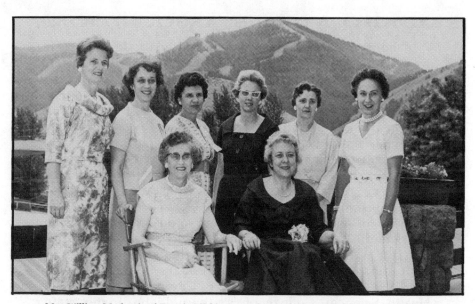

Mrs. William Mackersie of Detroit, Michigan, was honored at several events when she made an official visit as President of the American Medical Association Auxiliary to the Auxiliary of the Idaho Medical Association in 1961. This photo, taken from the deck at the Sun Valley Lodge with the Idaho officers has Mrs. Mackersie seated beside IMAA president Mary (Mrs. V. Ellis) Knight of Kimberly. *Standing, left to right:* Lorene Gorton of Pocatello; Judy Carlsson of Nampa; Phyllis Ann Miller of Pocatello; Enid Husted of Coeur d' Alene; Mrs. Mark Baum of Idaho Falls.

(Courtesy Marie Whitesell)

Frank Freeman, a collector of early American glass, displays a handcut vase to four members of the Ada County Medical Auxiliary. *(left to right)* Mr. Freeman, Mrs. J.M. Taylor, Mrs. Frank Minas, Mrs. Theodore Florentz, and Mrs. Ida Smithson.
(Courtesy late Irene Jones)

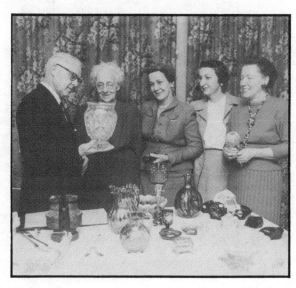

IDAHO NURSES ASSOCIATION

Idaho nurses cut such a wide swath across Idaho that it would take an entire book to tell of their activities. Their value to society has been demonstrated time and again and it is fortunate that they number more than all other health care providers combined. It has also been well demonstrated that nurses are motivated by a caring for people. Despite the difficult problems faced, America's and Idaho's nurses maintain high standards and code of ethics. Idaho nurses look to the future and sponsor funds for education, research, scholarships, loans and continuing public awareness on health issues.

Nurse of the Year is a program sponsored by various districts of the I.N.A. Others include awards for contribution to nursing, student nurse of the year, cooperation with nursing programs at North Idaho College, Lewis-Clark State College, Boise State University (College of Health Science), College of Southern Idaho, Idaho State University, and community awards.

Presidents of INA include:

1909-11	Iva Long	1946	Dorothy Collard
1912-14	Gertrude Creigon	1947	Viola Vreeland
1915-16	Anna Daly	1948-52	Frances Vassar
1917	Gertrude Creigon and Anna Daly	1953-56	Eldora King
		1957-60	Marj Schlotterbeck
1918-19	Alice Taylor	1961-64	Dorothy Smylie
1920-22	Emma Amack (Meier)	1965	Aileen Atwood
1923	Mary Brown-Lewers	1966-67	Marjorie Roose
1923-24	Barbara Williams	1968-70	Johnette Braga
1925-26	Beatrice Reichert	1971-72	Lorraine Barr
1927	Ethel Rogerson	1973	Mildred Burt
1928-29	Helen Smith	1974-75	Amy Savage
1930	Florence Johnson	1976-77	Pat Jory
1931	Jean Thomson	1978-81	Rosie Acton
1932-33	Helen Wolfe	1981-83	Mary Griffith
1934-35	Beulah Patteson	1983-85	Verlene Kaiser
1936-38	Minnie Rasmason	1985-86	Nancy Heyer
1939-40	Helen Smith	1986-87	Cheryl Juntunsen
1941-42	Katherine McCabe	1987-89	Marilyn Haynes
1943	Garnet Gilbertson	1989-90	Lynn Williams
1944	Edna Pickle	1990-92	Barb Allerton
1945	Lynn Wigen		

IDAHO DIETETIC ASSOCIATION

Organized in Boise in 1948 with eight members, the Idaho Dietetics Association has grown to more than two-hundred. Ambitious programs by the dietitians have brought Idaho standardized dietary procedures, forming of local associations, workshops for hospital cooks, better work hours in dietary departments, community nutrition seminars, diets for homes for the aged, grants for internships and scholarships, development of film and slide files, nutrition classes and continuing education, legislative action, nutrition fairs, and working on campaign to end childhood hunger.

Presidents of the association include:

1950-52	Sister Alicia Marie	1972-73	Mary Decker
1952-53	Viola Fisher	1973-74	Becky Ulray
1953-54	Helen Chase Walter	1974-75	Mary Echo
1954-55	Shirley Newcomb	1975-76	Mary Sugden
1955-56	Agnes Bahlert	1976-66	Bernice Morin
1956-57	Ethel Tuman	1977-78	Sally Howell
1957-58	Patricia Gilbertson	1978-79	Clara Day
1958-59	Eula Tombaugh	1979-80	Joy Burke
1959-60	Alice Henry	1980-81	Elaine Long
1960-61	Shirley Newcomb	1981-82	Arlene Jonas
1961-62	Helen Allen	1982-83	Marilyn Swanson
1962-63	Margaret Ritchie	1983-84	Becky Swartz
1963-64	Peggy Stanfield	1984-85	Sue Hagerman
1964-65	Ethel Helm	1985-86	Luan York
1965-66	Goldah Anderson	1986-87	Laura Ringe
1966-67	Eula Tombaugh	1987-88	Mary Lou Beck
1967-68	Sister Cora Marie	1988-89	Judi Schuerman
1968-69	Beverly Moorer	1989-90	Audrey Buck
1969-70	Judy Stanton	1990-91	Denise Carter
1970-71	Agnes Foley	1991-92	Kathe Gabel
1971-72	June Yearington	1992-93	Ruth Schneider

HOSPITALS

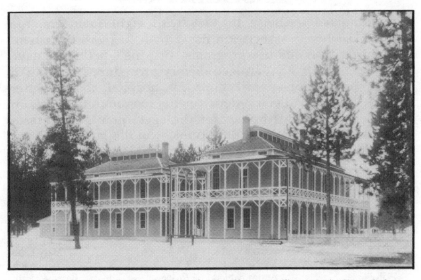

One of the most attractive hospitals was the Fort Sherman military one in Coeur d'Alene. Later, when the Fort was disbanded, a part of the building was used as a school by the Immaculate Heart of Mary Academy.

(National Archives photo)

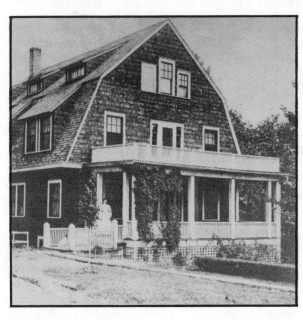

It is probably Dr. Ethel Page Westwood standing in the entryway of the old City Hospital in Sandpoint. She is still talked of with admiration in the area.

(Courtesy Penny Armstrong)

Note the jaunty nurse's cap and chef's headgear in this photo of the staff and mobile patients at the old Bonners Ferry Hospital on North Hill above the town. The Steve "Slim" Allured family lived in the building from 1935 until early 1980s. Now owned by Ray and Beth Holmes, they have added a Victorian tower in the area where the people are.

(Courtesy Jack and Arlene Allured)

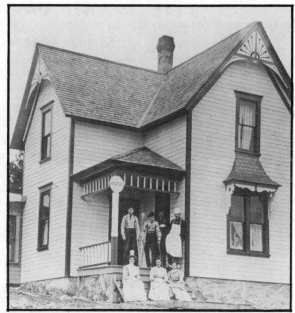

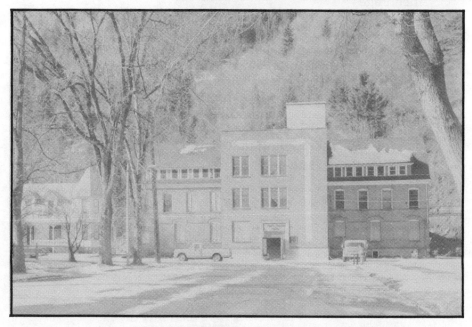

The modern Wallace hospital filled a long-felt need in that mining community. Mining is a hazardous occupation and physicians who practiced here were kept busy.

(Courtesy Paula Stephenson)

THE WAMI PROGRAM

It is often suggested that Idaho should have its own Medical College, despite a population that now hovers just above the million mark. Medical schools are expensive and Idaho's neighboring state of Washington had internships and hospital-based medical education for forty years before a medical school. The University of Washington School of Medicine began after World War II, and has become the site of the regional education program for Washington, Alaska, Montana and Idaho.

WAMI guarantees fifteen seats to Idaho students in each entering class. The students take the first year of medical studies at the University of Idaho, where the President, Elizabeth Zinser, has a background in nursing (Stanford, 1964) and educational psychology (University of California, Berkeley, 1972), and worked with the WAMI program developing community clinical units in Pocatello, Boise, Billings, Missoula, Omak, Wenatchee, Kodiak and Anchorage.

Dr. Roy Schwarz, founder and director of WAMI and a former resident of American Falls, returned to Idaho in August 1992, as WAMI celebrated its 20th anniversary. He reported that, "The program is making a medical difference for the people of the rural northwest. It remains Idaho's best hope for securing a more adequate supply of physicians in its rural communities."

Dr. Michael Laskowski is the current director of the Idaho program. Preceding him were Drs. Art Rourke, Mark DeSantis and Tom McKean.

BIBLIOGRAPHY

I. BOOKS

Arnold, R. Ross. *Indian Wars of Idaho*. Caldwell, Idaho: The Caxton Printers, Ltd., 1932.

Bailey, Robert G. *River of No Return*. Lewiston, Idaho: R.G. Bailey Printing Company, 1935-1947. (out of print)

Beal, Merrill D., Ph.D., and Wells, Merle W., Ph.D. *History of Idaho*, Volumes I, II, and III. New York: Lewis Historical Publishing Co., Inc., 1959.

Brosnan, Cornelius J. *History of the State of Idaho*. Revised edition. New York: Charles Scribner's Sons, 1935.

Defenbach, Byron. *The State We Live In: Idaho*. Caldwell, Idaho: The Caxton Printers, Ltd., 1933.

Eisensohn, Sister M. Alfreda. *Pioneer Days in Idaho County*, Vol. 1. Caldwell, Idaho: Caxton Printers, Ltd., 1947.

Idaho Department of Commerce and Development. *The Idaho Territorial Almanac*. Boise, Idaho: Syms-York Company, 1963.

Federal Writers Project, W.P.A. *The Idaho Encyclopedia*. Caldwell, Idaho: The Caxton Printers, Ltd.

Hailey, John. *History of Idaho*. Boise, Idaho: Syms-York Company, Inc., 1910.

Hawley, James H., editor. *History of Idaho, the Gem of the Mountains*, Vol. 1. Chicago: S.J. CLarke Publishing Co., 1920.

Lewis, Meriwether, and William Clark. *History of the Expedition under the command of Captains Lewis and Clark to the Sources of the Missouri, thence across the Rocky Mountains and down the River Columbia to the Pacific Ocean, during the Years 1804-5-6 by Order of the Government of the United States*, Vols. I, II, and III. New York: Allerton Book Company, 1922.

Lindsley, Margaret Hawkes, and Andrew Henry. *Mine and Mountain Major*. Laramie, Wyoming: Jelm Mountain Publications, 1990.

Mills, Nellie Ireton. *All Along the River*. Montreal, Canada: B.C. Payette Radio Limited, 1963.

Peterson, Keith C. *Company Town.* Moscow, Idaho: Latah County Historical Society, and Pullman, Washington: Washington State University Press, 1987.

Pitts, Elaine and Maitland, Joanna. *Women In America,* booklet. New York: Sperry and Hutchinson, 1967.

Rees, John E. *Idaho Chronology, Nomenclature, Bibliography.* Chicago: W.B. Conkey, 1918.

Schwantes, Carlos A. *In Mountain Shadows, A History of Idaho.* Lincoln and London: University of Nebraska Press, 1991.

Smith, Robert S., M.D. *Idaho Surgeon, An Autobiography,* Boise, Idaho: Syms-York Company, 1974.

Spencer, Betty Goodwin. *The Big Blowup, The Northwest's Great Fire.* Caldwell, Idaho: The Caxton Printers, Ltd., 1958.

Scott, Orland A. *Pioneer Days on the Shadowy St. Joe.* Printed and Bound by Caxton Printers, Ltd., Caldwell, Idaho 1967.

Ward, Betty Penson. *Idaho Women in History,* Volume I. Boise, Idaho: Legendary Publishing Company, 1990.

Yarber, Esther, with Edna and Arthur McGowan. *Land of the Yankee Fork.* Denver, Colorado: Sage Books, 1963.

Lanham, John M., M.D. *The Making of a Medicare Doctor.* New York: Vantage Press, Inc., 1977.

UNPUBLISHED MATERIAL

Fox, Mrs. E.R.W. (Ellen). *Fifty Years* (1928–1978), IMA Auxiliary.

Maxey, E.E. *History of the Idaho State Medical Association.*

Robins, C.A., M.D. *To My Daughters, History of His Life.*

Weston, Julie Whitesell. *Bitterroot,* Historical novel.

NEWSPAPERS

The *Coeur d'Alene Press*

The *Idaho Semi-Weekly Herald*

The *Idaho Daily and Sunday Statesman*

The *Kellogg Evening News*

The *Lewiston Tribune*

The *Owyhee Avalanche*

The *Post Register, Idaho Falls*

The *Spokesman-Review*

The *Twin Falls Times-News*

The *Wallace Miner*

PAMPHLETS

Quarterly Newsletters, Museum of North Idaho